Health Reference Series

Second Edition

Dental Care
and Oral Health
SOURCEBOOK

*Basic Consumer Health Information about Dental Care,
Including Oral Hygiene, Dental Visits, Pain Management,
Cavities, Crowns, Bridges, Dental Implants, and Fillings,
and Other Oral Health Concerns, Such as Gum Disease,
Bad Breath, Dry Mouth, Genetic and Developmental
Abnormalities, Oral Cancers, Orthodontics, and
Temporomandibular Disorders*

*Along with Updates on Current Research in Oral
Health, a Glossary, a Directory of Dental and Oral Health
Organizations, and Resources for People with
Dental and Oral Health Disorders*

Edited by
Amy L. Sutton

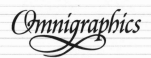

Omnigraphics

615 Griswold Street • Detroit, MI 48226

Bibliographic Note

Because this page cannot legibly accommodate all the copyright notices, the Bibliographic Note portion of the Preface constitutes an extension of the copyright notice.

Edited by Amy L. Sutton

Health Reference Series

Karen Bellenir, *Managing Editor*
David A. Cooke, MD, *Medical Consultant*
Elizabeth Barbour, *Permissions Associate*
Dawn Matthews, *Verification Assistant*
Laura Pleva Nielsen, *Index Editor*
EdIndex, Services for Publishers, *Indexers*

* * *

Omnigraphics, Inc.

Matthew P. Barbour, *Senior Vice President*
Kay Gill, *Vice President—Directories*
Kevin Hayes, *Operations Manager*
Leif Gruenberg, *Development Manager*
David P. Bianco, *Marketing Consultant*

* * *

Peter E. Ruffner, *Publisher*

Frederick G. Ruffner, Jr., *Chairman*

Copyright © 2003 Omnigraphics, Inc.

ISBN 0-7808-0634-4

Library of Congress Cataloging-in-Publication Data

Dental care and oral health sourcebook : basic consumer health information about dental
  care, including oral hygiene, dental visits, pain management, cavities, crowns, bridges,
  dental implants, and fillings, and other oral health concerns, such as gum disease, bad
  breath, dry mouth, genetic and developmental abnormalities, oral cancers, orthodontics,
  and temporomandibular disorders; along with updates on current research in oral health, a
  glossary, a directory of dental and oral health organizations, and resources for people with
  dental and oral health disorders / edited by Amy L. Sutton. -- 2nd ed.
    p. cm. -- (Health reference series)
  Previous edition published under title: Oral health sourcebook, 1998.
  Includes bibliographical references and index.
  ISBN 0-7808-0634-4 (alk. paper)
    1. Dentistry--Popular works. 2. Mouth--Diseases. 3. Mouth--Care and hygiene. I.
Sutton, Amy L. II Oral health sourcebook. III Series.

RK61.O66 2003
617.5'22--dc22

2003058485

Table of Contents

Part II: You and Your Dentist

Part III: Routine Dental Concerns

Part IV: Surgical, Orthodontic, and Other Specialized Procedures

Part V: Health Conditions That Affect Oral Care

Part VI: Disorders of the Mouth

Part VII: Current Research in Dental and Oral Health

Part VIII: Additional Help and Information

Preface

About This Book

Oral health can have a significant impact on overall wellness. Disorders, such as cavities and gum disease are progressive, and their impact on general health compounds over time. They can affect nutrition by influencing food choices and the ability to eat; they can undermine self-esteem by changing how a person looks and communicates; and they can cause considerable pain.

A hundred years ago, most Americans lost their teeth by middle age. Advances in dental care, including the discovery of fluoride, increased knowledge about the impact of tobacco use and dietary choices, and the adoption of personal hygiene habits such as brushing and flossing, led to dramatic improvements in oral health. Today, most middle-aged and younger Americans expect to retain their natural teeth for their lifetimes.

Despite the progress, however, many Americans still suffer from dental and oral health concerns. For example:

- Tooth decay, a largely preventable condition, remains the most common chronic disease of children aged 5–17 years. By age 17, 78% of children will have at least one cavity or filling.

- Employed adults lose more than 164 million hours of work each year due to dental disease or dental visits.

- 27% of middle-aged adults and 30% of older adults suffer from untreated tooth decay.

- Most adults show signs of periodontal or gingival diseases. Severe periodontal disease affects about 14% of adults aged 45–54 and 23 percent of those aged 65–74.

- Despite the importance of tooth and gum care, only 65% of persons ages 18 to 64, and even fewer seniors—only 56%—visit the dentist annually.

- Oral and pharyngeal cancers are diagnosed in about 30,000 Americans every year.

- Public opinion surveys reveal that 46% of adults avoid visiting the dentist when they have no immediate condition requiring dental treatment.

- Barriers to dental care include cost, time, fear of pain, and a lack of awareness regarding the importance of oral health.

This book provides information about dental care and oral health at all stages of life. It includes facts about mouth hygiene, home care products, routine dental concerns, periodontal disease, orthodontic treatment, oral surgery, cosmetic dentistry, and other specialized procedures. Information about dental problems caused by health conditions such as diabetes, cancer, arthritis, and hemophilia, is included, along with facts about oral cancer, Sjögren's syndrome, dry mouth, fever blisters, canker sores, bad breath (halitosis), and other mouth disorders. Current research initiatives are also described. A glossary and directory of additional resources guide readers seeking further help and information.

How to Use This Book

This book is divided into parts and chapters. Parts focus on broad areas of interest. Chapters are devoted to single topics within a part.

Part I: General Information about Dental Care and Oral Health describes oral health needs and preventive dental care in infancy, childhood, adolescence, and adulthood. It explains mouth hygiene, home dental care products, fluoride, and the relationship between nutrition and oral health.

Part II: You and Your Dentist defines the different dental specialties, offers tips for finding a practitioner, and discusses dental anxiety. Other concerns that may accompany a dental visit, such as exposure to lead and radiation or the prophylactic use of antibiotics, are also addressed.

Part III: Routine Dental Concerns offers information about preventing, diagnosing, and treating common dental problems, including plaque, cavities, cracked teeth, gum disease, and dental injuries.

Part IV: Surgical, Orthodontic, and Other Specialized Procedures describes such treatments as root canals, extractions, oral surgery, and cosmetic dentistry. The use of orthodontics (braces) during childhood and adulthood is explained, and dental devices such as crowns, bridges, implants, and dentures are discussed. Other topics include disorders of the jaw and bruxism (grinding the teeth).

Part V: Health Conditions That Affect Oral Care addresses the relationship between oral health and conditions such as arthritis, cancer, cleft lip and cleft palate, diabetes, hemophilia and other bleeding disorders, latex allergies, and respiratory diseases.

Part VI: Disorders of the Mouth presents facts about the symptoms, treatment, and prevention of oral disorders, including dry mouth, halitosis (bad breath), fever blisters, canker sores, oral cancer, and taste and smell disorders.

Part VII: Current Research in Dental and Oral Health reviews areas of recent and current investigation in oral health, including current efforts to reduce oral health disparities.

Part VIII: Additional Help and Information includes a glossary of important terms and a directory of dental and oral health care organizations. Resource directories for people with dental and oral disorders and sources for charitable and accessible dental care are also included.

Bibliographic Note

This volume contains documents and excerpts from publications issued by the following U.S. government agencies: Centers for Disease Control and Prevention (CDC); U.S. Food and Drug Administration (FDA); National Women's Health Information Center; National Cancer Institute (NCI); National Institute of Arthritis and Musculoskeletal and Skin Diseases; National Institute of Child Health and Human Development; National Institute of Dental and Craniofacial Research

(NIDCR)/National Oral Health Information Clearinghouse; National Institute of Diabetes and Digestive and Kidney Disorders (NIDDK); National Institute on Aging; National Institute on Deafness and Other Communication Disorders; National Institutes of Health (NIH); and the Office of the U.S. Surgeon General.

In addition, this volume contains copyrighted documents from the following organizations and individuals: About Cosmetic Dentistry; Academy of General Dentistry (AGD); American Academy of Pediatric Dentistry (AAPD); American Academy of Periodontology (AAP); American Association of Endodontists (AAE); American Association of Oral and Maxillofacial Surgeons (AAOMS); American Association of Orthodontists (AAO); American Dental Association (ADA); American Dental Hygienists' Association (ADHA); Arthritis Foundation; British Dental Health Foundation; California Dental Association; Cleft Palate Foundation; DentalZone, Inc./SaveYourSmile.com; Dentistinfo.com; Dystonia Medical Research Foundation; Gale Group; Hemophilia Galaxy/Baxter Healthcare Corporation; HIVdent; Kimberly A. Loos, DDS; Nemours Foundation/KidsHealth.org; Quackwatch, Inc.; Society for Office-Based Anesthesia; and the University at Buffalo (SUNY) School of Dental Medicine.

Full citation information is provided on the first page of each chapter. Every effort has been made to secure all necessary rights to reprint the copyrighted material. If any omissions have been made, please contact Omnigraphics to make corrections for future editions.

Acknowledgements

Thanks go to the many organizations, agencies, and individuals who have contributed materials for this *Sourcebook* and to medical consultant Dr. David Cooke, verification assistant Dawn Matthews, and document engineer Bruce Bellenir. Special thanks go to managing editor Karen Bellenir and permissions specialist Liz Barbour for their help and support.

Note from the Editor

This book is part of Omnigraphics' *Health Reference Series*. The *Series* provides basic information about a broad range of medical concerns. It is not intended to serve as a tool for diagnosing illness, in prescribing treatments, or as a substitute for the physician/patient relationship. All persons concerned about medical symptoms or the possibility of disease are encouraged to seek professional care from an appropriate health care provider.

Our Advisory Board

The *Health Reference Series* is reviewed by an Advisory Board comprised of librarians from public, academic, and medical libraries. We would like to thank the following board members for providing guidance to the development of this *Series*:

Dr. Lynda Baker,
Associate Professor of Library and Information Science,
Wayne State University, Detroit, MI

Nancy Bulgarelli,
William Beaumont Hospital Library, Royal Oak, MI

Karen Imarisio,
Bloomfield Township Public Library, Bloomfield Township, MI

Karen Morgan,
Mardigian Library, University of Michigan-Dearborn,
Dearborn, MI

Rosemary Orlando,
St. Clair Shores Public Library, St. Clair Shores, MI

Medical Consultant

Medical consultation services are provided to the *Health Reference Series* editors by David A. Cooke, MD. Dr. Cooke is a graduate of Brandeis University, and he received his M.D. degree from the University of Michigan. He completed residency training at the University of Wisconsin Hospital and Clinics. He is board-certified in Internal Medicine. Dr. Cooke currently works as part of the University of Michigan Health System and practices in Brighton, MI. In his free time, he enjoys writing, science fiction, and spending time with his family.

Health Reference Series *Update Policy*

The inaugural book in the *Health Reference Series* was the first edition of *Cancer Sourcebook* published in 1989. Since then, the *Series* has been enthusiastically received by librarians and in the medical community. In order to maintain the standard of providing high-quality health information for the layperson the editorial staff at Omnigraphics felt it was necessary to implement a policy of updating volumes when warranted.

Medical researchers have been making tremendous strides, and it is the purpose of the *Health Reference Series* to stay current with the most recent advances. Each decision to update a volume will be made on an individual basis. Some of the considerations will include how much new information is available and the feedback we receive from people who use the books. If there is a topic you would like to see added to the update list, or an area of medical concern you feel has not been adequately addressed, please write to:

Editor
Health Reference Series
Omnigraphics, Inc.
615 Griswold Street
Detroit, MI 48226
E-mail: editorial@omnigraphics.com

Part One

General Information about Dental Care and Oral Health

Chapter 1

The Mouth and Teeth

Your smile, formed by your mouth at your brain's command, is often the first thing people notice when they look at you. It's the facial expression that most engages others, and one smile often elicits another.

Your mouth also forms your frown, which has the opposite effect on others, and myriad other expressions that show on your face.

The mouth is the body part through which food is taken in and words are brought forth. Inside the mouth, at the entrance of the alimentary canal, are your teeth—the hardest bones in the body. Long after the body's flesh and other bones have dissolved and disintegrated, teeth remain in perfect condition. A body that's been burned or disfigured beyond recognition can often be identified by dental records.

How Are the Mouth and Teeth Necessary for Living?

The mouth houses the tongue, which enables us to form words when we speak and allows us to taste. The lips that line the outside of the mouth both help hold food in while we chew and pronounce words when we talk. They open wide when we scream or yawn and are closed when we are not speaking, eating, or drinking.

This information was provided by KidsHealth, one of the largest resources online for medically reviewed health information written for parents, kids, and teens. For more articles like this one, visit www.KidsHealth.org or www.Teens Health.org. © 2001 The Nemours Center for Children's Health Media, a division of The Nemours Foundation.

3

Without our teeth, we'd have to live on a liquid diet, or possibly a diet of soft, mashed food. Teeth are necessary for chewing or mastication, the process by which we tear, cut, and grind food in preparation for swallowing and digestion. Chewing allows enzymes and lubricants released in the mouth to further break down food.

The mouth and teeth play a large role in speech. Words exit through our mouths. With the lips and tongue, teeth help form words by controlling air flow out of the mouth. The tongue strikes the teeth as certain words are pronounced. The th sound, for example, is produced by the tongue being placed against the upper row of teeth. If your tongue touches your teeth when you say words with the s sound, you may have a lisp. Teeth also provide structural support for face muscles, and they play a role in your smile and other facial expressions.

Basic Anatomy

The entrance to the digestive tract, the mouth is lined with mucous membranes. Its roof is called the palate. The front consists of a bony, membrane-covered portion called the hard palate, and a soft rear part called the soft palate. The hard palate divides the mouth and the nasal passages. The soft palate forms a curtain between the mouth and pharynx, and contains the uvula, a free-hanging projection at the rear of the mouth.

A bundle of muscles extends from the floor of the mouth to form the tongue. The upper surface of the tongue is covered with tiny projections called papillae. These contain tiny pores that are our taste buds. Four kinds of taste buds are grouped together on certain areas of the tongue—those that sense sweet, salty, sour, and bitter tastes. Three pairs of salivary glands secrete saliva, which contains amylase, a digestive enzyme that starts the breakdown of carbohydrates even before food enters the stomach.

The lips are covered with skin on the outside and mucous membranes on the inside. The major lip muscle, the orbicularis oris, allows for the lips' mobility. The reddish tint of the lips comes from underlying blood vessels. Each lip is connected to the gum within the mouth by a small fold of membrane called the frenulum.

Humans are diphyodont, meaning that they develop two sets of teeth. The first set of 20 deciduous teeth are also called the milk, primary, temporary, falling-off, or baby teeth. They begin to develop before birth and fall out when a child is around 6 years old. They are replaced by a set of 32 permanent teeth, which are also called secondary or adult teeth.

Around the 8th week after conception, cellular oval-shaped tooth buds form in the embryo. These begin to harden about the 16th week. At birth, teeth are not visible, but below the gums both the primary and permanent teeth are beginning to form. The crown, or the hard enamel-covered part that is visible in the mouth, develops first, and when the crown is fully grown, the root begins to develop.

Between the ages of 6 months and 1 year, the primary teeth begin to appear. This process is called eruption or teething. At this point, the crown is complete and the root is almost fully formed. By the time a child is 3 years old, he has a set of 20 deciduous teeth, 10 in the lower and 10 in the upper jaw. Each jaw has four incisors, two canines, and four molars. The incisors and canine teeth are used to bite into food, and the molars grind food.

The primary teeth help the permanent teeth erupt in their normal positions; most of the permanent teeth form close to the roots of the primary teeth. When a primary tooth is preparing to fall out, its root begins to dissolve. This root has completely dissolved by the time the permanent tooth below it is ready to erupt.

When a child is about 6 years old, the roots of the baby teeth dissolve as the permanent teeth push them up and out. This begins a transitional phase of tooth development that lasts over the next 15 years. The jaw develops toward its adult form, and from age 6 to 9, the permanent incisors, canines, and molars erupt. The bicuspids come through from age 10 to 12, and the second molars by age 13. The wisdom teeth erupt between the ages of 18 and 21.

Human teeth are comprised of four different types of tissue: pulp, dentin, enamel, and cementum. The pulp is the inner layer of the tooth. It consists of connective tissue, nerves, and blood vessels, which nourish the tooth. It has two parts, the pulp chamber, which lies in the crown, and the root canal, which is in the root of the tooth. Blood vessels and nerves enter the root through a small hole in its tip, and extend through the canal into the pulp chamber.

Dentin surrounds the pulp. A hard yellow substance consisting mostly of mineral salts and water, it makes up most of the tooth, and it's hard as bone. It is the dentin that gives teeth their yellowish tint. Enamel, the hardest tissue in the body, covers the dentin and forms the outermost layer of the crown. It enables the tooth to withstand the pressure of chewing and protects it from harmful bacteria and changes in temperature from hot and cold foods. Both the dentin and pulp extend into the root. A bony layer of cementum covers the outside of the root, under the gum line, and holds the tooth in place within the jawbone. It's also as hard as bone.

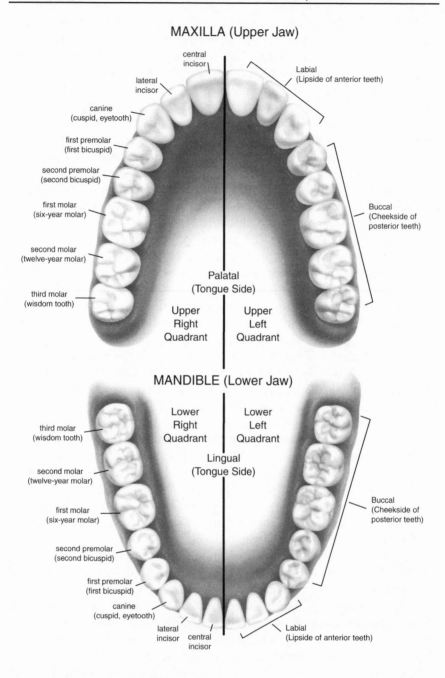

Figure 1.1. Anatomy of the mouth. © American Academy of Periodontology. Reprinted with permission.

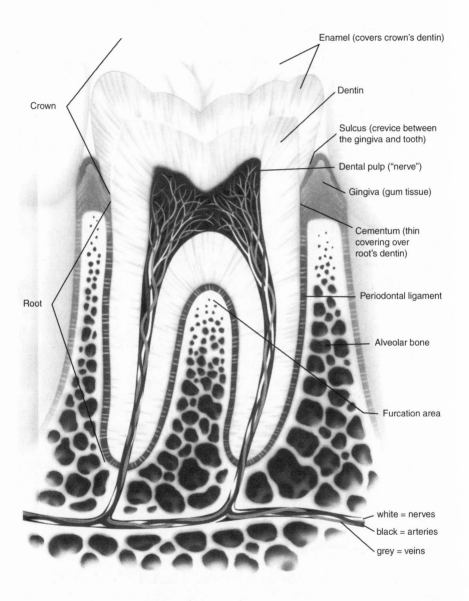

Enamel (covers crown's dentin)

Dentin

Crown

Sulcus (crevice between the gingiva and tooth)

Dental pulp ("nerve")

Gingiva (gum tissue)

Cementum (thin covering over root's dentin)

Periodontal ligament

Root

Alveolar bone

Furcation area

white = nerves

black = arteries

grey = veins

Figure 1.2. Anatomy of a tooth. © American Academy of Periodontology. Reprinted with permission.

There are several types of temporary and permanent teeth. Incisors are the squarish, sharp edged teeth in the front of the mouth. There are four on the bottom and four on the top. On either side of the incisors are the sharp canines. The upper canines are sometimes called eyeteeth. Behind the canines are the flat bicuspids, or premolars. There are two sets, or four bicuspids, in each jaw.

The molars, situated behind the bicuspids, have points and grooves. There are 12 molars; three sets in each jaw, called the first, second, and third molars. Third molars are the wisdom teeth, developed thousands of years ago when human diets consisted of mostly raw foods that required extra chewing power. But because they can crowd out the other teeth, sometimes a dentist will need to remove these teeth.

Normal Physiology

The first step of digestion involves the mouth and teeth. Food enters the mouth and is immediately broken down into smaller pieces by our teeth. Each type of tooth serves a different function in the chewing process.

Incisors cut foods when you bite into them. Canines, the upper set of which are also known as eyeteeth, tear food. The flat bicuspids, or premolars, grind and mash food. Molars, with their points and grooves, are responsible for the most vigorous chewing. All the while, the tongue helps to push the food up against our teeth.

As we chew, salivary glands in the walls and floor of the mouth secrete saliva, which moistens the food and helps break it down further. Saliva makes it easier to chew and swallow foods (especially dry foods), and it contains enzymes that aid in the digestion of carbohydrates.

Once food has been converted into a soft, moist mass, it's pushed into the pharynx at the back of the mouth and is swallowed. When we swallow, the soft palate closes the nasal passages from the throat to prevent food from entering the nose.

Diseases, Conditions, Disorders, and Dysfunctions

Dental care is essential to maintaining healthy teeth and avoiding tooth decay and gum disease. A good diet, proper and frequent cleaning of the teeth after eating, and regular dental checkups are all necessary for proper care. Some common mouth and dental diseases and conditions are listed below.

Disorders of the Mucous Membranes of the Mouth

Aphthous stomatitis (canker sores). A common form of mouth ulcer, canker sores occur in women more often than in men. Ulcers may develop in response to a mouth injury or when the tongue or cheek is bitten. Stress, dietary deficiencies, menstrual periods, hormonal changes, or food allergies can also trigger them. They usually appear on the inner surface of the cheeks, lips, tongue, soft palate, or the base of the gums, and begin with a tingling or burning sensation followed by a red spot or bump that ulcerates. Pain spontaneously decreases in 7 to 10 days, with complete healing in 1 to 3 weeks.

Periodontal disease. The gums and bones supporting the teeth are subject to disease. A common periodontal disease is gingivitis, an inflammation characterized by red, swollen, and/or bleeding gums. The accumulation of tartar (a hardened film of food particles and bacteria that builds up on teeth) usually causes this condition, and it is almost always the result of inadequate brushing and flossing. When gingivitis isn't treated, it leads to periodontitis, in which the gums loosen around the teeth and pockets of bacteria and pus form, affecting the supporting bone and resulting in tooth loss. A rare but severe form of gingivitis is called trench mouth. Also known as Vincent's infection, trench mouth gets its name from World War I, when it was a common disorder among soldiers. Trench mouth usually affects young adults between 15 and 35 years and may be caused by viruses that allow bacteria in the mouth to overgrow. Several factors can contribute to the development of trench mouth, including poor nutrition; throat, tooth, or mouth infections; smoking; fatigue; and emotional stress.

Herpetic stomatitis (oral herpes). Babies and children can get the herpes simplex virus, which is responsible for oral herpes, from an adult who has it. The resulting painful, clustered blisters can make it difficult to drink or eat, which can lead to dehydration especially in a young child.

Enteroviral stomatitis is an infection caused by enterovirus, including the coxsackie virus, which causes hand, foot, and mouth disease. This infection results in small, painful ulcers in the mouth that may decrease a child's desire to eat and drink and put him at risk for dehydration.

Disorders of the Teeth

Malocclusion. The failure of the teeth in the upper and lower jaws to meet properly, malocclusions include overbite, underbite, and crowding. Most conditions can be corrected with braces. Braces are metal or clear ceramic brackets bonded to the front of each tooth. Wires connect them; these are tightened periodically to force the teeth to move into the right position.

Cavities and tooth decay. When bacteria and food particles stick to saliva on the teeth, plaque forms. The bacteria digest the carbohydrates and produce acid, which dissolves the tooth's enamel and causes a cavity. If the cavity is not treated, the decay process progresses to the dentin. The most common ways to treat cavities and more serious tooth decay problems are filling the cavity with silver amalgam; performing root canal therapy, involving the removal of the pulp of a tooth; crowning a tooth with a cap that looks like a tooth made of metal, porcelain, or plastic; or removing or replacing the tooth. A common cause of tooth decay in toddlers is "milk bottle mouth," which occurs when a child goes to sleep with a milk or juice bottle in his mouth and his teeth are exposed to sugary liquid for an extended period of time. To avoid tooth decay and cavities, teach your child good dental habits—including proper tooth brushing techniques—at an early age.

Developmental Disorders

Cleft lip and palate are birth defects in which the tissues of the mouth or lip don't form properly during fetal development. Children born with these disorders may have trouble feeding immediately after birth. Reconstructive surgery in infancy corrects the anatomical defects and helps prevent speech disorders from occurring later on in development.

Glossary

amylase: A digestive enzyme that starts the breakdown of food before it begins the digestion process.

bicuspid: Premolar used for grinding and mashing food.

canine: One of four pointed teeth near the front of the mouth used for tearing food.

cementum: Bone-like material that covers the outside of the root of a tooth.

crown: Top part of a tooth that shows above the gums.

deciduous teeth: The first set of human teeth; also called milk, primary, temporary, falling-off, or baby teeth.

dentin: Hard yellow substance that makes up most of a tooth.

diphyodont: A species that develops two sets of teeth.

enamel: Hard surface of a tooth covering the dentin.

frenulum: Small fold of membrane that connects the lip to the gum within the mouth.

hard palate: The bony, membrane-covered front part of the roof of the mouth.

incisor: Sharp, square tooth at the front of the mouth used for cutting food.

mastication: The process by which food is torn, cut, and grinded by teeth in preparation for swallowing and digestion.

molar: Tooth at the back of the mouth used for grinding and mashing food.

orbicularis oris: Major lip muscle.

papillae: Tiny projections that cover the upper surface of the tongue that contain the taste buds.

pulp: Soft, inner layer of a tooth.

soft palate: The soft rear part of the roof of the mouth.

uvula: A free-hanging projection at the rear of the mouth.

Note: All information on KidsHealth is for educational purposes only. For specific medical advice, diagnoses, and treatment, consult your doctor.

Chapter 2

Infant and Toddler Oral Health

Chapter Contents

Section 2.1

How to Prevent Baby Bottle Tooth Decay

Every year thousands of infants and young children suffer from extensive tooth decay. Surprisingly, the major culprits are milk and other liquids from the baby's bottle.

Bacteria—Your Baby's Enemies

Just like an adult's mouth, a baby's mouth is full of bacteria. These bacteria feed on sugars found in the liquids we drink and in the foods we eat. These bacteria produce acid as a byproduct of their feasting. It is this acid that attacks the tooth enamel and causes cavities.

Many parents put their children to sleep with a bottle. They often find that this helps the baby settle down. Unfortunately, studies show that babies fall asleep with the baby bottle nipples in their mouths, allowing fluid from the bottle to pool around teeth.

Sugar present in the fluid continually nourishes the bacteria that are in the baby's mouth. Using this constant source of sugar, bacteria multiply and create a steady stream of tooth-damaging acid. Night after night of acid attack results in cavity formation and extensive tooth decay. In some cases, the entire tooth can be eaten away by bacterially produced acid.

It is especially important to be vigilant against baby bottle tooth decay because baby teeth are more susceptible to tooth decay than adult teeth. Additionally, constant sugar in the mouth can lead to a buildup of bacteria to a point where more harmful types of bacteria start becoming predominant. These bacteria cause gingivitis by invading gum tissue and releasing toxins. In severe cases, the bacteria and their toxins can attack bone structures supporting the teeth (periodontal disease), resulting in permanent damage.

Protecting Your Child

What can parents do to protect their children's teeth? We suggest that after every bottle feeding you take a wet cloth or gauze pad and gently wipe your child's gums and teeth. This will remove any bacteria-containing plaque and excess sugar that may have built up.

What liquid should you put in your baby's bedtime bottle? Natural juices such as grape juice or apple juice contain natural sugars that bacteria can use to create acids. Milk contains a sugar called lactose which bacteria can also use to create acid.

If you give you child a bedtime bottle, the liquid of choice inside of the baby's bottle is water. Water contains no sugar and cannot be used by bacteria to produce acid.

Finally, never give your baby a pacifier dipped in any type of substance containing large amounts of sugar. Many parents, for example, give their children pacifiers dipped in honey. This can be very bad for the baby's teeth. [Note: Feeding honey to infants under 1 year of age may also put an infant at risk of infant botulism.]

When you protect your child from baby bottle tooth decay, you ensure that his or her smile will last a lifetime.

Section 2.2

Thumb, Finger, and Pacifier Habits

Reprinted with permission from the American Academy of Pediatric Dentistry, www.aapd.org. © 2002.

Why Do Children Suck on Fingers, Pacifiers, or Other Objects?

This type of sucking is completely normal for babies and young children. It provides security. For young babies, it's a way to make contact with and learn about the world. In fact, babies begin to suck on their fingers or thumbs even before they are born.

Are These Habits Bad for the Teeth and Jaws?

Most children stop sucking on thumbs, pacifiers, or other objects on their own between two and four years of age. No harm is done to their teeth or jaws. However, some children repeatedly suck on a finger, pacifier, or other object over long periods of time. In these children, the upper front teeth may tip toward the lip or not come in properly.

When Should I Worry about a Sucking Habit?

Your pediatric dentist will carefully watch the way your child's teeth come in and jaw develops, keeping the sucking habit in mind at all times. For most children there is no reason to worry about a sucking habit until the permanent front teeth are ready to come in.

What Can I Do to Stop My Child's Habit?

Most children stop sucking habits on their own, but some children need the help of their parents and their pediatric dentist. When your child is old enough to understand the possible results of a sucking habit, your pediatric dentist can encourage your child to stop, as well as talk about what happens to the teeth if your child doesn't stop. This advice, coupled with support from parents, helps most children quit. If this approach doesn't work, your pediatric dentist may recommend a mouth appliance that blocks sucking habits.

Are Pacifiers a Safer Habit for the Teeth than Thumbs or Fingers?

Thumb, finger, and pacifier sucking all affect the teeth essentially the same way. However, a pacifier habit is often easier to break.

Section 2.3

Teething Tots

This information was provided by KidsHealth, one of the largest resources online for medically reviewed health information written for parents, kids, and teens. For more articles like this one, visit www.KidsHealth.org, or www.TeensHealth.org. © 2002 The Nemours Center for Children's Health Media, a division of The Nemours Foundation.

An old wives' tale links a baby's mental development to how early teething starts. Does this mean that your 5-month-old, who has already begun cutting her second tooth, is going to be the next Einstein? The truth is, teething is not related to mental development, so parents need not worry even if their baby hasn't begun teething in the first year. Teething can start as early as 3 months and continue until a child's third birthday.

Typically between the ages of 4 and 7 months, you will notice your child's first tooth pushing through the gum line. The first teeth to appear are usually the two bottom front teeth, also known as the central incisors.

These are usually followed 4 to 8 weeks later by the four front upper teeth (central and lateral incisors). About 1 month later, the lower lateral incisors (the two teeth flanking the bottom front teeth) will appear. Next to break through the gum line are the first molars (the back teeth used for grinding food), then finally the eyeteeth (the pointy teeth in the upper jaw). Most children have all 20 of their primary teeth by their third birthday. (This is a general rule; if your child experiences significant delay, speak to your child's doctor.)

Rarely, children will be born with one or two teeth or will have a tooth emerge within the first few weeks of life. Unless the teeth interfere with feeding or are loose enough to pose a choking risk, this is usually not a cause for concern.

Easing Teething

Whenever your child begins teething, it generally will be a process marked by increased drooling and the desire to chew on things. For most babies, teething is painless. Others may experience brief periods of irritability, and some may seem cranky for weeks, experiencing crying episodes and disrupted sleeping and eating patterns. Teething can be uncomfortable, but if your baby seems very irritable, contact your child's doctor.

Although tender and swollen gums could cause your baby's temperature to be a little higher than normal, teething, as a rule, does not cause high fever or diarrhea. If your baby does develop a fever during the teething phase, it is probably due to something else and your child's doctor should be contacted.

Here are some tips to keep in mind when your baby is teething:

- Wipe your baby's face often with a cloth to remove the drool and prevent rashes from developing.

- Place a clean, flat cloth under the baby's head during sleep to catch the drool. This way, you'll only have to change the cloth when it gets wet, not the whole sheet.

- Give your baby something to chew on. Make sure it's big enough so that she can't swallow it and that it can't break into small pieces. A wet washcloth placed in the freezer for 30 minutes makes a handy teething aid—just be sure to wash it after each use. A cool spoon works well, too. Rubber teething rings are also good, but avoid the ones with liquid inside because they may break. If you use a teething ring, be sure to take it out of the freezer before it becomes rock hard—you don't want to bruise those already swollen gums!

- Rub your baby's gums with a clean finger.

- Never tie a teething ring around a baby's neck, as it could get caught on something and strangle the baby.

- If your baby seems irritable, acetaminophen (such as Tylenol) may help—but always consult your child's doctor first. Never place an aspirin against the tooth, and don't rub whiskey on your baby's gums.

Baby Teeth Hygiene

The care and cleaning of your baby's teeth is important for long-term dental health. Even though the first set of teeth will fall out, tooth decay can hasten this process and leave gaps before the permanent teeth are ready to come in. The remaining primary teeth may then crowd together to attempt to fill in the gaps, which may cause the permanent teeth to come in crooked and out of place.

Daily dental care should begin even before your baby's first tooth emerges. Wipe your baby's gums daily with a clean, damp washcloth or gauze, or brush them gently with a soft, infant-sized toothbrush and water (no toothpaste!). As soon as the first tooth appears, brush them with water. Not only does this help prevent tooth decay, it also shows your child the importance of regular dental care.

Toothpaste is OK to use on your child's teeth once she gets old enough to spit it out—usually around age 3. Choose one with fluoride and use only a pea-sized amount or less in younger children. Don't let your child swallow the toothpaste or eat it out of the tube because an overdose of fluoride can be harmful for children.

By the time all her baby teeth are in, you should be brushing your child's teeth twice a day—after breakfast and before bed. It's also a good idea to get your child used to flossing early on. A good time to start flossing is when two teeth start to touch. Talk to your child's dentist for advice on flossing those tiny teeth. You can also get your toddler interested in the routine by letting her watch and imitate you as you brush and floss on a regular basis. Be sure to help your child brush and floss until she's able to do it herself.

Another important tip for preventing tooth decay: don't let your baby fall asleep with a bottle. The milk or juice can pool in her mouth and cause tooth decay and plaque.

It used to be that regular dental checkups weren't recommended until after age 3 or when all 20 primary teeth came in. Now there are two schools of thought on early dental care. The American Academy of Pediatrics recommends that before age 3, your child's doctor should check for dental problems at regular medical checkups and refer your child to a dentist if necessary. The American Dental Association and the American Academy of Pediatric Dentists recommend that children see a dentist by age 1, when six to eight teeth are in place, to spot any potential problems and advise parents about preventive care. Whichever you choose, your ultimate goal should be to make good dental care habits a lifelong goal for your child.

Note: All information on KidsHealth is for educational purposes only. For specific medical advice, diagnoses, and treatment, consult your doctor.

Chapter 3

Oral Health in Children

Chapter Contents

Section 3.1

Keeping Your Child's Teeth Healthy

This information was provided by KidsHealth, one of the largest resources online for medically reviewed health information written for parents, kids, and teens. For more articles like this one, visit www.KidsHealth.org or www.TeensHealth.org. © 2001 The Nemours Center for Children's Health Media, a division of The Nemours Foundation.

When should I schedule my child's first trip to the dentist? Should my 3-year-old be flossing? How do I know if my child needs braces? Many parents have a difficult time judging how much dental care their children need. They know they want to prevent cavities, but they don't always know the best way to do so.

When Should I Start Caring for My Child's Teeth?

Proper dental care begins even before a baby's first tooth appears. Remember that just because you can't see the teeth doesn't mean they aren't there. Teeth actually begin to form in the second trimester of pregnancy. At birth your baby has 20 primary teeth, some of which are fully developed in the jaw.

Running a damp washcloth over your baby's gums following feedings can prevent buildup of damaging bacteria. Once your child has a few teeth showing, you can brush them with a soft child's toothbrush or rub them with gauze at the end of the day.

Even babies can have problems with dental decay when parents do not practice good feeding habits at home. "Putting your baby to sleep with a bottle propped in his mouth may be convenient in the short term—but it is bad news for the baby's teeth," explains pediatric dentist Garrett B. Lyons, DDS.

When the sugars from juice or milk remain on a baby's teeth for hours, they may eat away at the enamel, creating a condition known as bottle mouth. Pocked, pitted, or discolored front teeth are signs of bottle mouth. Severe cases result in cavities and the need to pull all the front teeth until the permanent ones grow in. Parents and child care providers should also help young children develop set times for drinking during the day as well because sucking on a bottle throughout the day can be equally damaging to young teeth.

What Kind of Dentist Should My Child See?

You may want to take your child to a dentist who specializes in treating children. Pediatric dentists are trained to handle the wide range of issues associated with your child's dental health. They also know when to refer you to a different type of specialist, such as an orthodontist to correct an overbite or an oral surgeon for jaw realignment.

A pediatric dentist's primary goals are prevention, heading off potential oral health problems before they occur, and maintenance, ensuring through routine checkups and proper daily care that teeth and gums stay healthy.

How Can I Prevent Cavities?

The American Dental Association recommends that your child's first visit to the dentist take place by her first birthday. At this visit, your child's dentist will explain proper brushing and flossing techniques (you need to floss once your baby has two teeth that touch) and conduct a modified exam while your baby sits on your lap. Such visits can help in the early detection of potential problems. Your child also will become accustomed to visiting the dentist, which means she'll have less fear as she grows older.

When all of your child's primary teeth have come in (usually around age 2 1/2) your dentist may start applying topical fluoride during your child's visits. Fluoride hardens the tooth enamel, helping to ward off the most common childhood oral disease, dental caries, or cavities. Cavities are caused by bacteria and food that are left on the teeth after eating. When these are not brushed away, acid collects on a tooth, softening its enamel until a hole—or cavity—forms. Regular use of fluoride toughens the enamel, making it more difficult for acid to penetrate.

Although many municipalities require tap water to be fluoridated, other communities have no such regulations. "Parents must ask, especially when you move to a new community," Dr. Lyons says. If the water supply is not fluoridated, or if your family uses purified water, ask your dentist for fluoride supplements. Even though most toothpastes contain fluoride, toothpaste alone will not fully protect a child's mouth. Be careful, however, since too much fluoride can cause tooth discoloration. Check with your dentist before supplementing.

Discoloration can also occur as a result of prolonged use of antibiotics. "Some children's medications are almost 75% sugar," says Dr. Lyons. He suggests that parents encourage children to brush after they take their medicine, particularly if the prescription will be long term.

Brushing at least twice a day and routine flossing will help maintain a healthy mouth. Children as young as age 2 or 3 can begin to use toothpaste when brushing, as long as they are supervised. "Children should not ingest large amounts of toothpaste—a pea-sized amount for toddlers is just right," Dr. Lyons suggests. He cautions parents to make sure that the child spits the toothpaste out, instead of swallowing.

As your child's permanent teeth grow in, her dentist can help seal out decay by applying a thin wash of resin to the back teeth, where most chewing occurs. Known as a sealant, this protective coating keeps bacteria from settling in the hard-to-reach crevices of the molars. "Most kids can benefit from sealants, unless the tops of their molars are unusually smooth and flat," explains Constance Killian, DDS, a pediatric dentist and trustee of the American Academy of Pediatric Dentistry.

Although dental research has resulted in increasingly sophisticated preventative techniques, including fillings and sealants that seep fluoride, a dentist's care is only part of the equation. Follow-up at home plays an equally important role. For example, the sealants on a child's teeth do not mean that she can eat sweets uncontrollably or slack off on the daily brushing and flossing. "We can only do so much at the office—parents must work with children to teach good oral health habits," says Dr. Killian.

What Should I Do If My Child Has a Problem?

If you are prone to tooth decay or gum disease, your child may be at higher risk as well. "Dental caries is an infectious disease, so if the parents carry high levels of the disease in their mouths, the kids are at higher risk," Dr. Killian says. Therefore, sometimes even the most diligent brushing and flossing will not prevent a cavity. Be sure to call your dentist if your child complains of pain in her teeth. The pain could be a sign of a cavity that needs to be treated.

New materials have given the pediatric dentist more filling and repair options than ever before. Silver remains the substance of choice for the majority of fillings in permanent teeth. Other materials, such as composite resins, also are gaining popularity. "The beauty of the composite resins is that they bond to the teeth, so the filling won't pop out," Dr. Killian says. "They can be used to rebuild teeth damaged through injury or conditions such as cleft palate."

Tooth-colored resins are also more attractive. But in cases of fracture, extensive decay, or malformation of baby teeth, dentists often opt for stainless steel crowns. "A small amount of decay will destroy a baby tooth very quickly. The crown maintains the tooth while preventing the decay from spreading," Dr. Killian says.

As your child grows older, you may be concerned about her bite and the straightness of her teeth. Orthodontic treatment begins earlier now than it once did. What once was a symbol of preteen anguish—a mouth filled with metal wires and braces—has become a relic of the past. Kids as young as age 7 are now sporting corrective appliances. Efficient, plastic-based materials have replaced old-fashioned metal contraptions.

Dentists now understand that manipulation of teeth at a younger age can be easier and more effective in the long run. Younger children's teeth can be positioned with relatively minor orthodontia, thus preventing major orthodontia later on.

In some rare instances, usually when a more complicated dental procedure is to be performed, a dentist will recommend general anesthesia to put the child to sleep. "When there is a severe behavioral problem, for instance, or a child has multiple lesions in the mouth, we will use anesthesia," Dr. Lyons explains.

Parents should make sure that the professional who administers the medicine is a trained anesthesiologist or oral surgeon before agreeing to the procedure. Don't be afraid to question the dentist. "General anesthesia use is relatively safe, as long as licensed, trained professionals follow proper guidelines and maintain appropriate equipment," Dr. Killian says. Giving your child an early start on checkups and good dental hygiene is an effective way to help prevent this kind of extensive dental work. Encouraging your child to use a mouth guard during sports can also prevent serious dental injuries.

As your child grows, plan on routine dental checkups anywhere from once every 3 months to once a year, depending on her dentist's recommendations. Limiting intake of sugary foods and regular brushing and flossing all contribute to your child's dental health. Your partnership with your child's dentist will help keep your child's teeth healthy and her smile beautiful.

Note: All information on KidsHealth is for educational purposes only. For specific medical advice, diagnoses, and treatment, consult your doctor.

Section 3.2

Diet, Snacking, and Your Child's Dental Health

Reprinted with permission from the American Academy of Pediatric Dentistry, www.aapd.org. © 2002.

What Is a Healthy Diet for My Child?

A healthy diet is a balanced diet that naturally supplies all the nutrients your child needs to grow. And what's a balanced diet? One that includes the following major food groups every day: fruits and vegetables; breads and cereals; milk and dairy products; meat, fish and eggs.

How Does My Child's Diet Affect Her Dental Health?

She must have a balanced diet for her teeth to develop properly. She also needs a balanced diet for healthy gum tissue around the teeth. Equally important, a diet high in certain kinds of carbohydrates, such as sugar and starches, may place your child at extra risk of tooth decay.

How Do I Make My Child's Diet Safe for His Teeth?

First, be sure he has a balanced diet. Then, check how frequently he eats foods with sugar or starch in them. Foods with starch include breads, crackers, pasta, and such snacks as pretzels and potato chips. When checking for sugar, look beyond the sugar bowl and candy dish. A variety of foods contain one or more types of sugar, and all types of sugars can promote dental decay. Fruits, a few vegetables, and most milk products have at least one type of sugar.

Sugar can be found in many processed foods, even some that do not taste sweet. For example, a peanut butter and jelly sandwich not only has sugar in the jelly, but may have sugar added to the peanut butter. Sugar is also added to such condiments as catsup and salad dressings.

Should My Child Give up All Foods with Sugar or Starch?

Certainly not! Many provide nutrients your child needs. You simply need to select and serve them wisely. A food with sugar or starch is safer for teeth if it's eaten with a meal, not as a snack. Sticky foods, such as dried fruit or toffee, are not easily washed away from the teeth by saliva, water, or milk. So they have more cavity-causing potential than foods more rapidly cleared from the teeth. Talk to your pediatric dentist about selecting and serving foods that protect your child's dental health.

Does a Balanced Diet Assure That My Child Is Getting Enough Fluoride?

No. A balanced diet does not guarantee the proper amount of fluoride for the development and maintenance of your child's teeth. If you do not live in a fluoridated community or have an ideal amount of naturally occurring fluoride in your well water, your child needs a fluoride supplement during the years of tooth development. Your pediatric dentist can help assess how much supplemental fluoride your child needs, based upon the amount of fluoride in your drinking water and your child's age and weight.

My Youngest Isn't on Solid Foods Yet. Do You Have Suggestions for Her?

Don't nurse your daughter to sleep or put her to bed with a bottle of milk, formula, juice, or sweetened liquid. While she sleeps, any unswallowed liquid in the mouth supports bacteria that produce acids and attack the teeth. Protect your child from severe tooth decay by putting her to bed with nothing more than a pacifier or bottle of water.

Final Advice

Here are tips for your child's diet and dental health.

- Ask your pediatric dentist to help you assess your child's diet.
- Shop smart! Do not routinely stock your pantry with sugary or starchy snacks. Buy fun foods just for special times.
- Limit the number of snack times; choose nutritious snacks.
- Provide a balanced diet, and save foods with sugar or starch for mealtimes.

- Don't put your young child to bed with a bottle of milk, formula, or juice.

- If your child chews gum or sips soda, choose those without sugar.

Section 3.3

Milk Matters for Your Child's Healthy Mouth

Excerpted from "Milk Matters for Your Child's Healthy Mouth!" a brochure produced by the National Institute of Child Health and Human Development, NIH Publications Number 99-4521, May 2000.

That's because milk and dairy foods have lots of calcium and other nutrients that make bones grow strong and healthy. Children and teenagers especially need the calcium and other bone building materials in milk because their bones are growing more than at any other time in their lives.

Studies show that most kids don't get the calcium they need. In fact, more than half of teenage boys and girls don't get the recommended amount of calcium.

Why Do Kids Need Calcium?

Calcium is a mineral found in many foods that does lots of good things for the body.

Calcium Makes Bones Strong

Bones may seem hard and lifeless. But they are actually growing and alive. Since bones grow most during the childhood and teenage years, these are especially important times to give them the calcium they need. By eating and drinking lots of foods with calcium, children and teens can help build their bone banks to store calcium to keep bones strong for the rest of their lives.

Calcium Helps Reduce the Risk of Osteoporosis

Osteoporosis is a condition that makes bones become weak and break more easily. Getting enough calcium as children or teens can help protect against osteoporosis. Although the effects of osteoporosis might not show up until we are adults, kids need to get enough calcium when they are young to help prevent it.

Calcium Makes the Whole Mouth Healthy

Calcium keeps teeth strong and healthy throughout life. Even before baby and adult teeth come in they need calcium to develop fully. And after teeth come in they stay strong and resist decay by taking in calcium. Calcium also makes gums healthy. Getting enough calcium as a young adult may help prevent gum disease later in life. And calcium makes jawbones strong and healthy, too. Bones also need exercise to become stronger. Playing sports, running, jumping, or dancing, for example, helps makes bones stronger.

Table 3.1. How Much Calcium Does My Child Need?

Age	Calcium Needed Each Day (in milligrams)
Birth to 6 months	210 mg
6 to 12 months	270 mg
1 to 3 years	500 mg
4 to 8 years	800 mg
9 to 18 years	1,300 mg
19 to 50 years	1,000 mg

Source: Dietary Reference Intakes for Calcium, National Academy of Sciences, 1997.

Where Can Kids Get Calcium?

Milk and other dairy foods, such as cheese and yogurt, are excellent sources of calcium. One 8-ounce glass of milk has about 300 milligrams (mg) of calcium. Just a few glasses can go a long way toward giving kids the calcium they need each day.

Milk also has other vitamins and minerals that are good for bones and teeth. One especially important nutrient is vitamin D, which helps the body to absorb more calcium.

Other sources of calcium include dark green, leafy vegetables, such as kale, and foods like broccoli, soybeans, tofu made with calcium, orange juice with calcium added, and other calcium-fortified foods.

Table 3.2. Where Is the Calcium?

Food	Serving Size	Calcium (in milligrams)	% Daily Value on Food Label
Plain yogurt, fat-free	1 cup	450	45%
Frozen yogurt, fat-free, calcium fortified	½ cup	450	45%
American cheese	2 ounces	350	35%
Ricotta cheese, part skim	½ cup	337	30%
Yogurt with fruit	1 cup	315	30%
Cheddar cheese	1 ounce	200	20%
Milk (fat-free, low-fat, whole, or lactose-free)	1 cup	300	30%
Orange juice with added calcium	1 cup	300	30%
Tofu (made with calcium sulfate)	½ cup	260	25%
Soy milk, calcium-fortified	1 cup	250–300	25%–30%
Cheese pizza	1 slice	220	20%
Macaroni and cheese	½ cup	180	18%
Corn tortilla	3 tortillas	132	10%
Broccoli, cooked or fresh	1 cup	90	9%
Soybeans, cooked	½ cup	90	9%
Almonds, dry roasted	1 ounce	80	8%
Bok choy, boiled	½ cup	80	8%
White bread	1 slice	30	3%

Note: Calcium content varies depending on the ingredients for many foods. % Daily Values have been rounded according to Food and Drug Administration guidelines.

Sources for Calcium Food Table: American Dietetic Association's Complete Food and Nutrition Guide, 1996; Bowes and Church's Food Values of Portions Commonly Used, 1998. Some values have been rounded.

Chapter 4

Oral Health in Adolescents

Chapter Contents

Section 4.1

Adolescent Dental Care

"Adolescent Care" is reprinted with permission from HIVdent, www. hivdent.org. © 2000 HIVdent. Available online at http://www. hivdent.org/_peag/faq-teen.htm; accessed May 2003.

Once your adolescent reaches the teen years, he or she should have all of the permanent teeth except for the four wisdom teeth (which appear around age 16.) A good appearance is especially important to preteens and teens, so it can be easy to motivate them to practice good oral care habits to ensure a healthy and beautiful smile.

Some preteens and teenagers may wear braces (orthodontic appliances) on their teeth. Orthodontics is the area of dentistry that involves the diagnosis, prevention, and treatment of teeth that are twisted, overlapping, or do not fit together properly.

Unless your teen continues to have problems with cavities, he or she will not require continued use of fluoride supplements after his or her permanent teeth completely appear as the teeth should be well protected from decay.

When Will My Teen Have All of His Permanent Teeth?

Your teen will begin to replace his baby teeth with permanent teeth from around age six until age 12 or 13. At this time he or she will have a complete set of 32 permanent teeth. The wisdom teeth are the last to appear at around age 16.

Should My Teen Be Receiving Additional Fluoride?

Unless your teen continues to have problems with cavities, he or she will not require continued use of fluoride supplements after his or her permanent teeth completely appear as the teeth should be well protected from decay.

My Teen's Teeth Are Crooked and Overlap. At What Age Should He Begin Wearing Braces?

Orthodontic treatment (wearing braces) usually begins around age 10 although braces can be worn at any age.

Made of metal or plastic, braces include brackets attached to the teeth and wires that connect them. Pressure to move the teeth is caused by adjusting the wires regularly.

The length of time a person wears braces depends on age, the severity of the problem, and the condition of the mouth. However, the average teen wears braces for 18-30 months. After the braces are removed, a removable retainer must be worn for several months to hold the teeth in their proper position until they're more secure.

What Is the Proper Way for My Teen to Brush and Floss?

Your teen should brush twice a day with a fluoride toothpaste and with a toothbrush that has soft bristles and a small head for those hard-to-reach back teeth. A thorough job of brushing removes plaque from the inner, outer, and chewing surfaces of his or her teeth.

Every teen should floss once a day to remove plaque from between teeth and under the gum line where a toothbrush cannot reach.

Section 4.2

Oral Piercings

"Oral Piercings Gaining Popularity, Critics," reprinted with permission from the American Dental Hygienists' Association Web site, www.adha.org. © 2003.

From the chin to the cheeks, tongue, and everything in between, millions of young people are expressing their individuality with oral piercings.

However, self-expression comes at a hefty cost for many as laws governing piercing studios vary from state to state, making it difficult to regulate the industry.

As a result, many piercees suffer serious infection, toxic shock syndrome, and even loss of taste resulting from a poorly placed piercing.

The mouth is the ideal environment for infection and bacteria, said Ann Naber, RDH, President of the American Dental Hygienists' Association (ADHA).

"It's well documented that there are fractures of teeth, periodontal disease (advanced gum disease), and trauma associated with the jewelry used in oral piercings," Naber said.

In general, "dental hygienists probably don't see as many cases of infection as we did when they first started, but the risk is very real," Naber said.

Other concerns Naber raised deal with the possibility of hepatitis, tetanus, and HIV infection.

Any piercing procedure should use equipment that has been properly sterilized utilizing an autoclave process, she said.

For the parents of young teens who are considering getting an oral piercing, Naber recommended consulting an oral health care professional beforehand.

In addition, make sure the body artist practices good hygiene and uses hypoallergenic equipment.

Chapter 5

Oral Health in Adults

Chapter Contents

Section 5.1

Oral Health and General Well-Being

Excerpted from "The Oral-Systemic Health Connection," a report pub-
lished by the National Institute of Dental and Craniofacial Research
(NIDCR), May 1999. Available online at www.nidcr.nih.gov/spectrum/
NIDCR2/2menu.htm. Accessed May 2003.

There is no doubt that oral health and general well-being are in-
extricably bound. Many conditions that plague the body are mani-
fested in the mouth, a readily accessible vantage point from which to
view the onset, progress, and management of numerous systemic diseases.

What does this mean for traditional dental research? It means that
perhaps this term is an anachronism, that it limits the field of inquiry
to only the teeth and surrounding tissues, that the word traditional
no longer applies.

In fact, there is nothing traditional about the science of the oral, dental, and craniofacial tissues. The teeth and gingiva (gums) are but one
vital part of a remarkably dynamic system that touches on virtually
every biomedical and behavioral discipline. Research in virology, immunology, genetics, biochemistry, developmental biology, and many
other fields is carried out by men and women whose names end in
PhD, DDS, and MD. They are laboratory researchers. They are patient-
oriented clinical scientists. They see the beauty and order of a world
at its molecular level. They engineer genes to correct nature's mis-
takes. Their educational backgrounds and training experiences are
as diverse as the diseases and systems they study. What these scientists share in common, however, is the recognition that oral health is
not an independent entity cut off from the rest of the body. Rather, it
is woven deeply into the fabric of overall health.

The Body's Silent Alarm

One human mouth is home to more microorganisms than there are
people on our planet earth. The wide array of habitat renders the
mouth a microbial paradise, offering preferred accommodations on the

cheek, or on the back of the tongue in an anaerobic crevice, or in the moist, oxygen-deprived area between the tooth surface and the adjacent periodontal tissues.

The mouth's microbial ecology, however, is extremely sensitive to the challenges that confront its human host throughout the lifespan and, therefore, can often change precipitously. From fetal life through senescence, the mouth's continued exposure to opportunistic infectious pathogens is in balance with host immunity; the balance between these profoundly important processes often serves as a mirror for the detection of not only oral pathology, but also major systemic diseases.

It is especially in the soft tissues that this relationship is played out. The lips, tongue, gums, salivary glands, and oral mucosa can all warn of trouble in our general health. Because of their exquisite positioning in the body, these tissues and their fluids form a protective barrier of mucosal immunity to the outside world that when breached, signal clinical disease. They tell of direct assaults by a broad range of systemic disorders such as diabetes, AIDS, and Sjögren's syndrome, as well as complications of treatments like cancer chemotherapy and radiation. For some disorders, particularly AIDS and diabetes, oral tissues may reveal lesions or pathology that are the first signs of systemic disease.

Oral Opportunistic Infections and Links to Systemic Diseases

The periodontium, comprised of the gingiva, bone, and other supporting tissues that anchor the teeth, plays a key role in the interplay between oral health and systemic disease. Infection in these tissues can initiate a series of inflammatory and immunologic changes leading to the destruction of connective tissue and bone. Long considered a localized infection, periodontal diseases are now linked to a variety of conditions with systemic implications.

Chronic Degenerative Diseases

Periodontitis, advanced infection of the periodontium that often causes tooth mobility and tooth loss, appears to share genetically determined risk factors with several other chronic degenerative diseases such as ulcerative colitis, juvenile arthritis, and systemic lupus erythematosus. Recent research points to specific genetic markers associated with increased production of the pro-inflammatory cytokines interleukin-1 and TNF as strong indicators of susceptibility to severe

37

periodontitis. This recent finding could lead to early identification of people at most risk for severe periodontal disease and initiation of appropriate therapeutic interventions.

Diabetes Mellitus

The destructive inflammatory processes that define periodontal disease are closely intertwined with diabetes. Persons with noninsulin-dependent diabetes mellitus (NIDDM) are three times more likely to develop periodontal disease than nondiabetic individuals. Add smoking to the mix, and the chances of developing periodontitis with loss of tooth-supporting bone are 20 times higher. An increased risk for destructive periodontal disease also holds for persons with insulin-dependent diabetes mellitus (IDDM).

Much of what is known about the periodontal complications of diabetes has been learned from the Pima Indians of Arizona, who have the highest reported rates of NIDDM in the world. NIDCR-supported research in the Pima community has shown that periodontal infection is more prevalent, more severe, and develops at an earlier age in this population than in nondiabetic persons. As diabetes increases in severity, the rate at which vital tooth-anchoring bone is lost accelerates. Pima Indians with NIDDM are 15 times more likely to be edentulous than those without diabetes.

Now there is evidence that a history of chronic periodontal disease can disrupt diabetic control, suggesting that periodontal infections may have systemic repercussions. The exact nature of this complex relationship is not clear. It is likely, however, that increased genetic susceptibility to infection, impaired host response, and the excessive production of collagenase found in periodontal disease may all play important roles in NIDDM. Similarities in the etiology of periodontal and other complications of diabetes have also emerged.

Studies have shown, for example, that hyperglycemia is the common basis for diabetic complications in the eyes, kidneys, and nerves. Glucose in high concentrations attaches to other molecules, stimulating chemical reactions that produce advanced glycosylation end products. These large molecules accumulate in tissues, causing damage and disrupting normal function. Scientists suspect that these cellular reactions figure as well in the tissue destruction seen in periodontal disease.

Investigators are also examining the interplay between periodontal infection and metabolic control. Acute viral and bacterial infections are known to induce insulin resistance, which disrupts blood glucose control. Factors including stress, fever, catabolism, and elevated levels of hormones antagonistic to insulin such as growth hormone, cortisol, and glucagon likely play a role in the development of insulin resistance during infection.

Their findings offer evidence that chronic infections such as periodontal disease worsen glycemic control and that eliminating these infections could enhance metabolic control in persons with diabetes. Additional large-scale studies are needed to further evaluate the effects of treating periodontitis on blood glucose levels. Future research should also examine, in other populations, the relationship between severe periodontal disease and poor glycemic control that has been evidenced in the Pima Indian community.

Heart Disease

A number of studies has shown that people with periodontitis are more likely to develop cardiovascular disease than individuals without periodontal infection. One such study suggests that the risk of fatal heart disease doubles for persons with severe periodontal disease.

Part of the link between these two diseases may be discovered through novel investigations of the opportunistic, infectious bacteria that colonize the mouth. Scientists theorize that certain types of these bacteria, which form biofilms and cause periodontal disease, also activate white blood cells in the body to release pro-inflammatory mediators that may contribute to heart disease and stroke.

To explore the underlying inflammatory responses common to both diseases, NIDCR grantees are examining periodontal disease measures (pocket depth where gingival tissues have pulled away from tooth surfaces and where there is loss of tissue) and biological responses in 14,000 people enrolled in an extensive study of heart disease sponsored by the National Heart, Lung and Blood Institute. Scientists will also analyze gingival crevicular fluid constituents that may contain pro-inflammatory mediators associated with heart disease, as well as blood samples to identify antibodies to periodontal pathogens.

The research team will compare these measures with clinical indicators of heart disease, ultrasound measures of carotid vessel thickening, and the occurrence of heart attacks, stroke, and death to determine if there is a correlation. Should the link between oral disease and heart disease be firmly established, future studies will focus on identifying the specific biological factors involved and transferring this knowledge to prevent disease.

Acquired Immunodeficiency Syndrome

The oral effects of systemic disease are by no means limited only to the periodontium. All of the tissues in the oral cavity are fair game for a variety of insults, either directly from infection, or indirectly as part of the systemic disease process. There is perhaps no better illustration of the involvement of oral tissues in systemic disease than the oral manifestations of AIDS.

A New Research Tradition

The identification of dental caries and periodontal disease as infectious diseases by the 1960's heralded the first revolution in dental research. We are now in the midst of a second revolution where oral health research is taking its place in an ever-changing scientific world driven by the need to understand health and disease through the intricate interactions of human behavior, environment, and biology.

What is emerging is a biology of complexity as we approach the 21st century. Infectious diseases that took the young lives of our ancestors have been replaced with chronic and degenerative diseases that victimize us in our old age. These changing patterns of disease and demographics now challenge science to shift its focus from its success in extending life to the challenge of improving the quality of life from before birth until death. To reach this goal, science cannot look at a single molecule, or cell, or system in isolation, but rather at how these act in concert with behavioral, environmental, and genetic influences to heighten or minimize one's risk of disease.

Once the grist of science fiction, today a human genetic book is in process that will eventually decode each of the 100,000 genes that comprise the human genome. We now know that virtually all human diseases have a genetic component, including inherited, infectious, neoplastic, and chronic disabling craniofacial-oral-dental diseases and disorders. We are learning about inherited susceptibility genes that predispose to disorders such as diabetes and severe periodontitis, and we are finding that some chronic diseases may share major genetic determinants and, perhaps, diagnostic and therapeutic approaches as well.

The oral and systemic health connection, then, lies in the many factors they hold in common. Fully integrated into the realm of biomedical research, oral health science is not only expanding our understanding of craniofacial-oral-dental diseases and disorders, but also is broadening the critical knowledge base of fundamental disease processes.

Section 5.2

Oral Health and Quality of Life

Centers for Disease Control and Prevention (CDC), www.cdc.gov.
Published May 2000; updated August 2002.

Diseases and disorders that damage the mouth and face can disturb well-being and self-esteem. The effect of oral health and disease on quality of life is a relatively new field of research that examines the functional, psychological, social, and economic consequences of oral disorders. Most of the research has focused on a few conditions: tooth loss, craniofacial birth defects, oral-facial pain, and oral cancer. The impact of oral health on an individual's quality of life reflects complex social norms and cultural values, beliefs, and traditions. There is a long tradition of determining character on the basis of facial and head shapes. Although cultures differ in detail, there appear to be overall consistencies in the judgment of facial beauty and deformity that are learned early in life. Faces judged ugly have been associated with defects in character, intelligence, and morals.

The Impact of Craniofacial-Oral-Dental Conditions on Quality of Life

Missing Teeth

People who have many missing teeth face a diminished quality of life. Not only do they have to limit food choices because of chewing problems, which may result in nutritionally poor diets, but many feel a degree of embarrassment and self-consciousness that limits social interaction and communication.

Craniofacial Birth Defects

Children with cleft lip or cleft palate experience not only problems with eating, breathing, and speaking, but also have difficulties adjusting socially, which affects their learning and behavior. The tendency to "judge a book by its cover" persists in the world today and accounts

41

for many of the psychosocial problems of persons affected by cranio-facial birth defects.

Oral-Facial Pain

The craniofacial region is rich in nerve endings sensitive to painful stimuli, so it is not surprising that oral-facial pain, especially chronic pain conditions where the cause is not understood and control is inadequate, severely affects quality of life. Conditions such as temporomandibular (jaw joint) disorders, trigeminal neuralgia, and postherpetic neuralgia (chronic pain following an attack of shingles affecting facial nerves) can disrupt vital functions such as chewing, swallowing, and sleep; interfere with normal activities at home or work; and lead to social withdrawal and depression.

Oral Cancer

Surgical treatment for oral cancer may result in permanent disfigurement as well as functional limitations affecting speaking and eating. Given the poor prognosis for oral cancer (the five-year survival rate is only 52 percent), it is not surprising that depression is common in these patients.

Economic Costs

- Recent estimates put the lifetime costs of the multiple surgeries and other medical, dental, and rehabilitation therapies for treating cleft lip or cleft palate at a minimum of $100,000.

- The overall cost of chronic pain conditions in America was estimated to be $79 billion a decade ago. Given the prevalence of temporomandibular disorders and headaches, the amount representing chronic oral-facial pain would certainly be in the billions.

- The Centers for Disease Control and Prevention estimated in 1988 that 16.2 years of life were lost per person dying of oral cancer. This exceeds the average for all cancer sites, which was 15.4 years lost.

Chapter 6

Pregnancy and Dental Care

Nutrition and Dental Care during Pregnancy

The foods you eat during your pregnancy affect every aspect of the health of your baby-to-be, including her teeth, and your own health. Here are some quick nutritional and dental tips.

Your baby's teeth begin to develop below the gums between the third and sixth months of pregnancy, so getting the right nutrients is especially important then. A sufficient amount of protein, calcium, phosphorus and vitamins A, C and D will all help ensure healthy teeth for your baby. A daily diet including the following foods should provide plenty of these nutrients:

- 6 or more servings of breads, cereals, and other grains

- 3 or more servings of vegetables

- 3 servings of dairy products

This chapter includes text from "Pregnancy and Dental Care," © 2001 California Dental Association. Reprinted with Permission. For more information, visit the website of the California Dental Association at www.cda.org. As a public service, the California Dental Association also maintains a consumer information website at www.smilecalifornia.org. This chapter also includes "The Effect of Dental Health on Birth Weight" excerpted from "The Oral-Systemic Health Connection," a report published by the National Institute of Dental and Craniofacial Research (NIDCR), May 1999. Available online at www.nidcr.nih.gov/spectrum/NIDCR2/2menu.htm; accessed May 2003.

- 2 to 3 servings of meat, fish, or poultry

- 2 or more servings of fruits

Talk to your doctor for specific advice about your diet, especially if there are certain food groups that give you difficulty (e.g., dairy products).

As far as your own dental health goes, as an expectant mother you're slightly more prone to cavities. This is due to the fact that you're eating more often, thereby accumulating more plaque on your teeth. To help prevent cavities, be sure to brush and floss after meals and snacks. This will also help combat gum disease, which can be brought on by the combination of excess plaque and the change in hormone levels that accompany pregnancy.

The Effect of Dental Health on Birth Weight

Emerging evidence may link severe periodontal disease in pregnant women to a sevenfold increase in the risk of delivering preterm low birth weight babies. NIDCR [National Institute of Dental and Craniofacial Research]-supported researchers estimate that as many as 18 percent of the 250,000 premature low-weight infants born in the United States each year may be attributed to infectious oral disease.

The emotional, social, and economic costs associated with these small babies are staggering. Hospital costs alone surpass $5 billion annually. When costs to society in terms of suffering and managing long-term disabilities often associated with prematurity are considered, this figure escalates dramatically.

In a recent study, mothers of preterm low-weight newborns were found to have significantly more severe periodontal disease than did mothers of full-term, normal weight babies. Investigators believe that the molecular pathogenesis may be similar to that characterized for other maternal, bacterial, opportunistic infections, such as genitourinary infections, that are associated with low-weight preterm births.

Scientists theorize that oral pathogens release toxins that reach the human placenta via the mother's blood circulation and interfere with fetal growth and development, which has been shown to occur in animal studies. The oral infection also prompts accelerated production of inflammatory mediators PGE2 and TNF that normally build to a threshold level throughout pregnancy, then cue the onset of labor. Instead, the elevated levels of these inflammatory mediators trigger premature delivery.

Taking into account all the known risk factors for premature birth, the researchers could identify no other reason for the relationship they had found between severe periodontal disease and preterm low-weight births. Additional research is needed to confirm this intriguing finding and to determine if treating and preventing periodontal disease would reduce the incidence of these high risk births.

Chapter 7

Aging and Oral Health

Chapter Contents

Section 7.1

The Oral Health of Aging Americans

Vargas CM, Kramarow EA, Yellowitz JA. "The Oral Health of Aging Americans," *Aging Trends*; No. 3. Hyattsville, Maryland: National Center for Health Statistics. 2001.

Overview

Oral health is an important and often overlooked component of an older person's general health and well-being. In the words of former Surgeon General C. Everett Koop: "You are not healthy without good oral health."[1] Oral health can affect general health in very direct ways. Oral health problems can cause pain and suffering as well as difficulty in speaking, chewing, and swallowing. These problems can also be a complication of certain medications used to treat systemic diseases. In addition, the treatment of systemic diseases can be complicated by oral bacterial infections.[2]

There are also associations between oral health and general health and well-being. For example, the loss of self-esteem is associated with loss of teeth[3] and untreated disease (caries and periodontal diseases) as well as the economic burden of dental care due to the paucity of dental insurance programs for the elderly. Although oral health problems are not usually associated with death, oral cancers result in nearly 8,000 deaths each year, and more than half of these deaths occur among persons 65 years of age and older.

This chapter focuses on the oral health needs of older adults. Using data from several national surveys, this chapter describes the current status of oral health among the elderly, how these older Americans use dental health services, and what the future holds for the oral health of older Americans. Some of the findings reported are from newly tabulated data, and some are from published data.

Highlights of the Oral Health of Older Americans

- More older people are keeping their natural teeth than ever before. However, there are sharp differences by race and socioeconomic status.

- Nearly one-third of persons 65 years of age and older have untreated dental caries.

- Oral cancer increases with age. Mortality rates from oral cancer are higher among black men than among black women or white persons.

- Slightly more than one-half of noninstitutionalized persons 65 years of age and older in 1997 had a dental visit in the past year. The percent of persons with dental visits varied by race, education, and whether they had their natural teeth.

- Only 22 percent of older persons were covered by private dental insurance in 1995; most elderly dental expenses were paid out of pocket.

Monitoring the Health of Our Aging Population

Older Americans can expect to live longer than ever before. Under existing conditions, women who live to age 65 can expect to live about 19 years longer, men about 16 years longer. Whether the added years at the end of the life cycle are healthy, enjoyable, and productive depends, in part, upon preventing and controlling a number of chronic diseases and conditions.

This chapter is one in a series undertaken by the National Center for Health Statistics, with support from the National Institute on Aging, to help meet the challenge of extending and improving life. By monitoring the health of the elderly, using information compiled from a variety of sources, we hope to help focus research on the most effective ways to use resources and craft health policy.

What Is the State of Oral Health among Older Americans?

Answering this question requires examining how oral health affects an older person's quality of life, as well as looking at the diseases that are related to oral health.

How Oral Health Affects Quality of Life

Oral health problems can hinder a person's ability to be free of pain and discomfort, to maintain a satisfying and nutritious diet, and to enjoy interpersonal relationships and a positive self-image. Overall, oral health problems are more frequently found in an older adult population for whom other health problems are often a priority.

Oral Pain

Oral pain is a sign of an advanced problem in a tooth or in the gingival (gum) tissues. Although pain may dissipate with time, professional attention is needed to effectively manage the affected tooth or tissue.

National data indicate that 7 percent of adults 65 years and older reported having tooth pain at least twice during the past 6 months. Older adults who belonged to racial/ethnic minorities or who had a low level of education were more likely to report dental pain than older adults who were white or better educated. Older men and older women showed no difference in their likelihood of reporting tooth pain.[4]

Difficulty Eating

Oral health problems, whether from missing teeth, ill-fitting dentures, cavities, gum disease, or infection, can cause difficulty eating and can force people to adjust the quality, consistency, and balance of their diet. For example, edentulous people (those with no natural teeth) tend to eat fewer raw vegetables, salads, and fresh fruits than people who have their own natural teeth. To date, however, available data do not show that these changes result in a diet of poor nutritional quality.[5]

Edentulism (Total Tooth Loss)

Edentulism can have obvious negative esthetic and functional (speech, chewing/eating) consequences. In 1993 one-third of noninstitutionalized adults 65 years of age and older reported having lost all their natural teeth.

Although there was no difference in the proportion of men and women who had lost all of their teeth, there were large differences in the prevalence of edentulism by socioeconomic status. Persons with family incomes below the poverty line were almost twice as likely to be edentulous as persons with family incomes at or above the poverty line. Similarly, edentulism was higher among black persons than among white persons.[6] In 1995-97, 52 percent of nursing home residents 75 years of age and older were edentulous.

The prevalence of total tooth loss also varied by state, ranging from 14 percent in Hawaii and 16 percent in Oregon and California to 48 percent in West Virginia and 44 percent in Kentucky.[7]

As a result of a more preventive approach toward oral health from the community and the dental profession, the proportion of older adults who have lost all of their teeth has declined.

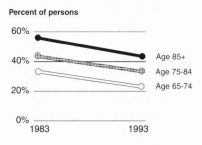

Percent of persons

Figure 7.1. Prevalence of edentulism (total tooth loss) among persons 65 years of age and older by age. Source: National Health Interview Survey, 1983, 1993.

Use of Dental Prostheses

Quality dental prostheses (dentures) can help persons who have lost some or all of their natural teeth improve their quality of life by restoring lost function and esthetics.

Overall in 1988-94, 92 percent of the edentulous noninstitutionalized adults 65 years of age and older had both an upper and a lower denture. However, in this group, 24 percent of black persons and 19 percent of Hispanic persons did not usually use their denture(s). Among elderly nursing home residents in 1995-97, 80 percent of those who had lost all of their natural teeth had both dentures; however, 18 percent did not usually use them.

Multiple Medications

Because chronic diseases are so prevalent among older adults, many take multiple prescriptions and over-the-counter medications. It is not unusual for at least one of these medications to have a side effect that is detrimental to their oral health.

For example, antihistamines, diuretics, antipsychotics, and anti-depressants can reduce salivary flow. This can result in dry mouth, one of the most common side effects of both prescription and over-the-counter medications. Having a dry mouth can cause difficulty chewing, speaking, and swallowing. It also increases the risk of developing cavities and soft tissue problems. Dry mouth may also decrease the ability to wear dentures.

Diseases Related to the Mouth

Dental Caries

Dental cavities (caries), an infection of the teeth, represent another physiological burden, especially important for those whose systems are already weakened by diseases and aging. In 1988-94 nearly one-third of adults 65 years of age and older with natural teeth had untreated dental cavities in either the crown or the root of their teeth.

Decay untreated by a dentist usually gets worse, resulting in pain and the potential loss of teeth. Dental caries is one of the main causes of tooth loss for both young and old adults.

Although the prevalence of dental caries has declined in the U.S. overall, declines have not occurred among the most socially disadvantaged groups of older adults. The percent of older black persons and poor persons with untreated caries increased between 1971-74 and 1988-94.

Periodontal Diseases

Periodontal diseases (gum diseases) are infections of the supporting structures of the teeth. When not treated, periodontal diseases can result in the loss of teeth. The prevalence of periodontal diseases increases with age, from 6 percent among persons 25-34 years to 41 percent among those 65 years and older.[8]

This increase is not necessarily due to older persons being more susceptible to periodontal diseases, but rather to the consequences of these diseases (i.e., bone loss and gingival recession), which accumulate over time and are thus more evident in the elderly.[9] Preventing periodontal diseases is particularly relevant because recent studies have shown a possible association between these diseases and diabetes and cardiovascular diseases, which are major causes of death among the elderly population.[10]

Oral Cancer

Oral cancer, which includes lip, oral cavity, and pharynx cancer, is of particular concern for persons 65 years of age and older because they are 7 times more likely to be diagnosed with oral cancer than persons under 65 years of age.[11] In 1997, 4,775 people 65 years and older died as a result of oral cancer. More older adults died from oral cancer than from skin cancer (3,978).

Although the occurrence of new cases (incidence) of oral cancer is slightly higher among white adults than among black adults, mortality from oral cancer is substantially higher among black men than among white men.

As with other cancers, survival improves when the cancer is diagnosed at an early stage rather than at a later, more advanced stage. Because patients with an early stage of oral cancer rarely have pain or other symptoms, detecting an early oral cancer is primarily dependent upon the clinician providing a comprehensive oral cancer examination.[12] One possible explanation of the higher mortality from oral cancers among older black men is that they are less likely than older white men to use dental and medical services.

Incidence Rate

	Total	Male	Female
All races	44	68	27
White	45	69	28
Black	40	65	21

Death Rate

	Total	Male	Female
All races	14	21	9
White	14	20	9
Black	17	30	9

Figure 7.2. Oral cancer incidence and death rates among persons 65 years of age and older by sex and race, 1993-1997 (rate per 100,000 persons). Note: Rates are age adjusted to the 1970 U.S. standard population. Source: Ries LAG, Eisner MP, Hosary CL, et al. 2000.

How Do Older People Use Dental Care Services?

Visiting a dentist is the most basic use of dental care services. Whether elderly persons get needed dental care is closely related to whether they have dental insurance.

Dental Visits

A visit to the dentist allows for a comprehensive evaluation of teeth, gums, and soft tissues, and for prevention, early detection, and treatment of oral health problems. It is also an opportunity for the dental professional to review home care practices. A visit in the previous year is considered the standard measure of appropriate utilization of dental care, independent of the presence or absence of teeth.

For edentulous persons, a dental visit will include a comprehensive evaluation of soft tissues as well as an evaluation and possible adjustment of prostheses. In 1997, edentulous persons were much less likely to report having visited the dentist in the previous year than were dentate persons (persons with their natural teeth). When asked how often they went to the dentist, 75 percent of edentulous persons selected "when needed," compared with 37 percent of dentate persons.

In general, socioeconomic characteristics played a significant role in who received dental care. Overall, persons with more than a high school education were twice as likely to have visited the dentist in the past year than were persons with less than a high school education. Non-Hispanic whites were also much more likely to have visited a dentist than were racial/ethnic minorities.

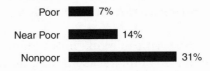

Figure 7.3. *Percent of persons 65 years of age and older with private dental insurance by poverty status, 1995. Source: National Health Interview Survey.*

Dental Insurance

Dental insurance is an important predictor of dental care utilization.[13] Because dental insurance is usually acquired as part of a job benefit package, most persons lose their dental insurance coverage when they retire. In some states, Medicaid provides limited coverage for routine dental care for low income and disabled elderly persons. Medicare, on the other hand, does not cover routine dental care for older adults, but provides a few, very limited services considered to be "medically necessary."

With only 22 percent of the adults 65 years and older covered by private dental insurance in 1995, most dental care expenses for the elderly were paid out of pocket. Only 10 percent of dental expenditures were paid by private insurance, and 79 percent were paid out of pocket.[14]

What Does the Future Hold for the Oral Health of Older Americans?

The trend in improved oral health status among persons 65 years of age and older is expected to continue as the new cohorts of older persons continue to be better educated, more affluent, and more likely to keep their natural teeth. This positive change in oral health status shows that oral diseases and tooth loss are not inevitable with aging, and that teeth can be expected to last in good condition for all of a person's life.

However, the fact that the coming generations of elderly are maintaining their teeth poses a challenge for satisfying their dental care needs. As more people keep their teeth, more will be at risk for dental diseases and will need more preventive, restorative, and periodontal services.

Unfortunately, financing dental care for older persons is particularly difficult compared with other age groups, in part, because there are no Federal or State dental insurance programs that cover routine dental services, and only 22 percent of older persons are covered by private dental insurance. Consequently, dental care is unreachable for many older persons living on a fixed income. Yet adequate oral health care is important for all older adults, as it is for other age groups.

Another challenge arises in providing dental care for older persons because their care is often more complex than dental care for younger adults. This complexity comes from the many changes associated with aging. Considering that caries and periodontal diseases, the most common oral health problems, are cumulative, older persons often endure the consequences of their oral health experience from earlier years, such as missing teeth, large fillings, and the loss of tooth support. These problems can be complicated by their decreased ability to care for their oral health. The elderly may also have multiple physical and psychological ailments that affect their treatment and require the dentist to have good medical knowledge and management skills.

Furthermore, there is noticeable social inequality in the oral health of older adults. Older persons who live below the poverty line were almost 3 times as likely to report unmet dental needs as those who live at or above the poverty line (11 and 4 percent, respectively).[15] Persons from lower socioeconomic groups are also more likely to report having untreated cavities.[16] The greater need for dental care among older persons at low socioeconomic levels is coupled with their lower level of private insurance coverage, which leaves this group at a significant disadvantage compared with those at a higher socioeconomic level.

One additional challenge to caring for older persons is that the actual number of practicing dentists and the proportion of dentists relative to the population are expected to decline.[17] The decline in the dentist-to-population ratio will particularly affect the elderly because they are the fastest growing segment of the population and because their special needs will require specialized dental skills. Optimally, the elderly should receive care from specialists in geriatric dentistry or general dentists with a good understanding of the medical, pharmacologic, and cognitive changes associated with the older adult population.

Conclusion

During the past 50 years, the oral health and use of dental services among older adults have improved.[18] Although this trend is expected to continue as the population of older adults grows and increasingly maintains their natural teeth, continued improvement will also be dependent on access to appropriate dental care.

References

1. Koop CE. Oral Health 2000. Second National Consortium Advance Program, 2, 1993.

2. U.S. Department of Health and Human Services. *Oral Health in America: A Report of the Surgeon General*. Rockville, MD: U.S. Department of Health and Human Services, National Institute of Dental and Craniofacial Research, National Institutes of Health, 2000.

3. Davis DM, Fiske J, Scott B, and Radford DR. The emotional effects of tooth loss: a preliminary quantitative study. *British Dental Journal*. 188(9):503–506, May 13, 2000.

4. Vargas CM, Macek MD, Marcus SE. Sociodemographic correlates of tooth pain among adults: United States, 1989. *Pain*. 85:87–92, 2000.

5. Krall E, Hayes C, Garcia R. How dentition status and masticator function affect nutrient intake. *JADA.* 129:1261–1269, 1998.

6. Kramarow E, Lentzner H, Rooks R, Weeks J, Saydah S. *Health and aging chartbook.* Health United States, 1999. Hyattsville, MD: National Center for Health Statistics. 1999.

7. Centers for Disease Control and Prevention. Total tooth loss among persons aged greater than or equal to 65 years—selected states, 1995-1997. *MMWR.* 48(10): 206–210, 1999.

8. Brown L, Brunelle JA, Kingman A. Periodontal status in the United States, 1988-91: prevalence, extent, and demographic variation. *Journal of Dental Research.* 75 (Spec Is):672–683, 1996.

9. Page RC. Periodontal diseases in the elderly: a critical evaluation of current information. *Gerodontology.* 1:63–70, 1984.

10. U.S. Department of Health and Human Services. Oral Health in America: A report of the Surgeon General—Executive summary. Rockville, MD: U.S. Department of Health and Human Services, National Institute of Dental and Craniofacial Research, National Institutes of Health, 2000.

11. Ries LAG, Eisner MP, Kosary CL, Hankey BF, Miller BA, Clegg L, Edwards BK (eds). SEER Cancer Statistics Review, 1973–1997, National Cancer Institute. Bethesda, MD, 2000.

12. Yellowitz JA. The Oral Cancer Examination, Chapter 3 of *Oral Cancer, The Dentist's Role in Diagnosis, Management Rehabilitation, and Prevention.* Quintessence Books, Quintessence Publishing Company, Inc. Illinois. 2000.

13. Isman R, Isman B. Oral Health America white paper: Access to oral health services in the United States 1997 and beyond. Chicago, IL: Oral Health America. 1997.

14. Manski RJ, Moeller JF, Maas WR. Dental services: use, expenditures, and sources of payment, 1987. *Journal of the American Dental Association.* 130:500–508, 1999.

15. Cohen RA, Bloom B, Simpson G, and Parsons PE. Access to health care. Part 3: Older adults. National Center for Health Statistics. Vital Health Stat. 10(198), 1997.

16. National Center for Health Statistics, Health, United States, 2000 with Adolescent Health Chartbook, Hyattsville, Maryland. Table 81, 2000.

17. U.S. Department of Health and Human Services. *Oral Health in America: A Report of the Surgeon General.* Rockville, MD: U.S. Department of Health and Human Services, National Institute of Dental and Craniofacial Research, National Institutes of Health, 2000.

18. Ibid.

Section 7.2

Taking Care of Your Teeth and Mouth as You Age

"Taking Care of Your Teeth and Mouth," from the National Institute on Aging, *Age Pages*, January 2002. Available online at www.nia.nih.gov/ health/agepages/teeth.htm; accessed May 2003.

No matter what your age, you need to take care of your teeth and mouth. When your mouth is healthy, you can easily eat the foods you need for good nutrition. Smiling, talking, and laughing with others also are easier when your mouth is healthy.

Tooth Decay (Cavities)

Teeth are meant to last a lifetime. By taking good care of your teeth and gums, you can protect them for years to come. Tooth decay is not just a problem for children. It can happen as long as you have natural teeth in your mouth.

Tooth decay ruins the enamel that covers and protects your teeth. When you don't take good care of your mouth, bacteria can cling to your teeth and form a sticky, colorless film called dental plaque. This plaque can lead to tooth decay and cavities. Gum disease can also cause your teeth to decay.

Fluoride is just as helpful for adults as it is for children. Using a fluoride toothpaste and mouth rinse can help protect your teeth. If you have a problem with cavities, your dentist or dental hygienist may give you a fluoride treatment during the office visit. The dentist also may prescribe a fluoride gel or mouth rinse for you to use at home.

Gum Diseases

Gum diseases (sometimes called periodontal or gingival diseases) are infections that harm the gum and bone that hold teeth in place. When plaque stays on your teeth too long, it forms a hard, harmful covering, called tartar, that brushing doesn't clean. The longer the plaque and tartar stay on your teeth, the more damage they cause. Your gums may become red, swollen, and bleed easily. This is called gingivitis.

If gingivitis is not treated, over time it can make your gums pull away from your teeth and form pockets that can get infected. This is called periodontitis. If not treated, this infection can ruin the bones, gums, and tissue that support your teeth. In time, it can cause loose teeth that your dentist may have to remove.

Here's how you can prevent gum disease:

- Brush your teeth twice a day (with a fluoride toothpaste).

- Floss once a day.

- Make regular visits to your dentist for a checkup and cleaning.

- Eat a well-balanced diet.

- Don't use tobacco products.

Cleaning Your Teeth and Gums

Knowing how to brush and floss the right way is a big part of good oral health. Here's how: every day gently brush your teeth on all sides with a soft-bristle brush and fluoride toothpaste. Small round motions and short back-and-forth strokes work best. Take the time to brush carefully and gently along the gum line. Lightly brushing your tongue also helps.

Along with brushing, clean around your teeth with dental floss to keep your gums healthy.

Careful flossing will remove plaque and leftover food that a toothbrush can't reach. Rinse after you floss.

If brushing or flossing causes your gums to bleed or hurt your mouth, see your dentist.

Your dentist also may prescribe a bacteria-fighting mouth rinse to help control plaque and swollen gums. Use the mouth rinse in addition to careful daily brushing and flossing. Some people with arthritis or other conditions that limit motion may find it hard to hold a toothbrush. It may help to attach the toothbrush handle to your hand with a wide elastic band. Some people make the handle bigger by taping it to a sponge or Styrofoam ball. People with limited shoulder movement may find brushing easier if they attach a long piece of wood or plastic to the handle. Electric toothbrushes can be helpful.

Dentures

Dentures (sometimes called false teeth) may feel strange at first. When you are learning to eat with them, it may be easier if you:

- Start with soft non-sticky food;
- Cut your food into small pieces; and
- Chew slowly using both sides of your mouth.

Dentures may make your mouth less sensitive to hot foods and liquids. They also may make it harder for you to notice harmful objects such as bones, so be careful. During the first few weeks you have dentures, your dentist may want to see you often to make sure they fit. Over time, your mouth changes and your dentures may need to be replaced or adjusted. Be sure to let your dentist handle these adjustments.

Keep your dentures clean and free from food that can cause stains, bad breath, or swollen gums. Once a day, brush all surfaces with a denture care product. When you go to sleep, take your dentures out of your mouth and put them in water or a denture cleansing liquid.

Take care of partial dentures the same way. Because bacteria can collect under the clasps (clips) that hold partial dentures, be sure to carefully clean that area.

Dental Implants

Dental implants are small metal pieces placed in the jaw to hold false teeth or partial dentures in place. They are not for everyone. You need a complete dental and medical checkup to find out if implants are right for you. Your gums must be healthy and your jawbone able to support the implants. Talk to your dentist to find out if you should think about dental implants.

Dry Mouth

Doctors used to think that dry mouth (xerostomia) was a normal part of aging. They now know that's not true. Older, healthy adults shouldn't have a problem with saliva.

Dry mouth happens when salivary glands don't work properly. This can make it hard to eat, swallow, taste, and even speak. Dry mouth also can add to the risk of tooth decay and infection. You can get dry mouth from many diseases or medical treatments, such as head and neck radiation therapy. Many common medicines also can cause dry mouth.

If you think you have dry mouth, talk with your dentist or doctor to find out why. If your dry mouth is caused by a medicine you take, your doctor might change your medicine or dosage.

To prevent the dryness, drink extra water. Cut back on sugary snacks, drinks that have caffeine or alcohol, and tobacco. Your dentist or doctor also might suggest that you keep your mouth wet by using artificial saliva, which you can get from most drugstores. Some people benefit from sucking hard candy.

Oral Cancer

Oral cancer most often occurs in people over age 40. It's important to catch oral cancer early, because treatment works best before the disease has spread. Pain often is not an early symptom of the disease.

A dental checkup is a good time for your dentist to look for early signs of oral cancer. Even if you have lost all your natural teeth, you should still see your dentist for regular oral cancer exams. See your dentist or doctor if you have trouble with swelling, numbness, sores, or lumps in your mouth, or if it becomes hard for you to chew, swallow, or move your jaw or tongue. These problems could be signs of oral cancer.

Here's how you can lower your risk of getting oral cancer: don't smoke; don't use snuff or chew tobacco; if you drink alcohol, do so in moderation; use lip cream with sunscreen; and eat lots of fruits and vegetables.

Section 7.3

Nursing Home Oral Health Care

Elderly people who live in nursing homes are at greater risk for oral health problems compared to elderly people who live independently, according to a study published in the July/August 2002 issue (Volume 50, Number 4) of *General Dentistry*, the peer-reviewed journal of the Academy of General Dentistry (AGD), an organization of general dentists dedicated to continuing education.

Thanks in part to widespread fluoridation, more people than ever before are keeping their teeth throughout their lives. But as people age, medical complications and other factors can negatively affect oral health. Evidence shows that older Americans are at risk for greater oral health problems than other groups because of age and the inability to get to a dentist's office due to an existing medical condition or lack of transportation.

"Oral health of frail elders residing in long-term care facilities is very poor, probably because access to dental services is limited," says Francesco Chiappelli, Ph.D., co-author of the study. "Most of the care at nursing homes is medical care and nursing care, and sometimes the oral health needs are overlooked."

Children or relatives should take an active role in the oral health needs of elderly people residing in nursing homes. "Assisting with brushing, flossing, and looking around the mouth for canker sores and abscesses can help ensure an elderly relative maintains their oral health which in turn helps maintains one's overall health. All oral health problems should be reported to the nursing staff for proper diagnosis and treatment," Dr. Chiappelli says.

According to the report, greater awareness among health care providers and caregivers can do much to ensure the elderly receive good oral health, primarily through assessments of the patient's mouth.

Before choosing a nursing home for an elderly person, relatives and loved ones should inquire about the quality and consistency of dental care at the facility, according to Trey L. Petty, DDS, FAGD, spokesperson for the AGD. Important questions include:

- Does the home have on-call dentists?
- Is nursing home staff trained in basic mouth care?
- Is the nursing home staff trained to recognize oral pathology?
- Does nursing home staff emphasize mouth care at least once a day?

"If the staff or home administrator can't say 'yes' to each of these questions, then a red flag should go up," he says.

Chapter 8

Mouth Hygiene

Chapter Contents

Section 8.1

Proper Brushing and Flossing Techniques

This section includes text from "Proper Brushing" © 2003 American Dental Hygienists' Association, and "Proper Flossing," © 2003 American Dental Hygienists' Association. Reprinted with permission from the American Dental Hygienists' Association Website, www.adha.org. Figures 8.1 and 8.2 © American Academy of Periodontology.

Proper Brushing Instructions

Proper brushing is essential for cleaning teeth and gums effectively. Use a toothbrush with soft, nylon, round-ended bristles that will not scratch and irritate teeth or damage gums.

- Place bristles along the gum line at a 45-degree angle. Bristles should contact both the tooth surface and the gum line.

- Gently brush the outer tooth surfaces of two to three teeth using a vibrating back-and-forth, rolling motion. Move brush to the next group of two to three teeth and repeat.

- Maintain a 45-degree angle with bristles contacting the tooth surface and gum line. Gently brush using a back-and-forth, rolling motion along all of the inner tooth surfaces.

- Tilt brush vertically behind the front teeth. Make several up-and-down strokes using the front half of the brush.

- Place the brush against the biting surface of the teeth and use a gentle back-and-forth scrubbing motion. Brush the tongue from back to front to remove odor-producing bacteria.

Remember to replace your toothbrush every three to four months. Researchers have established that thousands of microbes grow on toothbrush bristles and handles. Most are harmless, but others can cause cold and flu viruses, the herpes virus that causes cold sores, and bacteria that can cause periodontal infections.

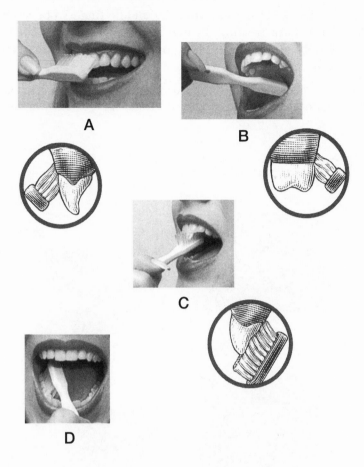

Figure 8.1. How to brush.

Proper Flossing Instructions

Flossing is an essential part of the tooth-cleaning process because it removes plaque from between teeth and at the gum line, where periodontal disease often begins.

If you find using floss awkward or difficult, ask your dental hygienist about the variety of dental floss holders or interdental cleaning devices that are available.

- Wind 18 inches of floss around the middle fingers of each hand. Pinch floss between thumbs and index fingers, leaving a 1- to 2-inch length in between. Use thumbs to direct floss between upper teeth.

- Keep a 1- to 2-inch length of floss taut between fingers. Use index fingers to guide floss between contacts of the lower teeth.

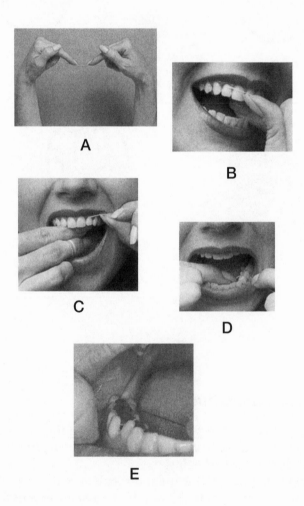

Figure 8.2. How to floss.

- Gently guide floss between the teeth by using a zigzag motion. Do not snap floss between your teeth. Contour floss around the side of the tooth.

- Slide floss up and down against the tooth surface and under the gum line. Floss each tooth thoroughly with a clean section of floss.

Section 8.2

Five Steps to a Better Smile

"5 Steps to a Great Smile—Little Known Secrets for a Celebrity Smile," reprinted with permission from www.saveyoursmile.com. © 2003 Dental Zone, Inc., dentalzone@aol.com.

Ever wonder why some people possess beautiful smiles whereas others try but can never achieve the same result? Believe it or not, the secrets to a great smile are simple steps that each and every one of us can take. Below are five steps that will lead you to a brighter and better smile.

#1: Take a Little Extra Time to Give Your Teeth the Care They Deserve.

Did you know that it takes two to three minutes to adequately brush your teeth but that most people spend less than 30 seconds brushing? Why is brushing this long so important?

It all has to do with bacteria. Millions of bacteria live, work, and play in our mouths. They feed on food left on our teeth after we eat. Acid is a byproduct of this bacterial feasting. It is this acid that destroys enamel-creating cavities.

Brushing removes bacteria from our teeth so they can no longer make acid. It is important, however, to remove bacteria from all tooth surfaces. This takes two to three minutes.

#2: Do a Little Flossing. It Just Might Save Your Teeth.

OK, so you've heard that you need to floss at least once a day. But has anyone ever told you why? You see it all has to do with bacteria again. These crafty critters like to hide between teeth to escape the wrath of the toothbrush. Here they continue to feed on food, spewing out cavity-causing acid.

If allowed to remain for a long time, these bacteria invade and destroy gum tissue as well as the bones and ligaments that support teeth. Flossing removes these bacteria from between teeth so they can no longer cause problems.

#3: It's Not Just the Candy That Is Dangerous to Your Smile.

Did you know that many foods other than candy promote tooth decay? Bacteria feed on the sugar of candy, creating cavity causing acid. Bacteria, however, not only use candy to create acid but can also use any food that contains sugars and other carbohydrates. This includes fruits, peanut butter, crackers, potato chips, popcorn, and other foods.

Especially harmful can be foods like raisins and peanut butter that stick to teeth where they provide a constant source of energy for bacteria. What can you do to protect yourself? Brushing after meals helps by removing both the bacteria and the leftover food particles that the bacteria feast on. If you cannot brush, try washing food down with liquids ensuring that less food remains on teeth. Chewing sugarless gum also helps because this stimulates saliva flow. Saliva acts as a natural plaque fighting substance.

#4: Stop Brushing So Hard.

Incredibly, nearly two out of three people damage their own teeth by brushing too hard! It takes very little pressure to remove bacteria, food, and plaque. Unfortunately, most people apply three to four times the necessary brushing pressure causing damage to teeth and gums. This damage includes: receding gums, sensitive teeth, notched teeth, and root cavities.

#5: Reduce Your Dependency on Coffee.

Believe it or not, coffee is one of the most dangerous threats to your smile. Coffee stains teeth destroying your naturally white smile. Worst yet, because most people sip coffee throughout the day, bacteria are provided with a constant source of sugar from which to produce cavity-causing acid.

If that wasn't bad enough, coffee can cause small fractures in teeth called crazes. These occur when the teeth are forced to expand and contract as a result of being exposed to hot foods or liquids. These hot and cold cycles occur when we drink hot coffee. Over a prolonged period of time, this will create crazes in the teeth.

Section 8.3

Improving Oral Health

Centers for Disease Control and Prevention (CDC), www.cdc.gov, March 5, 2003. Available online at www.cdc.gov/nccdphp/bb_oralhealth/ index.htm; accessed May 2003.

Each year in the United States, 500 million dental visits occur. Despite that large number, however, many U.S. children and adults do not have access to dental care and, therefore, receive none. Tooth decay is one of the most common infectious diseases among U.S. children.

Effects of Tooth Decay

This preventable health problem begins early: 17% of 2- to 4-year-olds, 52% of 8-year-olds, and 78% of 17-year-olds already have tooth decay. Among low-income children, almost 50% of tooth decay is untreated, and may cause pain, dysfunction, poor appearance, and underweight—problems that greatly reduce a child's capacity to succeed.

Adults also have serious oral health problems. Almost 1 in 3 adults have untreated tooth decay. More than 25% of adults older than 65 years have lost all of their teeth because of tooth decay or gum disease. Each year, about 30,000 cases of oral and pharyngeal (throat) cancer are diagnosed, and more than 8,000 people die of these diseases.

Costs

Nearly $64 billion is spent on dental services each year. In 1998, $53.8 billion was spent on dental care—48% was paid by dental insurance, 4% by government programs, and 48% was paid out-of-pocket. More than 108 million Americans do not have dental insurance. For each child without medical insurance, 2.6 are without dental insurance; for each adult without medical insurance, three are without dental insurance.

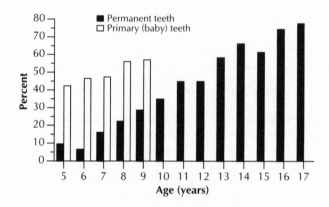

Figure 8.3. *Percentage of children who have experienced dental decay. Source: CDC, National Center for Health Statistics, Third National Health and Nutrition Examination Survey, 1988–1994.*

CDC Goals

- To support state and community programs to prevent oral disease.

- To promote oral health nationwide in communities, schools, and health care settings.

- To evaluate the cost-effectiveness of selected preventive strategies.

Effectiveness of Measures to Reduce Oral Disease

Proven preventive measures (e.g., water fluoridation, dental sealants, smoking prevention programs) can reduce oral and dental diseases. However, these measures are often unavailable to those who need them most.

Community water fluoridation prevents cavities and saves money, both for families and the health care system. In fact, for large communities of more than 20,000 people where it costs about 50¢ per person to fluoridate the water, every $1 invested in this preventive measure yields $38 savings in dental treatment costs.

Examples of CDC Activities

- In 2001, CDC provided $2.3 million to oral health programs in 19 states and Palau.

- Provides grants to 10 states and 1 American Indian tribe to assist with community water fluoridation systems.

- Builds and supports the infrastructure of state oral health programs.

- Five states and one territory now have funding to build core capacity to improve oral health.

- Promotes and supports the integration of oral health components into coordinated school health programs.

- Supports intervention and dissemination research to strengthen the scientific evidence of the benefits of oral disease prevention programs in communities.

- Influences oral health practice and policy by developing and distributing guidelines based on scientific research.

Examples of State Activities

Maine, Rhode Island, South Carolina, and Wisconsin: One proven strategy for reaching children at high risk for dental disease is through school programs that are linked with dental care professionals in the community. In 2001, CDC funded programs through the state education agencies in these four states to develop and implement models for improving access to oral health education, prevention, and treatment services for school-aged children who are at high risk for oral disease. CDC will evaluate the applicability of these models to other states.

Wisconsin: Healthy Smiles for Wisconsin is a statewide program, supported by CDC, to improve the oral health of Wisconsin children through school and community partnerships. By the 2001 school year, this program enabled 40 new dental sealant programs to be set up in communities. More than 5,500 school children in 40 counties across Wisconsin received dental sealants through this program in 2001.

Chapter 9

Nutrition and Oral Health

Chapter Contents

Section 9.1

Diet and Dental Health

Reprinted with permission of the American Dental Association. © 2003 American Dental Association. For additional information, visit www. ada.org.

How Does the Food You Eat Cause Tooth Decay?

When you eat, food passes through your mouth. Here it meets the germs, or bacteria, that live in your mouth. You may have heard your dentist talk about plaque. Plaque is a sticky film of bacteria.

These bacteria love sugars and starches found in many foods. When you don't clean your teeth after eating, plaque bacteria use the sugar and starch to produce acids that can destroy the hard surface of the tooth, called enamel. After a while, tooth decay occurs. The more often you eat and the longer foods are in your mouth, the more damage occurs.

How Do I Choose Foods Wisely?

Some foods that you would least expect contain sugars or starches. Some examples are fruits, milk, bread, cereals, and even vegetables.

The key to choosing foods wisely is not to avoid these foods, but to think before you eat. Not only what you eat but when you eat makes a big difference in your dental health. Eat a balanced diet and limit between-meal snacks. If you are on a special diet, keep your physician's advice in mind when choosing foods. For good dental health, keep these tips in mind when choosing your meals and snacks.

What Are Tips for Better Dental Health?

- To get a balanced diet, eat a variety of foods. Choose foods from each of the five major food groups: breads, cereals, and other grain products; fruits; vegetables; meat, poultry, and fish; and milk, cheese, and yogurt.

- Limit the number of snacks that you eat. Each time you eat food that contains sugars or starches, the teeth are attacked by acids for 20 minutes or more.

- If you do snack, choose nutritious foods, such as cheese, raw vegetables, plain yogurt, or a piece of fruit.

- Foods that are eaten as part of a meal cause less harm. More saliva is released during a meal, which helps wash foods from the mouth and helps lessen the effects of acids.

- Brush twice a day with a fluoride toothpaste that has the American Dental Association Seal of Acceptance.

- Clean between your teeth daily with floss or interdental cleaners.

- Visit your dentist regularly. Your dentist can help prevent problems from occurring and catch those that do occur while they are easy to treat.

Section 9.2

How Does What I Eat Affect My Oral Health?

© 2003 Academy of General Dentistry. Reprinted with permission from the Academy of General Dentistry. For additional oral health topics, toll free access to a directory of members in your zip code area and other consumer services, see page 557 of this *Sourcebook* or contact the Academy of General Dentistry, 211 E. Chicago Avenue, Suite 900, Chicago, IL 60611, 312-440-4300, or visit their website at www.agd.org.

You may be able to prevent two of the most common diseases of modern civilization, tooth decay (caries) and periodontal disease, simply by improving your diet. Decay results when the hard tissues are destroyed by acid products from oral bacteria. Certain foods and food combinations are linked to higher levels of cavity-causing bacteria. Although poor nutrition does not directly cause periodontal disease, many researchers believe that the disease progresses faster and is more severe in patients whose diet does not supply the necessary nutrients. Periodontal disease affects the supporting tissues of the teeth and is the leading cause of tooth loss in adults.

Poor nutrition affects the entire immune system, thereby increasing susceptibility to many disorders. People with lowered immune systems have been shown to be at higher risk for periodontal disease. Additionally, today's research shows a link between oral health and systemic conditions, such as diabetes and cardiovascular disease. So eating a variety of foods as part of a well-balanced diet may not only improve your dental health, but increasing fiber and vitamin intake may reduce the risk of other diseases.

How Can I Plan My Meals and Snacks to Promote Better Oral Health?

Eat a well-balanced diet characterized by moderation and variety. Develop eating habits that follow the recommendations from reputable health organizations such as the American Dietetic Association and the National Institutes of Health. Choose foods from the four basic food groups: fruits and vegetables, breads and cereals, milk and dairy products, meat, chicken, fish, or beans. Avoid fad diets that limit or eliminate entire food groups, which usually result in vitamin or mineral deficiencies.

Always keep your mouth moist by drinking lots of water. Saliva protects both hard and soft oral tissues. If you have a dry mouth, supplement your diet with sugarless candy or gum to stimulate saliva.

Foods that cling to your teeth promote tooth decay. So when you snack, avoid soft, sweet, sticky foods, such as cakes, candy, and dried fruits. Instead, choose dentally healthy foods such as nuts, raw vegetables, plain yogurt, cheese, and sugarless gum or candy.

When you eat fermentable carbohydrates, such as crackers, cookies, and chips, eat them as part of your meal, instead of by themselves. Combinations of foods neutralize acids in the mouth and inhibit tooth decay. For example, enjoy cheese with your crackers. Your snack will be just as satisfying and better for your dental health. One caution: malnutrition (bad nutrition) can result from too much nourishment as easily as too little. Each time you eat, y ou create an environment for oral bacteria to develop. Additionally, studies are showing that dental disease is just as related to overeating as heart disease, obesity, diabetes, and hypertension. So making a habit of eating too much of just about anything, too frequently, should be avoided.

When Should I Consult My Dentist or Dietitian about My Nutritional Status?

Always ask your dentist if you're not sure how your nutrition (diet) may affect your oral health. Conditions such as tooth loss, pain, or joint dysfunction can impair chewing and are often found in elderly people, those on restrictive diets and those who are undergoing medical treatment. People experiencing these problems may be too isolated or weakened to eat nutritionally balanced meals at a time when it is particularly critical. Talk to your dental health professional about what you can do for yourself or someone you know in these circumstances.

Section 9.3

The Role of Vitamins and Minerals in Good Oral Health

"You, and Your Mouth, Are What You Eat" © 2003 Academy of General Dentistry. Reprinted with permission from the Academy of General Dentistry. For additional oral health topics, toll free access to a directory of members in your zip code area and other consumer services, see page 557 of this *Sourcebook* or contact the Academy of General Dentistry, 211 E. Chicago Avenue, Suite 900, Chicago, IL 60611, 312-440-4300, or visit their website at www.agd.org.

Your mouth can say a lot about what you're eating, and your dentist may be the first person to spot potential nutritional imbalances, according to a recent study in *General Dentistry*, the peer-reviewed journal of the Academy of General Dentistry (AGD), an organization of general dentists dedicated to continuing education.

Nutritional deficiencies result when there is an imbalance between what the body needs and what it is getting, according to Robert Dorsky, DMD, author of the report. And those imbalances are particularly reflected in the oral cavity, where soft tissue renews very quickly—often as little as three to seven days. The sensitivity of oral tissue can be particularly telling regarding deficiencies in folic acid, zinc, and iron, which can show up as gum disease. Other conditions, such as diabetes and infection, can also show symptoms in the mouth.

As such, your dentist may be the first member of your health care team to notice potential nutritional problems. "The mouth is a mirror of overall nutritional health," says Academy spokesperson Bruce Burton, DMD, MAGD. "Health care is a team enterprise," Dr. Burton continued. "It is important that patients keep all members of their health care team well informed on their medical histories, lifestyle and eating habits, so they can work together to identify any risks." According to Dr. Dorsky, nutritional deficiencies limit the body's ability to fight disease; and in many cases the mouth is the first line of defense. Healthy gum tissue and saliva are crucial in fending off invading pathogens, Dr. Dorsky said.

Patients can improve their oral health and reduce the risk of periodontal disease by eating a balanced diet based on the well-known Food Guide Pyramid, which recommends eating a variety of foods from the five food groups-grain, fruit, vegetables, milk and meat. Vitamin and mineral supplements also can help preserve periodontal health and boost overall health and well-being. Milk, which contains high

Table 9.1. Vitamins Needed for Oral Health

Vitamins	Promotes	Deficiency
Vitamin A	Improved wound healing	Increases periodontal pockets
Vitamin C (Ascorbic Acid)	Healthy gums; essential for smokers and patients with diabetes	Loss of gum tissue, gum bleeding, tooth mobility
Vitamin D	Strong teeth and jaw bones	Bone resorption in the jaws, tooth loss
Vitamin E	Protects against oral leukoplakia	Prolongs wound healing
Vitamin B2 (Riboflavin), Vitamin B6 (Pyridoxine), Vitamin B12	Healthy gums; decreases redness and bleeding gums	Redness; bleeding gums; cheilitis (dryness/sores in the corner of lips); inflamed tongue (red, painful and smooth)
Folic Acid	Promotes good oral health	None known

levels of calcium, is important for oral health and strong teeth and bones.

Minerals vital to good oral health:

- Zinc
- Phosphorous
- Potassium
- Magnesium
- Iron
- Iodine
- Fluoride
- Copper

Section 9.4

The Relationship between Oral Problems, Disease, and Nutritional Health

"Interrelationship between Oral Problems, Disease, and Nutritional Health" reprinted with permission from the American Dental Hygienists' Association Website, www.adha.org. © 2003.

The links between oral problems, specific diseases and conditions, and nutritional health are becoming clearer, allowing for early and more effective intervention.

Osteoporosis

Aging is associated with a loss of bone mass and an increased risk of oral and systemic bone loss. Systemic osteoporosis can result in bone fractures, especially of the spine and hip, with the characteristic spinal curvature and loss of height often seen in osteoporotic postmenopausal women. Oral signs of osteoporosis include loss of teeth due to resorption of tooth supporting alveolar bone. Because alveolar bone of the jaws is thought to undergo resorption prior to other bones, changes in jaw structure and loose teeth may be early signs of osteoporosis.[1] Evidence suggests that calcium and vitamin D supplementation aimed at slowing the rate of bone loss from various parts of the skeleton can also affect oral bone and, in turn, support tooth retention.[2]

It has been suggested that factors responsible for osteoporotic bone loss may also combine with local factors, such as periodontal diseases, to increase rates of alveolar bone loss.[3-5] However, additional studies are needed to confirm this and the potential implications of this association in identifying individuals at risk. A closer look at the therapies designed to enhance bone mineral density, such as hormone replacement and biphosphonate therapy, will help to determine if these therapies can also aid in tooth retention and a slower loss of alveolar bone.[4]

Eating Disorders

Eating disorders such as anorexia nervosa, bulimia nervosa, and binge eating disorder are a serious concern in women's oral health and present unique challenges to oral health care professionals.[6] Each type of eating disorder presents with unique patterns of psychological, medical, and oral characteristics. Oral signs of eating disorders may include erosive tooth wear, low unstimulated salivary flow, and moderate to severe dental caries.[7] Patients may also complain of sensitivity to hot and cold temperatures and dental pain, and may express concern about the appearance of their teeth.[1] The extent of oral tissue damage depends on the frequency of purging—as seen in bulimia, binge eating disorder, and in some cases of anorexia—and the cariogenicity of the diet. Because oral health professionals are often the first health care providers to see these patients, early diagnosis and intervention may be possible.

Appropriate dental treatment should be coordinated with the primary health care provider, which may include psychological, nutritional, and medical treatment. Patients should be informed about the effects of purging on the mouth and teeth. They should be cautioned against brushing immediately after vomiting to prevent further erosion of enamel. Instead, a sodium bicarbonate or magnesium hydroxide rinse is recommended to neutralize mouth acids.[1] Patients should also be counseled to limit intake of acidic fruit juices, such as orange, grapefruit, and cranberry juices, and to avoid sticky, sweet foods between meals. If dry mouth is a problem, patients can be instructed to try sugarless chewing gum or sugar-free lemon drops to help stimulate saliva flow.

Diabetes

Diabetes is a chronic metabolic disease with oral health implications, including dental caries, periodontal disease, and tooth loss.[8-10] Dry mouth is a common complaint among patients with diabetes, especially among those who also smoke. The decreased salivary flow is associated with poorly controlled diabetes and the subsequent development of neuropathy.[11] Xerostomia and its consequent reduced salivary flow is also linked to an altered sense of taste and burning mouth syndrome. When diabetes is poorly controlled, hard candies may be used frequently to treat hypoglycemia. This habit, combined with reduced salivary flow common to diabetes, can significantly increase risk for dental caries and periodontal disease. Because of the importance of saliva in maintaining oral health, patients with diabetes should be evaluated for reduced salivary flow and treated accordingly, along with a regimen of controlled diet, oral hygiene, and topical fluoride when indicated.[12]

HIV Infection

The evaluation of oral health is an important, but often overlooked, part of the care of patients with HIV and AIDS. Oral infections, mouth ulcers, and other severe dental problems are associated with HIV infections.[13] These conditions can impair the desire and ability to eat, limiting the intake of nutrients at a time when nutrition is essential. Usually, palliative oral care and appropriate food choices, such as bland, soft foods and nutrition supplement beverages, can help to maintain adequate nutrition. However, when oral conditions are not treated either prophylactically or when problems first arise, nutritional status can be undermined, thus contributing further to progression of the disease as well as the oral manifestations.[1] Oral health care professionals are in a position to identify and help treat problems early on that may interfere with nutrient intake. Dental intervention in conjunction with nutrition management is an essential component of care at the earliest stages of HIV infection.

Oral and Pharyngeal Cancer

From a diet perspective, the most consistent factors in the development of oral and pharyngeal cancer are the protective effect of high fruit and vegetable consumption and the carcinogenic effect of alcohol intake. Although use of vitamin supplements in reducing risk for oral cancers has been explored, evidence is lacking that specific nutrients in isolation can prevent development of oral cancer. More likely, the protective effects of fruits and vegetables stem from the interaction of nutrients, including vitamins, minerals, and phytochemicals that occur naturally in these foods.

Cancer treatment, including radiation therapy and surgical intervention, can have significant oral implications. Radiation to the oropharyngeal area can lead to painful stomatitis, xerostomia, fibrosis of the muscles used for chewing, taste changes, and tooth loss.[14] These side effects often lead to reduced nutrient intake at a time when nutritional intake is essential to fight disease and promote healing. Surgical treatment, including reconstruction, may result in changes in chewing and swallowing ability and increased energy and nutrient needs for healing.[15]

References

1. DePaola DP, Faine MP, Palmer CA: Nutrition in Relation to Dental Medicine. In: Shils ME, Olson JA, Shike M, Ross AC, eds: *Modern Nutrition in Health and Disease, 9th ed.* Baltimore, Md: Williams & Wilkins, 1999:1099–1124.

2. Krall EA, Wehler C, Garcia RI, et al: Calcium and vitamin D supplements reduce tooth loss in the elderly. *Am J Med* 2001;111:452–6.

3. Hildebolt CF: Osteoporosis and oral bone loss. *Dentomaxillofac Radiol* 1997;26:3–15.

4. Jeffcoat MK: Osteoporosis: a possible modifying factor in oral bone loss. *Ann Periodontol* 1998;3:312–21.

5. Loza JC, Carpio LC, Dziak R: Osteoporosis and its relationship to oral bone loss. *Curr Opin Periodontol* 1996;3:27–33.

6. Studen-Pavlovich D, Elliott MA: Eating disorders in women's oral health. *Dent Clin North Am* 2001;45:491–511.

7. Ohrn R, Enzell K, Angmar-Mansson B: Oral status of 81 subjects with eating disorders. *Eur J Oral Sci* 1999;107:157–63.

8. Moore PA, Wyant RJ, Mongelluzzo MB, et al: Type 1 diabetes mellitus and oral health: assessment of periodontal disease. *J Periodontol* 1999;70:409–17.

9. Moore PA, Wyant RJ, Mongelluzzo MB, et al: Type 1 diabetes mellitus and oral health: assessment of coronal and root caries. *Community Dent Oral Epidemiol* 2001;29: 183–94.

10. Moore PA, Wyant RJ, Mongelluzzo MB: Type 1 diabetes mellitus and oral health: assessment of tooth loss and edentulism. *J Public Health Dent* 1998;58:135–42.

11. Moore PA, Guggenheimer J, Etzel KR, et al: Type 1 diabetes mellitus, xerostomia, and salivary flow rates. *Oral Surg Oral Med Oral Pathol Oral Radiol Endod* 2001;92:281–91.

12. Touger-Decker R, Sirois D. Dental care of the patient with diabetes. In: Powers MA, ed. *Handbook of Diabetes Nutrition Management.* 2nd ed. Rockville, MD: Aspen, 1996.

13. Heslin KC: Oral health is important, but often overlooked. *Aids Alert* 2001;16:72–73.

14. Oral health and nutrition: position of the American Dietetic Association. *J Am Diet Assoc* 1996;96:184–189.

15. Kyle UG: The patient with head and neck cancer. In: Bloch AS, ed. *Nutrition Management of the Cancer Patient.* Rockville, Md: Aspen; 1990:53–64.

Chapter 10

Products for Home Dental Care

Chapter Contents

Section 10.1

Flosses and Oral Irrigation Devices

"Flosses and Waterpicks" © 2003 Academy of General Dentistry. Reprinted with permission from the Academy of General Dentistry. For additional oral health topics, toll free access to a directory of members in your zip code area and other consumer services, see page 557 of this *Sourcebook* or contact the Academy of General Dentistry, 211 E. Chicago Avenue, Suite 900, Chicago, IL 60611, 312-440-4300, or visit their website at www.agd.org.

Plaque is a sticky layer of material containing germs that accumulates on teeth, including places where toothbrushes can't reach. This can lead to gum disease. The best way to get rid of plaque is to brush and floss your teeth carefully every day. The toothbrush cleans the tops and sides of your teeth. Dental floss cleans in between them. Some people use oral irrigation devices, but floss is the best choice.

Should I Floss?

Yes. Floss removes plaque and debris that adhere to teeth and gums in between teeth, polishes tooth surfaces, and controls bad breath.

Floss is the single most important weapon against plaque, perhaps more important than the toothbrush. Many people just don't spend enough time flossing or brushing and many have never been taught to floss or brush properly. When you visit your dentist or hygienist, ask to be shown.

Why Should I Floss?

Flossing is the one most important step in oral care that people forget to do or claim they don't have time for. By flossing your teeth daily, you increase the chances of keeping your teeth a lifetime and decrease your chance of having periodontal or gum disease. Flossing cleans away the plaque from between your teeth, decreases the chance of interproximal decay, and increases blood circulation in the gums.

Which Type of Floss Should I Use?

Dental floss comes in many forms: waxed and unwaxed, flavored and unflavored, wide and regular. Wide floss, or dental tape, may be helpful for people with a lot of bridgework. Tapes are usually recommended when the spaces between teeth are wide. They all clean and remove plaque about the same. Waxed floss might be easier to slide between tight teeth or tight restorations. However, the unwaxed floss makes a squeaking sound to let you know your teeth are clean. Bonded unwaxed floss does not fray as easily as regular unwaxed floss, but does tear more than waxed floss.

How Should I Floss?

There are two flossing methods: the spool method and the loop method. The spool method is suited for those with manual dexterity.

Take an 18-inch piece of floss and wind the bulk of the floss lightly around the middle finger. (Don't cut off your finger's circulation!) Wind the rest of the floss similarly around the same finger of the opposite hand. This finger takes up the floss as it becomes soiled or frayed. Maneuver the floss between teeth with your index fingers and thumbs. Don't pull it down hard against your gums or you will hurt them. Don't rub it side to side as if you're shining shoes. Bring the floss up and down several times forming a C shape around the tooth being sure to go below the gum line.

The loop method is suited for children or adults with less nimble hands, poor muscular coordination or arthritis. Take an 18-inch piece of floss and make it into a circle. Tie it securely with three knots.

Place all of the fingers, except the thumb, within the loop. Use your index fingers to guide the floss through the lower teeth, and use your thumbs to guide the floss through the upper teeth, going below the gum line forming a C on the side of the tooth.

How Often Should I Floss?

At least once a day. To give your teeth a good flossing, spend at least two or three minutes.

What Are Floss Holders?

You may prefer a prethreaded flosser or floss holder, which often looks like a little hacksaw. Flossers are handy for people with limited dexterity, for those who are just beginning to floss, or for caretakers who are flossing someone else's teeth.

Is It Safe to Use Toothpicks?

In a pinch, toothpicks are effective at removing food between teeth, but for daily cleaning of plaque between teeth, floss is recommended. Toothpicks come round and flat, narrow and thick. When you use a toothpick, don't press too hard as you can break off the end and lodge it in your gums.

Do I Need an Irrigating Device?

Don't use oral irrigation devices (such as a Waterpik) as a substitute for toothbrushing and flossing—but they are effective around orthodontic braces that retain food in areas a toothbrush cannot reach. However, they do not remove plaque.

Oral irrigation devices are frequently recommended by dentists for persons with gum disease. Solutions containing antibacterial agents like chlorhexidine or tetracycline, available through a dentist's prescription, can be added to the reservoir.

Section 10.2

Mouth Rinses

"What Are the Differences in Rinses?" © 2003 Academy of General Dentistry. Reprinted with permission from the Academy of General Dentistry. For additional oral health topics, toll free access to a directory of members in your zip code area and other consumer services, see page 557 of this *Sourcebook* or contact the Academy of General Dentistry, 211 E. Chicago Avenue, Suite 900, Chicago, IL 60611, 312-440-4300, or visit their website at www.agd.org.

Rinses are generally classified by the U.S. Food and Drug Administration (FDA) as either cosmetic or therapeutic, or a combination of the two. Cosmetic rinses are commercial over-the-counter (OTC) products that help remove oral debris before or after brushing, temporarily suppress bad breath, diminish bacteria in the mouth, and refresh the mouth with a pleasant taste. Therapeutic rinses have the benefits of their cosmetic counterparts, but also contain an added active ingredient that helps protect against some oral diseases. Therapeutic rinses are regulated by the FDA and are voluntarily approved by the American Dental Association (ADA). Therapeutic rinses also can be categorized into types according to use: antiplaque/antigingivitis rinses and anticavity fluoride rinses.

Should I Use a Rinse?

That depends upon your needs. Most rinses are, at the very least, effective oral antiseptics that freshen the mouth and curb bad breath for up to three hours. Their success in preventing tooth decay, gingivitis (inflammation of the gingival gum tissue), and periodontal disease is limited, however. Rinses are not considered substitutes for regular dental examinations and proper home care. Dentists consider a regimen of brushing with a fluoride toothpaste followed by flossing, along with routine trips to the dentist, sufficient in fighting tooth decay and periodontal disease.

Which Type Should I Use?

Again, that depends upon your needs. While further testing is needed, initial studies have shown that most over-the-counter antiplaque rinses and antiseptics aren't much more effective against plaque and periodontal disease than rinsing with plain water. Most dentists are skeptical about the value of these antiplaque products, and studies point to only a 20 to 25 percent effectiveness, at best, in reducing the plaque that causes gingivitis.

Many dentists consider the use of fluoride toothpaste alone to be more than adequate protection against cavities. Dentists will prescribe certain rinses for patients with more severe oral problems such as caries, periodontal disease, gum inflammation, and xerostomia (dry mouth). Patients who've recently undergone periodontal surgery are often prescribed these types of rinses. Likewise, many therapeutic rinses are strongly recommended for those who can't brush due to physical impairments or medical reasons.

What Is the Best Mouth Rinse?

Anticavity rinses with fluoride have been clinically proven to fight up to 50 percent more of the bacteria that cause cavities. However, initial studies have shown that most over-the-counter antiplaque rinses and antiseptics are not much more effective against plaque and gum disease than rinsing with water. Most rinses are effective in curbing bad breath and freshening the mouth for up to three hours.

When and How Often Should I Rinse?

If it's an anticavity rinse, dentists suggest the following steps, practiced after every meal: brush, floss, then rinse. Teeth should be as clean as possible before applying an anticavity rinse to reap the full preventive benefits of the liquid fluoride. The same steps can be followed for antiplaque rinses, although Plax brand recommends rinsing before brushing to loosen more plaque and debris, a measure which has not been clinically proven to be effective. If ever in doubt, consult your dentist or follow the instructions on the bottle or container. Be sure to heed all precautions listed.

What Is the Proper Way to Rinse?

First, take the proper amount of liquid as specified on the container or as instructed by your dentist into your mouth. Next, with the lips closed and the teeth kept slightly apart, swish the liquid around with as much force as possible using the tongue, lips, and sucking action of the cheeks. Be sure to swish the front and sides of the mouth equally.

Many rinses suggest swishing for 30 seconds. Finally, rinse the liquid from your mouth thoroughly.

Are There Any Side Effects to Rinsing?

Yes, and they vary depending on the type of rinse. Habitual use of antiseptic mouthwashes containing high levels of alcohol (ranging from 18 to 26 percent) may produce a burning sensation in the cheeks, teeth, and gums. Many prescribed rinses with more concentrated formulas can lead to ulcers, sodium retention, root sensitivity, stains, soreness, numbness, changes in taste sensation and painful mucosal erosions. Most anticavity rinses contain sodium fluoride, which if taken excessively or swallowed, can lead over time to fluoride toxicity. Because children tend to accidentally swallow mouthwash, they should only use rinses under adult supervision. If you experience any irritating or adverse reactions to a mouth rinse, discontinue its use immediately and consult your dentist.

Section 10.3

How Do I Choose and Use a Toothbrush?

© 2003 Academy of General Dentistry. Reprinted with permission from the Academy of General Dentistry. For additional oral health topics, toll free access to a directory of members in your zip code area and other consumer services, see page 557 of this *Sourcebook* or contact the Academy of General Dentistry, 211 E. Chicago Avenue, Suite 900, Chicago, IL 60611, 312-440-4300, or visit their website at www.agd.org.

Angled heads, raised bristles, oscillating tufts, and handles that change colors with use: you name it, toothbrushes come in all shapes, colors, and sizes, promising to perform better than the rest. But no body of scientific evidence exists yet to show that any one type of toothbrush design is better at removing plaque than another. The only thing that matters is that you brush your teeth.

Many just don't brush long enough. Most people brush less than a minute, but to effectively reach all areas and scrub off cavity-causing bacteria, it is recommended to brush for two to three minutes.

Which Toothbrush Is Best?

In general, a toothbrush head should be small (1 inch by ½ inch) for easy access to all areas of the mouth, teeth, and gums. It should have a long, wide handle for a firm grasp. It should have soft nylon bristles with rounded ends so you won't hurt your gums.

When Should I Change My Toothbrush?

Be sure to change your toothbrush, or toothbrush head (if you're using an electric toothbrush) before the bristles become splayed and frayed. Not only are old toothbrushes ineffective, but they may harbor harmful bacteria that can cause infection such as gingivitis and periodontitis.

Toothbrushes should be changed every three to four months. Sick people should change their toothbrush at the beginning of an illness and after they feel better.

How Do I Brush?

Place the toothbrush beside your teeth at a 45-degree angle and rub back-and-forth gently. Brush outside the teeth, inside the tooth, your tongue, and especially brush on chewing surfaces and between teeth. Be sure to brush at least twice a day, especially after meals.

How Long Should I Brush My Teeth?

You should brush your teeth at least two to three minutes twice a day. Brush your teeth for the length of a song on the radio, the right amount of time to get the best results from brushing. Unfortunately, most Americans only brush for 45 to 70 seconds twice a day.

Electric versus Manual Toothbrushes

Electric toothbrushes don't work that much better than manual toothbrushes, but they do motivate some reluctant brushers to clean their teeth more often. The whizzing sounds of an electric toothbrush and the tingle of the rotary tufts swirling across teeth and gums often captivates people who own electric toothbrushes. They are advantageous because they can cover more area faster.

Electric toothbrushes are recommended for people who have limited manual dexterity, such as a disabled or elderly person and those who wear braces. Sometimes, it takes more time and effort to use an electric toothbrush because batteries must be recharged, and it must be cleaned after every use. Most electric toothbrushes have rechargeable batteries that take 10 to 45 minutes to recharge. The gearing in an electric toothbrush occasionally must be lubricated with water. Prices range from $30 to $99.

How Do Electrics Work?

Electric toothbrushes generally work by using tufts of nylon bristles to stimulate gums and clean teeth in an oscillating or rotary motion. Some tufts are arranged in a circular pattern, while others have the traditional shape of several bristles lined up on a row. When first using an electric toothbrush, expect some bleeding from your gums. The bleeding will stop when you learn to control the brush and your gums become healthier. Children under 10 should be supervised when using an electric toothbrush. Avoid mashing the tufts against your teeth in an effort to clean them. Use light force and slow movements, and allow the electric bristle action to do its job.

How Long Have Toothbrushes Been Used?

The first toothbrush was invented in China in 1000 A.D. It was an ivory-handled toothbrush with bristles made from a horse's mane. Toothbrushes became popular in the 19th century among the Victorian affluent. Mass marketing and the advent of nylon bristles in the 20th century made toothbrushes inexpensive and available to everyone.

Don't Forget

Visit your dentist regularly because toothbrushing and flossing is most effective with periodic checkups and cleanings.

Section 10.4

Are Power Toothbrushes Better?

"Are Power Toothbrushes Better? Cochrane Group Reviews Controlled Trials," reprinted with permission of the American Dental Association. © 2003 American Dental Association. For additional information, visit www.ada.org.

Scientists reviewing how well toothbrushes work said January 11 [2003] that rotational oscillation power toothbrushes are more effective than manual or other powered toothbrushes.

The results of the Cochrane Oral Health Group review were announced at the Evidence Into Action conference sponsored by the Forsyth Center for Evidence-Based Dentistry.

According to the findings, toothbrush heads that rotate in one direction and then the other are more effective in both removing plaque and reducing gingivitis than manual toothbrushes and power toothbrushes that use side-to-side action, circular action, sonic and ultrasonic action, or unknown action.

"Rotational oscillation toothbrushes removed up to 11 percent more plaque and reduced gingival bleeding by up to 17 percent more than did manual or other power toothbrushes," said co-coordinating editor William Shaw, Ph.D., MScD.

Dr. Richard Niederman, director of Forsyth, added that this study was "one of the most comprehensive independent reviews of powered toothbrushes ever conducted."

"While this information can be useful to a practitioner," said Dr. Kenneth Burrell, director of the ADA Council on Scientific Affairs, "he or she has to take into account the oral health status of an individual patient. We already know that some patients do benefit from the power toothbrushes cited in the study. We also know that many patients do just as well with manual or other types of power toothbrushes."

Dr. Burrell noted that because the study has not been published, the dental community has not had the opportunity to review its contents in depth. "We will certainly be interested in reading the study to determine its clinical relevance."

Researchers reviewed data from 29 clinical trials conducted between 1964 and 2001, involving a total of 2,547 participants in North

America, Europe, and Israel. According to the study release, the trials compared the effectiveness of all forms of manual and six types of power toothbrushes with mechanically moving heads for periods of one month and up to three months.

Dr. Shaw emphasized the results do not indicate that tooth brushing is only worthwhile with rotational oscillation action. All tooth brushing reduces gingivitis and may prevent periodontitis, "whether the brush is manual or powered," he said.

The powered toothbrushes studied were the Braun Oral B Plaque Remover (rotational oscillation); the Philips Sonicare (sonic side-to-side action); the Interplak (counter oscillation); the Teledyne Aqua Tech (circular action); the Ultrasonex brush (ultrasonic side-to-side action); and the Rowenta Dentiphant, Rowenta and Plaque Dentacontrol Plus (unknown actions).

The review will appear in the January issue of *The Cochrane Library*, a quarterly electronic collection of evidence-based systematic reviews of data from health care studies prepared by the Cochrane Collaboration.

Section 10.5

Toothbrush Infection Control

"Recommended Toothbrush Care/Toothbrushing in Group Settings: The Use and Handling of Toothbrushes," published by the Centers for Disease Control and Prevention (CDC), www.cdc.gov. Published January 2002; updated August 2002.

Toothbrushing with a fluoride toothpaste is a simple, widely recommended, and widely practiced method of caring for one's teeth. When done routinely and properly, toothbrushing can reduce the amount of plaque which contains the bacteria associated with gum disease and tooth decay, as well as provide the cavity-preventing benefits of fluoride.

To date, the Centers for Disease Control and Prevention is unaware of any adverse health effects directly related to toothbrush use, although people with bleeding disorders and those severely immunodepressed may suffer trauma from toothbrushing and may need to seek alternate means of oral hygiene. The mouth is home to millions of microorganisms (germs). In removing plaque and other soft debris from the teeth, toothbrushes become contaminated with bacteria, blood, saliva, oral debris, and toothpaste.

Because of this contamination, a common recommendation is to rinse one's toothbrush thoroughly with tap water following brushing. Limited research has suggested that even after being rinsed visibly clean, toothbrushes can remain contaminated with potentially pathogenic organisms. In response to this, various means of cleaning, disinfecting, or sterilizing toothbrushes between uses have been developed. To date, however, no published research data documents that brushing with a contaminated toothbrush has led to recontamination of a user's mouth, oral infections, or other adverse health effects.

Recommended Toothbrush Care

• Do not share toothbrushes. The exchange of body fluids that such sharing would foster places toothbrush sharers at an increased risk for infections, a particularly important consideration for persons with compromised immune systems or infectious diseases.

• After brushing, rinse your toothbrush thoroughly with tap water to ensure the removal of toothpaste and debris, allow it to air dry, and store it in an upright position. If multiple brushes are stored in the same holder, do not allow them to contact each other.

• It is not necessary to soak toothbrushes in disinfecting solutions or mouthwash. This practice actually may lead to cross-contamination of toothbrushes if the same disinfectant solution is used over a period of time or by multiple users.

• It is also unnecessary to use dishwashers, microwaves, or ultraviolet devices to disinfect toothbrushes. These measures may damage the toothbrush.

• Do not routinely cover toothbrushes or store them in closed containers. Such conditions (a humid environment) are more conducive to bacterial growth than the open air.

• Replace your toothbrush every 3-4 months, or sooner if the bristles appear worn or splayed. This recommendation of the American Dental Association is based on the expected wear of the toothbrush and its subsequent loss of mechanical effectiveness, not on its bacterial contamination.

- A decision to purchase or use products for toothbrush disinfection requires careful consideration, as the scientific literature does not support this practice at the present time.

Toothbrushing Programs in Schools and Group Settings

Toothbrushing in group settings should always be supervised to ensure that toothbrushes are not shared and that they are handled properly. The likelihood of toothbrush cross-contamination in these environments is very high, either through children playing with them or toothbrushes being stored improperly. In addition a small chance exists that toothbrushes could become contaminated with blood during brushing. Although the risk for disease transmission through toothbrushes is still minimal, it is a potential cause for concern. Therefore, officials in charge of toothbrushing programs in these settings should evaluate their programs carefully.

Recommended measures for hygienic toothbrushing in schools:

- Ensure that each child has his or her own toothbrush, clearly marked with identification. Do not allow children to share or borrow toothbrushes.

- To prevent cross contamination of the toothpaste tube, ensure that a pea-sized amount of toothpaste is always dispensed onto a piece of wax paper before dispensing any onto the toothbrush.

- After the children finish brushing, ensure that they rinse their toothbrushes thoroughly with tap water, allow them to air dry, and store them in an upright position so they cannot contact those of other children.

- Provide children with paper cups to use for rinsing after they finish brushing. Do not allow them to share cups, and ensure that they dispose of the cups properly after a single use.

Section 10.6

What Is the Most Effective Toothpaste?

"What Is the Most Effective Toothpaste?," by Kimberly A. Loos, D.D.S. © 2003 Kimberly Loos. For additional information, visit www.smiledoc. com.

Advertising can be a seductive force! This statement is especially true with respect to dentifrices (toothpastes). The proliferation of specialty toothpastes over the last 5 years has clogged pharmacy shelves and confused many consumers. This product diversification helped American toothpaste sales exceed 1.4 billion dollars in 1994, according to Information Resources Incorporated. Advertisements suggest that we need a tartar control toothpaste for removing tartar, a whitening toothpaste to brighten teeth, and even a gum care toothpaste to prevent gum disease. Is this all true?

Many toothpastes share common ingredients. The average toothpaste is about 75% humectants and water, 20% abrasive (silica or powdered calcium), 1-2% foaming and flavoring agents, 1-2% buffers, 1-1.5% coloring agents, binders and opacifiers, and 0.1-0.3% fluoride. Most fluoride toothpastes contain stannous fluoride, sodium fluoride, or monofluoride phosphate (MFP). So what is the most effective toothpaste?

Answer: Any toothpaste that contains fluoride and is applied to the teeth correctly is an effective cavity preventative. However, there are other factors to consider when using a toothpaste! The truth is that there may not be one single brand of toothpaste that is the best. I elaborate on different types of toothpastes in the sections below.

Tartar Control Toothpastes

Most studies suggest that tartar control toothpastes do not remove tartar. They do seem to prevent the accumulation of additional tartar, however. They do not reduce the tartar that forms below the gum line, which is the area where tartar can cause gum disease. This is why it is important for your dentist or hygienist to perform regular professional cleanings. Many companies, including Procter & Gamble, are currently working to formulate a tartar control dentifrice that also fights plaque and gingivitis.

Toothpastes versus Gels

While gels may seem less abrasive than pastes, this is not the case. Actually, gels can be more abrasive because of the silica (sand) used to make them. However, both are safe, effective cleaners—use whichever type you prefer.

Gum Care Toothpastes

Gum care toothpastes have questionable efficacy. This type of paste contains stannous fluoride as opposed to sodium fluoride found in other types of paste. While some studies show stannous fluoride may be helpful in reducing the incidence of gingivitis (a reversible form of gum disease), it has also been suggested that stannous fluoride is not as effective in protecting against cavities as sodium fluoride. Any toothpaste containing fluoride is recommended over nonfluoridated pastes.

Baking Soda Toothpastes

Baking soda toothpastes have mounted an incredible comeback in recent years. I have not seen any conclusive studies that prove baking soda toothpastes significantly reduce cavities compared to other toothpastes. Some people enjoy the taste and feel of baking soda or mint toothpastes. The attractive taste of baking soda and mint toothpastes may encourage people to brush longer. This is advantageous. However, many baking soda toothpastes may also contain peroxides, which can irritate and damage gum tissue. These peroxide formulas can be dangerous. Advertisers have conditioned people to believe that the fizzing action of the combined baking soda and peroxide clean teeth. People think they are getting extra cleaning action from the bubbling activity but there is no scientifically proven therapeutic activity! The American Dental Association (ADA) believes that the current levels of peroxide in toothpaste are safe. Still, peroxide toothpastes are controversial. Peroxide toothpastes are not sold in Canada.

Abrasive Smoker's Toothpastes

These toothpastes are not recommended as they can cause recession of the gums and abrasion (slow removal) of tooth structure. The best way to rid your teeth of smoking stains is to quit smoking and then have a professional cleaning by a dentist or dental hygienist.

Toothpastes for Sensitive Teeth

About 20% of all adults will experience sensitive teeth during their lifetime. You should have any sensitivity checked by your dentist first to be sure it is not a symptom of a more serious problem. Sensitive toothpastes work for the 80-85% of the population that regularly brush with them. Generally, they are needed when a patient has had gum recession, thereby exposing the root of the tooth. Once this exposure occurs, a tooth can be sensitive to hot or cold temperatures or sweet and sour foods. Sensodyne, Denquel, Protect, and Aquafresh for Sensitive Teeth are the major brands on the market. Now many more brands are jumping on the bandwagon. Some brands use different ingredients, including potassium nitrate, sodium citrate, or strontium, as their desensitizing agents. If one brand does not reduce sensitivity, try a different brand.

Whitening Toothpastes

Again, one must be careful when using these dentifrices due to their abrasive components. These should not be used exclusively but should be incorporated into a routine using a fluoride paste. Do not use a whitening paste every time you brush; use it only once every day or two. Certain brands can be more abrasive than others. Brands with sodium pyrophosphate are very abrasive. Rembrandt is one of the least abrasive whitening toothpastes. I question the effectiveness of whitening toothpastes. Some people claim to notice a brightening of tooth color, while others notice no change. This difference is partly due to variety in diet and tooth structure among people. If you are serious about whitening your teeth, you should discuss various options, including bleaching, with your dentist.

Bleaching Kits

It is highly recommended that you have your teeth whitened under the supervision of a qualified dentist. The at-home bleaching kits available over the counter in many drug stores can be dangerous. The trays that contain the bleaching agent are not custom made which often causes leakage of the peroxide or other whitening agent. Gum tissue can be irritated or damaged by these kits.

The Take-Home Message

Brush with a fluoride toothpaste for 2 minutes at least twice a day using a soft bristled toothbrush. Most people only brush their teeth for about 20 seconds on average! Your toothpaste should also bear the ADA (American Dental Association) seal of approval on the container, which means that adequate evidence for safety and efficacy have been demonstrated in controlled, clinical trials. The mechanical action employed using the proper brushing technique is more important than the brand of toothpaste you purchase. Contrary to what toothpaste commercials show, the amount of toothpaste or gel needed on your brush for effective cleaning should only be pea-sized. Flossing at least once a day is also very important because it removes food and plaque from between teeth where even the best toothbrush and toothpaste are ineffective. Studies suggest that plaque (bacteria) regrow on clean teeth about 4 hours after brushing. Brush and floss regularly!

Chapter 11

Fluoride for Cavity Prevention

Chapter Contents

Section 11.1

Facts about Fluoride

"Using Fluoride to Prevent and Control Dental Caries in the United States" is published by the Centers for Disease Control and Prevention, published August 2001; updated August 2002. Available online at www.cdc.gov/ Oralhealth/factsheets/fl-caries.htm; accessed May 2003.

The Centers for Disease Control and Prevention (CDC) has issued recommendations on using fluoride to prevent dental caries (tooth decay). The recommendations provide guidance to health care providers, public health officials, policymakers, and the general public on how to achieve maximum dental decay protection while efficiently using dental care resources and minimizing any cosmetic concerns. In 1999, CDC profiled the widespread practice of fluoridating community drinking water to prevent dental decay as one of 10 great public health achievements of the 20th century.

Fluoride Facts

- Fluorine, from which fluoride is derived, is the 13th most abundant element and is released into the environment naturally in both water and air.

- Fluoride is naturally present in all water. Community water fluoridation is the addition of fluoride to adjust the natural fluoride concentration of a community's water supply to the level recommended for optimal dental health, approximately 1.0 ppm (parts per million). One ppm is the equivalent of 1 mg/L, or 1 inch in 16 miles.

- Community water fluoridation is an effective, safe, and inexpensive way to prevent tooth decay. Fluoridation benefits Americans of all ages and socioeconomic status.

- Children and adults who are at low risk of dental decay can stay cavity-free through frequent exposure to small amounts of fluoride. This is best gained by drinking fluoridated water and using a fluoride toothpaste twice daily.

- Children and adults at high risk of dental decay may benefit from using additional fluoride products, including dietary supplements (for children who do not have adequate levels of fluoride in their drinking water), mouth rinses, and professionally applied gels and varnishes.

- Good scientific evidence supports the use of community water fluoridation and the use of fluoride dental products for preventing tooth decay for both children and adults.

- Fluoride was first used purposefully to prevent tooth decay in Grand Rapids, Michigan, in 1945 by adjusting the level of fluoride in drinking water. Fluoridation of drinking water has been used successfully in the United States for more than 50 years.

- Fluoridation of community water has been credited with reducing tooth decay by 50%-60% in the United States since World War II. More recent estimates of this effect show decay reduction at 18%-40%, which reflects that even in communities that are not optimally fluoridated, people are receiving some benefits from other sources (e.g., bottled beverages, toothpaste).

- Fluoride's main effect occurs after the tooth has erupted above the gum. This topical effect happens when small amounts of fluoride are maintained in the mouth in saliva and dental plaque (the film that adheres to tooth enamel).

- Fluoride works by stopping or even reversing the tooth decay process. It keeps the tooth enamel remain strong and solid by preventing the loss of (and enhancing the reattachment of) important minerals from the tooth enamel.

- Of the 50 largest cities in the United States, 43 have community water fluoridation. Fluoridation reaches 62% of the population on public water supplies—more than 144 million people.

- Water fluoridation costs, on average, 72 cents per person per year in U.S. communities (1999 dollars).

- Consumption of fluids—water, soft drinks, and juice—accounts for approximately 75 percent of fluoride intake in the United States.

- Children aged 6 years or less may develop enamel fluorosis if they ingest more fluoride than needed. Enamel fluorosis is a chalk-like discoloration (white spots) of tooth enamel. A common source of extra fluoride is unsupervised use of toothpaste in very young children.

- Fluoride also benefits adults, decreasing the risk of cavities at the root surface as well as the enamel crown. Use of fluoridated water and fluoride dental products will help people maintain oral health and keep more permanent teeth.

Section 11.2

Fluoride and Children

"Fluoride" is reprinted with permission from the American Academy of Pediatric Dentistry, www.aapd.org. © 2002.

How Does Fluoride Work?

When the element fluoride is used in small amounts on a routine basis it helps to prevent tooth decay. It encourages remineralization, a strengthening of weak areas on the teeth. These spots are the beginning of cavity formation. Fluoride occurs naturally in water and in many different foods, as well as in dental products such as toothpaste, mouth rinses, gels, varnish, and supplements. Fluoride is effective when combined with a healthy diet and good oral hygiene.

Will My Child Need Fluoride Supplements?

Children between the ages of six months and 16 years may require fluoride supplements. The pediatric dentist considers many different factors before recommending a fluoride supplement. Your child's age, risk of developing dental decay, and the different liquids your child drinks are important considerations. Bottled, filtered, and well waters vary in their fluoride amount, so a water analysis may be necessary to ensure your child is receiving the proper amount.

What Type of Toothpaste Should My Child Use?

Your child should use toothpaste with fluoride and the American Dental Association Seal of Acceptance. Young children, especially preschool aged children, should not swallow any toothpaste. Careful supervision and only a small pea-sized amount on the brush are recommended. If not monitored, children may easily swallow over four times the recommended daily amount of fluoride in toothpaste.

How Safe Is Fluoride?

Fluoride is documented to be safe and highly effective. Research indicates water fluoridation, the most cost effective method, has decreased the decay rate by over 50 percent. Only small amounts of fluoride are necessary for the maximum benefit. Proper toothpaste amount must be supervised, and other forms of fluoride supplementation must be carefully monitored in order to prevent a potential overdose and unsightly spots on the developing permanent teeth. Do not leave toothpaste tubes where young children can reach them. The flavors that help encourage them to brush may also encourage them to eat toothpaste.

What Is Topical Fluoride?

Topical fluoride comes in a number of different forms. Gels and foams are placed in fluoride trays and applied at the dental office after your child's teeth have been thoroughly cleaned. Fluoride varnish is one of the newer forms of topical fluoride applied at the dentist office. It has been documented to be safe and effective to fight dental decay through a long history of use in Europe.

The advantages of varnish are:

- Easily and quickly applied to the teeth.
- Decreases the potential amount of fluoride digested.
- Continues to soak fluoride into the enamel for approximately 24 hours after the original application.

This method is especially useful in young patients and those with special needs that may not tolerate fluoride trays comfortably.

Children who benefit the most from fluoride are those at highest risk for dental decay. Risk factors include a history of decay, high sucrose carbohydrate diet, orthodontic appliances, and certain medical conditions such as dry mouth.

Section 11.3

Community Water Fluoridation

"Frequently Asked Questions—Community Water Fluoridation," is published by the Centers for Disease Control and Prevention, March 2002. Available online at www.cdc.gov/nohss/guideFL.htm; accessed May 2003.

Most water supplies contain trace amounts of fluoride. Water systems are considered naturally fluoridated when the fluoride level is greater than 0.7 ppm (parts per million) under natural conditions. When a water system adjusts the level of fluoride upward to 0.7-1.2 ppm it is referred to as community water fluoridation. In 1945, Grand Rapids, Michigan, adjusted the fluoride content of their water supply to 1.0 ppm and became the first city to implement community water fluoridation. Today, approximately 65.8 percent of the U.S. population on public water supplies has access to fluoridated water systems.

How Does Fluoride Work?

Tooth decay is an infectious and transmissible bacterial disease. When a person eats sugar, or other refined carbohydrates, some oral bacteria produce acid that removes minerals from the surface of the tooth (demineralization). If the demineralization process continues for a period of time, a cavity is formed. If fluoride is available, the demineralization process can be reversed thereby preventing the formation of a cavity. In addition, fluoride reduces the ability of the oral bacteria to produce acid.

Will Community Water Fluoridation Benefit My Family?

It has been demonstrated that the action of fluoride in preventing tooth decay provides a benefit to both children and adults throughout their lives. The health benefits of fluoridation include a reduction in the frequency and severity of tooth decay, a decrease in the need for tooth extractions and fillings, a reduction in pain and suffering associated with tooth decay, and the obvious elevation of self-esteem that goes with improved functioning and appearance.

Is Community Water Fluoridation Safe?

Yes. Extensive research conducted over the past 50 years has shown that fluoridation of public water supplies is a safe and effective way to reduce tooth decay for all community residents. More recent reviews of the safety of water fluoridation include a comprehensive review of the scientific literature by the U.S. Public Health Service in 1991 and the University of York in 2000. The overall value and safety of community water fluoridation has been endorsed by the Centers for Disease Control and Prevention in 2001, by the U.S. Surgeon General's Report on Oral Health in 2000, and by the U.S. Task Force on Community Preventive Services in 2001. Community water fluoridation has also been endorsed by numerous public health and professional organizations, such as the American Dental Association, the American Medical Association, the American Association of Public Health, U.S. Public Health Service, and the World Health Organization, to name just a few.

How Much Does It Cost to Fluoridate the Water?

The per person cost of fluoridation varies by the size of the community population. The average cost of providing fluoridated water to communities with more that 20,000 residents is about 50 cents per year. For communities of 10,000-20,000 residents, the cost is about $1, and for those living in communities of less than 5,000, the cost is about $3 per year.

The information provided on this Web page is general background information and should not be construed as CDC recommended practice or guidelines, except where official recommendation or guideline documents are specifically mentioned.

Section 11.4

If You Drink Bottled Water, Don't Forget to Think about Fluoride

"Bottled Water: Better Than the Tap?", by Anne Christiansen Bullers, *FDA Consumer*, U.S. Food and Drug Administration, July 2002.

It's a rare day that Kelly Harrison, a mother of five from Tulsa, Oklahoma, doesn't find herself chauffeuring kids to some kind of sports practice or school activity. As she checks to see that each child is seat-belted into the family's minivan, Harrison also makes sure they've got the essentials: the right sports equipment, the right clothes, and what she considers to be the right drink—bottled water.

When she was growing up, Harrison, 34, might have grabbed a soft drink or juice on her way out the door. But for her kids, Harrison insists on what she thinks is a healthier choice—water. She says her children's young bodies need water as they play in the Oklahoma sun. Bottled water also contains no caffeine, no calories, and no sugar. Plus, bottled water comes in convenient bottles, easy to tote from home to wherever the busy family goes.

"I really think this is best for a lot of different reasons," says Harrison, who often tucks a bottle for herself into the basket in her minivan that contains other on-the-go mom necessities, such as a paperback book and her cell phone.

Once, most Americans got their water only from the tap. Now, like Harrison, they're often buying their water in a bottle. At work, after a workout, or just about any time, Americans are drinking bottled water in record numbers—a whopping 5 billion gallons in 2001, according to the International Bottled Water Association (IBWA), an industry trade group. That's about the same amount of water that falls from the American Falls at Niagara Falls in two hours.

Explosive growth in the industry for more than a decade has placed bottled water in nearly every supermarket, convenience store, and vending machine from coast to coast, where dozens of brands compete for consumers' dollars. In four years, industry experts anticipate that bottled water will be second only to soda pop as America's beverage of choice.

Water, of course, is essential to human health. Drinking enough water to replace whatever is lost through bodily functions is important. But surveys indicate that most of us might not be drinking enough. Is bottled water part of the answer? To decide, consumers need to arm themselves with knowledge about what they're buying before they grab the next bottle of Dasani, Evian, or Perrier off the shelf. "It really pays to do your homework," says Stew Thornley, a water quality health educator with the Minnesota Department of Health.

Different Varieties

Bottled water may seem like a relatively new idea—one born during the heightened awareness of fitness and potential water pollution during the last two or three decades. However, water has been bottled and sold far from its source for thousands of years. In Europe, water from mineral springs was often thought to have curative and sometimes religious powers. Pioneers trekking west across the United States during the 19th century also typically considered drinkable (potable) water a staple to be purchased in anticipation of the long trip across the arid West.

Today, of course, there are dozens of brands of bottled water and many different kinds, including flavored or fizzy, to choose from.

Federal Regulations

The Food and Drug Administration regulates bottled water products that are in interstate commerce under the Federal Food, Drug, and Cosmetic Act (FD&C Act).

Under the FD&C Act, manufacturers are responsible for producing safe, wholesome, and truthfully labeled food products, including bottled water products. It is a violation of the law to introduce into interstate commerce adulterated or misbranded products that violate the various provisions of the FD&C Act.

The FDA also has established regulations specifically for bottled water, including standard of identity regulations, which define different types of bottled water, and standard of quality regulations, which set maximum levels of contaminants (chemical, physical, microbial, and radiological) allowed in bottled water.

From a regulatory standpoint, the FDA describes bottled water as water that is intended for human consumption and that is sealed in bottles or other containers with no added ingredients, except that it may contain a safe and suitable antimicrobial agent. Fluoride may also be added within the limits set by the FDA.

High Standards

Is the extra expense of bottled water worth it? One thing consumers can depend on is that the FDA sets regulations specifically for bottled water to ensure that the bottled water they buy is safe, according to Henry Kim, Ph.D., a supervisory chemist at the FDA's Center for Food Safety and Applied Nutrition, Office of Plant and Dairy Foods and Beverages. Kim, whose office oversees the agency's regulatory program for bottled water, says that major changes have been made since 1974, when the Safe Drinking Water Act (SDWA) first gave regulatory oversight of public drinking water (tap water) to the U.S. Environmental Protection Agency (EPA). Each time the EPA establishes a standard for a chemical or microbial contaminant, the FDA either adopts it for bottled water or makes a finding that the standard is not necessary for bottled water in order to protect the public health.

"Generally, over the years, the FDA has adopted EPA standards for tap water as standards for bottled water," Kim says. As a result, standards for contaminants in tap water and bottled water are very similar.

However, in some instances, standards for bottled water are different than for tap water. Kim cites lead as an example. Because lead can leach from pipes as water travels from water utilities to home faucets, the EPA set an action level of 15 parts per billion (ppb) in tap water. This means that when lead levels are above 15 ppb in tap water that reaches home faucets, water utilities must treat the water to reduce the lead levels to below 15 ppb. In bottled water, where lead pipes are not used, the lead limit is set at 5 ppb. Based on FDA survey information, bottlers can readily produce bottled water products with lead levels below 5 ppb. This action was consistent with the FDA's goal of reducing consumers' exposure to lead in drinking water to the extent practicable.

Production of bottled water also must follow the current good manufacturing practices (CGMP) regulations set up and enforced by the FDA. Water must be sampled, analyzed, and found to be safe and sanitary. These regulations also require proper plant and equipment design, bottling procedures and recordkeeping.

The FDA also oversees inspections of the bottling plants. Kim says, "Because the FDA's experience over the years has shown that bottled water poses no significant public health risk, we consider bottled water not to be a high risk food." Nevertheless, the FDA inspects bottled water plants under its general food safety program and also contracts with the states to perform some bottled water plant inspections. In addition, some states require bottled water firms to be licensed annually.

Members of the IBWA also agree to adhere to the association's Model Code, a set of standards that is more stringent than federal regulations in some areas. Bottling plants that adopt the IBWA Model Code agree to one unannounced annual inspection by an independent firm.

The FDA also classifies some bottled water according to its origin.

- Artesian well water. Water from a well that taps an aquifer—layers of porous rock, sand, and earth that contain water—which is under pressure from surrounding upper layers of rock or clay. When tapped, the pressure in the aquifer, commonly called artesian pressure, pushes the water above the level of the aquifer, sometimes to the surface. Other means may be used to help bring the water to the surface. According to the EPA, water from artesian aquifers often is more pure because the confining layers of rock and clay impede the movement of contamination. However, despite the claims of some bottlers, there is no guarantee that artesian waters are any cleaner than ground water from an unconfined aquifer, the EPA says.

- Mineral water. Water from an underground source that contains at least 250 parts per million total dissolved solids. Minerals and trace elements must come from the source of the underground water. They cannot be added later.

- Spring water. Derived from an underground formation from which water flows naturally to the earth's surface. Spring water must be collected only at the spring or through a borehole tapping the underground formation feeding the spring. If some external force is used to collect the water through a borehole, the water must have the same composition and quality as the water that naturally flows to the surface.

- Well water. Water from a hole bored or drilled into the ground, which taps into an aquifer.

Bottled water may be used as an ingredient in beverages, such as diluted juices or flavored bottled waters. However, beverages labeled as containing sparkling water, seltzer water, soda water, tonic water, or club soda are not included as bottled water under the FDA's regulations, because these beverages have historically been considered soft drinks.

Some bottled water also comes from municipal sources—in other words—the tap. Municipal water is usually treated before it is bottled. Examples of water treatments include:

- Distillation. In this process, water is turned into a vapor. Since minerals are too heavy to vaporize, they are left behind, and the vapors are condensed into water again.

- Reverse osmosis. Water is forced through membranes to remove minerals in the water.

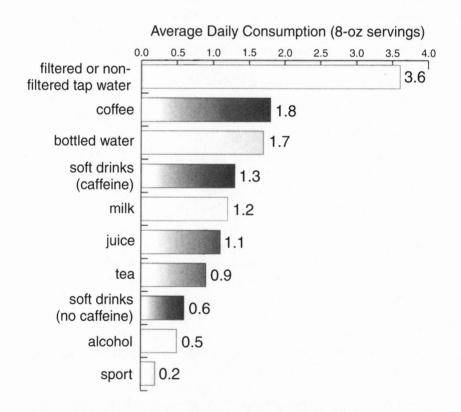

Figure 11.1. *What Americans are drinking in 2002. Source: International Bottled Water Association. Infographic by Renée Gordon.*

- Absolute 1 micron filtration. Water flows through filters that remove particles larger than one micron in size, such as *Cryptosporidium*, a parasitic protozoan.

- Ozonization. Bottlers of all types of waters typically use ozone gas, an antimicrobial agent, to disinfect the water instead of chlorine, since chlorine can leave residual taste and odor to the water.

Bottled water that has been treated by distillation, reverse osmosis, or other suitable process and that meets the definition of purified water in the *U.S. Pharmacopeia* can be labeled as purified water.

Bottled versus Tap

Whether bottled water is better than tap water, and justifies its expense, remains under debate. Stephen Kay, vice president of the IBWA, says member bottlers are selling the quality, consistency, and safety that bottled water promises, and providing a service for those whose municipal systems do not provide good quality drinking water.

"Bottled water is produced and regulated exclusively for human consumption," Kay says. "Some people in their municipal markets have the luxury of good water. Others do not."

Thornley, of the Minnesota Department of Health, agrees that consumers can depend on bottled water's safety and quality. But he says consumers should feel the same way about the quality of their tap water. Tap water may sometimes look or taste differently, he says, but that doesn't mean it's unsafe. In fact, the most dangerous contaminants are those that consumers cannot see, smell, or taste, he says. But consumers don't need to worry about their presence, he adds.

Municipal water systems serving 25 people or more are subject to the federal Safe Drinking Water Act. As such, the water constantly and thoroughly tested for harmful substances, he says. If there is a problem, consumers will be warned through the media or other outlets.

"In lieu of being told otherwise, consumers should feel confident of the safety of their water," Thornley says.

Dr. Robert Ophaug, a professor of oral health at the University of Minnesota School of Dentistry, notes that tap water has another advantage many people don't think about: It typically contains fluoride. Many communities have elected to add fluoride to drinking water to promote strong teeth and prevent tooth decay in residents, though some groups continue to oppose this practice and believe it's detrimental to health.

Ophaug says bottled water often does not have fluoride added to it. Or, if it has been purified through reverse osmosis or distillation, the fluoride may have been removed. People who drink mostly bottled water, especially those who have children, need to be aware of this, he says. They may need to use supplemental fluoride that is available by prescription from dentists or doctors. The supplements are usually recommended for children ages 7 to 16. Fluoride supplements cost around $15 for a three-month supply.

"At the least, inform the children's dentist or doctor that you are relying on bottled water," Ophaug says.

The IBWA says there are more than 20 brands of bottled water with added fluoride available to consumers today. When fluoride is added to bottled water, the FDA requires that the term "fluoridated," "fluoride added," or "with added fluoride" be used on the label. Consumers interested in how much fluoride bottled water contains can usually find out by contacting individual companies directly.

Surging Sales

Consumers don't appear ready to give up their bottled water any time soon. Younger, health-oriented people are driving the market's growth, according to industry officials. "They've grown up with bottled water, and it doesn't seem like such a stretch to them to buy water," says Kay.

Jeremy Buccellato, 31, of Ramsey, Minn., says he's heard the arguments that tap water is just as good if not better than bottled water. A glass from his own tap, however, provides water that's discolored, chlorinated, and tastes like "pool water." Buccellato says the extra money he spends on bottles of Dasani water is worth it.

"It tastes better and looks better, plus it's easy to take with me," says Buccellato. "What's not to like?"

Harrison agrees that there's nothing like a refreshing cool bottle of water to beat the heat during an Oklahoma summer.

"It's a product that fits our needs and our lifestyle," she says.

To Filter or Not to Filter?

Consumers can buy purified water. They also have the option of doing it at home. Numerous companies sell filtration systems. Some attach to the faucet and filter the water as it comes through the tap. Others are containers that filter the water in them. Among the best-known manufacturers are PUR and Brita.

Water purified with these products typically costs less than buying bottled water. According to Brita, its high-end faucet filter system provides water for 18 cents a gallon, a considerable saving from $1 or more typically charged for an 8- to 12-ounce bottle of water.

John B. Ferguson, communications manager/executive editor with the Water Quality Association, says that consumers can feel confident about the water quality provided by brand name home-filtration systems.

Stew Thornley of the Minnesota Department of Health agrees that home filtration systems can improve the taste or appearance of tap water at a minimal cost.

However, Thornley points out that consumers need to be careful about maintaining these filters. Typically, specific instructions are included with the purchase of the product. Without proper maintenance, he says, it's possible bacteria or other contaminants can build up in the products.

Anne Christiansen Bullers is a freelance writer in Prairie Village, Kansas.

Section 11.5

Too Much Fluoride: Enamel Fluorosis

"Enamel Fluorosis" reprinted with permission from the American Academy of Pediatric Dentistry, www.aapd.org. © 2002.

What Is Enamel Fluorosis?

A child may face the condition called enamel fluorosis if he or she gets too much fluoride during the years of tooth development. Too much fluoride can result in defects in tooth enamel.

Why Is Enamel Fluorosis a Concern?

In severe cases of enamel fluorosis, the appearance of the teeth is marred by discoloration or brown markings. The enamel may be pitted, rough, and hard to clean. In mild cases of fluorosis, the tiny white specks or streaks are often unnoticeable.

How Does a Child Get Enamel Fluorosis?

By swallowing too much fluoride for the child's size and weight during the years of tooth development. This can happen in several different ways. First, a child may take more of a fluoride supplement than the amount prescribed. Second, the child may take a fluoride supplement when there is already an optimal amount of fluoride in the drinking water. Third, some children simply like the taste of fluoridated toothpaste. They may use too much toothpaste, then swallow it instead of spitting it out.

How Can Enamel Fluorosis Be Prevented?

Talk to your pediatric dentist as the first step. He or she can tell you how much fluoride is in your drinking water. (Your local water treatment plant is another source of this information.) If you drink well water or bottled water, your pediatric dentist can assist you in getting an analysis of its fluoride content. After you know how much fluoride your child receives, you and your pediatric dentist can decide together whether your child needs a fluoride supplement. Watch your child's use of fluoridated toothpaste as the second step. A pea-sized amount on the brush is plenty for fluoride protection. Teach your child to spit out the toothpaste, not swallow it, after brushing.

Should I Just Avoid Fluorides for My Child Altogether?

No! Fluoride prevents tooth decay. It is an important part of helping your child keep a healthy smile for a lifetime. Getting enough—but not too much—fluoride can be easily accomplished with the help of your pediatric dentist.

Can Enamel Fluorosis Be Treated?

Once fluoride is part of the tooth enamel, it can't be taken out. But the appearance of teeth affected by fluorosis can be greatly improved by a variety of treatments in esthetic dentistry. If your child suffers from severe enamel fluorosis, your pediatric dentist can tell you about dental techniques that enhance your child's smile and self-confidence.

Part Two

You and Your Dentist

Chapter 12

Finding a Dental Practitioner

Chapter Contents

123

Section 12.1

Definitions of Dental Specialties

Reprinted with permission from www.dentistinfo.com.
© 2000 Ron Widen, D.D.S.

Endodontist

An endodontist is a dentist that strictly deals with the nerve of the tooth. They may perform simple to difficult root canal treatments as well as surgical root procedures. They may perform an apicoectomy (surgically removing the tip of the root) or a root amputation (removing a root on a multi-rooted tooth) also. They have usually 2 or more years of continuing education after graduating dental school, and most limit their practice to only endodontics.

Oral Surgeon

An oral surgeon is a dentist that performs many aspects of surgery in and about the head area. They can perform simple to extremely difficult extractions. They also perform biopsies and removal of tumors in the head and neck region. Most place implants in the jaw for future restorations and do complex jaw realignment surgeries. They have usually 4 or more years of continuing education after graduating dental school, and most limit their practice to only oral surgery.

Orthodontist

An orthodontist is a dentist that straightens teeth. They analyze the mouth and surrounding bone structures and determine where the teeth should be. If there is enough room they will manipulate the teeth and bone through the use of bands, wires, elastics, headgears, and other appliances to achieve a harmonious balance between facial muscles and teeth. If there is not enough room, teeth may have to be extracted to achieve the desired results. They treat children as well as adults, so don't be afraid that you are too old to have braces. They have usually 2 or more years of continuing education after graduating dental school, and most limit their practice to only orthodontics.

Pedodontist

A pedodontist is a pediatric dentist. They focus their dentistry to treating the younger patients. They will usually treat children as young as 1 or 2 years old to early adulthood. They can perform all aspects of dentistry on this population. They can detect early on if there are problems with decayed, missing, crowded, or malpositioned teeth and correct them as well as spot signs of child abuse. They have usually 2 or more years of continuing education after graduating dental school, and most limit their practice to only pedodontics.

Periodontist

A periodontist is a dentist that deals with the supporting structures of the teeth. They diagnose and treat gingivitis (inflammation of the gum tissue) as well as periodontitis (gum disease). They may perform simple cleanings to complicated bone surgeries. They perform bone grafting where indicated and do soft tissue grafts to treat gum recession. Most also place implants in the jaw for future restoration. They have usually 3 or more years of continuing education after graduating dental school, and most limit their practice to only periodontics.

Prosthodontist

A prosthodontist is a dentist that deals with simple to complicated full-mouth restorations. They may be crowns, fixed bridges, dentures, implant cases, or mixed implant and fixed bridge cases. They sometimes encompass the majority of the patient's remaining teeth. They also perform needed restorative procedures, such as obturators, after removal of cancerous portions of the mouth. They have usually 3 or more years of continuing education after graduating dental school, and most limit their practice to only prosthodontics.

These are the only official specialties in the field of dentistry. Cosmetic, aesthetic, geriatric, or implantology are not recognized specialties yet.

Section 12.2

Choosing a Dental Office

Reprinted with permission from the American Dental Hygienists'
Association Website, www.adha.org. © 2003.

To lessen some of the anxiety people often experience with oral
health care visits, it is important to select a dental office where you
feel comfortable. Choose a dental office that has a registered dental
hygienist on staff. Dental hygienists are highly educated and licensed
specialists whose job is to prevent periodontal disease and tooth decay.

Look for a dental office that is prevention-oriented. Your oral health
professional should allow time for you to ask questions about ways
to improve your oral health—from more effective brushing and flossing techniques to selecting oral health care products.

After finding the right office for you, be sure to work with your
dental hygienist to get the most out of your visits. Ask questions about
ways to improve your oral health—from more effective brushing and
flossing techniques to selecting oral health care products that meet
your specific needs.

Your complete medical and oral health history—including thorough
head and neck examinations—should be a part of your initial visit to
a dental office. You should be told about the exam results and recommended treatment (if any) as well as costs before treatment is started.

Infection Control in the Dental Office

While experts agree that the chance of transmitting infectious diseases during routine visits to a dental office is remote, be sure that
your dental office personnel follow the universal CDC and OSHA
safety standards:

- Use protective clothing, including gloves, masks, gowns or laboratory coats, and protective eyewear for all treatment procedures.

- Change gloves after each patient contact.

- Wash hands thoroughly before and after treating each patient.

- Heat sterilizes all nondisposable instruments and disinfects surfaces and equipment after treatment of each patient.

- Discard disposable needles, syringes, and other sharp instruments in puncture-resistant containers.

- Place all potentially infectious waste in closable, leak-proof containers or bags that are color-coded, labeled, or tagged in accordance with applicable federal, state, and local regulations.

Many offices do post a list of the infection control procedures they follow in a reception area or elsewhere. If you don't see this information, ask about it.

Section 12.3

Choosing a Dentist

"How to Choose a Dentist" © 2002 Quackwatch, Inc.
Reprinted with permission.

Dentists are licensed practitioners who hold either a doctor of dental surgery (D.D.S.) degree or the equivalent doctor of dental medicine (D.M.D.) degree.

Becoming a dentist requires a minimum of two years of predental college work followed by four years of dental school. However, almost all students entering dental school have a baccalaureate degree.

The first two years of dental school consist largely of basic and preclinical sciences. The last two years are spent primarily in dental practice under faculty supervision. State licensure is then acquired by passing national and state board examinations. Dentists who wish to specialize spend two or more years in advanced training. To become board-certified they must then pass an examination administered by a specialty board recognized by the American Dental Association. The eight recognized specialties are:

- Dental public health: Prevention and control of dental disease and promotion of community dental health

- Endodontics: Prevention and treatment of diseases of the root pulp and related structures (root canal therapy)

- Oral and maxillofacial pathology: Diagnosis of tumors, other diseases, and injuries of the head and neck

- Oral and maxillofacial surgery: Tooth extractions; surgical treatment of diseases, injuries, and defects of the mouth, jaw, and face

- Orthodontics and dentofacial orthopedics: Diagnosis and correction of tooth irregularities and facial deformities

- Pediatric dentistry: Dental care of infants and children

- Periodontics: Treatment of diseases of the gums and related structures

- Prosthodontics: Treatment of oral dysfunction through the use of prosthetic devices such as crowns, bridges, and dentures

Positive Signs

Good dentists take a personal interest in patients and their health. They are prevention-oriented but not faddists. They use x-ray films and probably suggest a full-mouth study unless suitable films are available from the patient's previous dentist.

A thorough dental examination includes inspection of the teeth, gums, tongue, lips, inside of the cheek, palate, and the skin of the face and neck, plus feeling the neck for abnormal lymph nodes and enlargement of the thyroid gland.

In adults a periodontal probe should be inserted between the gums and teeth to detect abnormally large crevices. Good dentists also chart their findings in detail.

Regular checkups can detect problems early. Routine tooth cleanings, bite evaluations, periodontal examinations, early interventions, and fluoride treatments can often avoid costly repairs. The frequency of maintenance care (including calculus removal and x-ray examinations) should be based on an assessment of the frequency of cavity formation, the rate of calculus formation, the condition of the gums, and any other special problem. Once current treatment has been completed, the patient should be placed on a recall schedule and notified when the next checkup is due.

High-quality dental work usually lasts a very long time, whereas low-quality work may fall out or decay out in a few years. The price of dental work is not the best way to judge quality; rather, pay attention to the time the dentist takes to do the work. High-quality dentistry cannot be done assembly-line style; it takes time and meticulous attention to detail.

Before embarking on treatment, get a clear understanding at your own level of what is to be done and what the outcome might be. Consider treatment options, because there may be more than one way to accomplish a goal. For example, a removable bridge, fixed bridge, or an implant may all be acceptable ways to replace a missing tooth; but they have different advantages, disadvantages, and cost.

Negative Signs

Be wary of flamboyant advertising, because it is likely to signify an emphasis on mass production rather than quality care When the fees charged per service are low, the number of services performed may be greater than needed, resulting in higher overall cost.[1]

Dentists whose ads overemphasize twilight sleep, cosmetic dentistry, and one-visit comprehensive treatment may not be interested in long-term maintenance care that does not generate high income.[1]

Routine use of intravenous sedation is another bad sign because it means that patients are exposed to unnecessary risks. Although general anesthesia can be appropriate for children,[2,3] adults with seizure disorders, and a few other situations, the vast majority of patients do not need it for routine dentistry.

A small percentage of dentists espouse or engage in unscientific practices. You should avoid any dentists who:

- Sell vitamins or other dietary supplements

- Automatically recommend replacement of amalgam fillings or removal of teeth that have root canals

- Specialize in treating headaches, backaches, myofascial pain, or TMJ problems

- Allege that fluoridation is dangerous

- Identify themselves as practicing holistic or biological dentistry

- Diagnose neuralgia-inducing cavitational osteonecrosis (NICO)

- Go beyond dentistry by diagnosing heavy metal toxicity or diseases other than those of the mouth, gums, teeth, and associated tissues.

Other Tips

It makes sense to become acquainted with a family dentist before an emergency arises. Suitable prospects can be identified by asking among friends, acquaintances, and local health professionals. Additional recommendations can be obtained from a local dental society or a dental school if one is located nearby.

A good first step is to schedule a get acquainted visit to see whether your personalities and philosophies of health care are a match. Ask about fees and payment plans. Most dentists prefer patients to initiate discussion of fees because patients know more about their own financial situation. Where large fees are involved for major work, it is best to have a written understanding of what fees will be charged and when payment will be due.

Consumers Research offers these questions for judging a dentist's skills after you have received treatment:

• How does your bite feel?

• Is any of the dental work irritating your gum?

• Does the treated tooth look like a tooth?

• Does dental floss or your tongue catch on the tooth?

• Did the dentist take time to polish your fillings?

• Do you feel pain when drinking hot or cold liquids?

• Was any debris left in your mouth after treatment?

• Does the dentist use a water spray to cool your teeth while drilling?[4]

Be cautious about dentists who recommend elaborate treatment plans. In 1996, a reporter on assignment for *Reader's Digest* visited 50 dentists in 28 states and found that their fees, examinations, and recommendations varied widely. The visits cost from $20 to $141. The reporter brought along his own x-ray films and told the dentists he had ample insurance coverage. Before embarking on the study, the reporter was checked by four dentists who agreed that he had only one immediate problem (one molar needed filling or a crown), and that work on another tooth might be advisable. Only 12 of the dentists agreed with this appraisal, and 15 failed to note a problem with the molar. One dentist recommended crowning all of the reporter's teeth, at a cost of $13,440. Other estimates ranged from $500 to $29,850.

The reporter also visited a dental school clinic where the student and a department chairman independently recommended capping both teeth, which would cost $460.[5]

In 1997, ABC-TV's *Prime Time Live* conducted a similar investigation in which, after evaluation by an expert panel, two patients with completely healthy mouths were examined by six dentists. One patient was given estimates for $645, $1175, $1195, $2220, $2323, and $2563. The other received proposals for $2135, $2410, $2829, $3140, $3190, $3700, $4061, and $7960. No program was broadcast, but the figures were made public by one of the review panel members.[6]

These investigations indicate that when extensive dental work is advised, a second opinion is often a good idea, preferably a dentist who is affiliated with a dental school. No practitioner should fear or resist having you get a second opinion. If a treatment plan is sound, particularly a major and/or expensive one, it should hold up to scrutiny by others.

References

1. Friedman JW and others. *Complete Guide to Dental Health: How to Avoid Being Overcharged and Overtreated.* New York, 1991, Consumer Reports Books.

2. Clinical guideline on the elective use of conscious sedation, deep sedation and general anesthesia in pediatric dental patients. American Academy of Pediatric Dentistry, revised May 1998.

3. Policy statement on the use of deep sedation and general anesthesia in the pediatric dental office. American Academy of Pediatric Dentistry, May 1999.

4. How to choose a dentist. *Consumers Research*, March 1997, pp. 20–24.

5. Ecenbarger W. How honest are dentists? *Reader's Digest*, February 1997, pp 50–56.

6. Dodes J. Coverage questioned (letter to the editor). *ADA News*, Sept 15, 1997.

Section 12.4

Holistic Dentistry: An Opposing Point of View

© 2002 Quackwatch, Inc. Reprinted with permission.

A significant number of dentists have gone overboard in espousing pseudoscientific theories, particularly in the area of nutrition. Holistic dentists typically claim that disease can be prevented by maintaining optimum overall health or wellness. In the dental office, this usually involves recommendations for expensive dietary supplements, a plastic bite appliance, and unnecessary replacement of amalgam fillings. John E. Dodes, D.D.S., an expert on dental quackery, has remarked that wellness is "something for which quacks can get paid when there is nothing wrong with the patient."

Historical Perspective

Much of holistic dentistry is rooted in the activities of Weston A. Price, D.D.S. (1870-1948), a dentist who maintained that sugar causes not only tooth decay but physical, mental, moral, and social decay as well. Price made a whirlwind tour of primitive areas, examined the natives superficially, and jumped to simplistic conclusions. While extolling their health, he ignored their short life expectancy and high rates of infant mortality, endemic diseases, and malnutrition. While praising their diets for not producing cavities, he ignored the fact that malnourished people don't usually get many cavities.

Price knew that when primitive people were exposed to modern civilization they developed dental trouble and higher rates of various diseases, but he failed to realize why. Most were used to feast or famine eating. When large amounts of sweets were suddenly made available, they overindulged. Ignorant of the value of balancing their diets, they also ingested too much fatty and salty food. Their problems were not caused by eating civilized food but by abusing it. In addition to dietary excesses, the increased disease rates were due to: (a) exposure to unfamiliar germs, to which they were not resistant; (b) the drastic change in their way of life as they gave up strenuous physical activities such as hunting; and (c) alcohol abuse.

Price also performed poorly designed studies that led him to conclude that teeth treated with root canal therapy leaked bacteria or bacterial toxins into the body, causing arthritis and many other diseases. This focal infection theory led to needless extraction of millions of endodontically treated teeth until well-designed studies, conducted during the 1930s, demonstrated that the theory was not valid.

Melvin Page, D.D.S., one of Price's disciples, coined the phrase "balancing body chemistry" and considered tooth decay an "outstanding example of systemic chemical imbalances." Page ran afoul of the Federal Trade Commission by marketing a mineral supplement with false claims that widespread mineral deficiencies were an underlying cause of goiter, heart trouble, tuberculosis, diabetes, anemia, high and low blood pressure, hardening of the arteries, rheumatism, neuritis, arthritis, kidney and bladder trouble, frequent colds, nervousness, constipation, acidosis, pyorrhea, overweight, underweight, cataracts, and cancer. Page also claimed that milk was unnatural and was the underlying cause of colds, sinus infections, colitis, and cancer.

The human body contains many chemicals, ranging from water and simple charged particles (ions) to complex organic molecules. The amounts vary within limits. Some are in solution and others are not. Legitimate medical practitioners may refer to a specific chemical or a balance between a few chemicals that can be measured. But the idea that body chemistry goes in and out of balance is a quack concept.

The Price-Pottenger Nutrition Foundation of La Mesa, California, is the repository for many of Price's manuscripts and photographs. It was founded in 1965 as the Weston Price Memorial Foundation and adopted its current name in 1972. Its newsletter, book catalog, and information service promote food faddism, megavitamin therapy, homeopathy, chelation therapy, and many other dubious practices.

Dubious Practices

Some practitioners use hair analysis, computerized dietary analysis, a blood chemistry screening test, or muscle-testing, as a basis for recommending supplements to "balance the body chemistry" of their patients. Hair analysis is not a reliable tool for measuring the body's nutritional state. Computer analysis can be useful for determining the composition of a person's diet and can be a legitimate tool for dietary counseling. Dentists receive training in the nutritional aspects of dental health. However, few are qualified to perform general dietary counseling, and computerized nutrient deficiency tests are not legitimate. The blood chemistry tests, usually obtained from a reputable laboratory, are legitimate but misinterpreted. Instead of accepting the laboratory's range of normal values, holistic dentists use a much narrower range and tell patients that anything outside that range means they are out of balance and need treatment. Muscle testing is a feature of behavioral kinesiology, a variant of applied kinesiology, a pseudoscientific system of diagnosis and treatment based on the notion every health problem can be related to a weak muscle and nutritional imbalances. In January 2000, the Holistic Dental Association had about 80 members listed online.

Disorders of the TMJ (jaw joint) and facial muscles can cause facial pain and restrict opening of the mouth. Clicking alone is not considered a problem. Allegations that TMJ problems can affect scoliosis, premenstrual syndrome, or sexual problems are not supported by scientific evidence. Scientific studies show that 80% to 90% of patients with TMJ pain will get better within three months if treated with nonprescription analgesics, moist heat, and exercises.

Correction of a bad bite can involve irreversible treatments such as grinding down the teeth or building them up with dental restorations. The most widespread unscientific treatment involves placing a plastic appliance between the teeth. These devices, called mandibular orthopedic repositioning appliances (MORAs), typically cover only some of the teeth and are worn continuously for many months or even years. When worn too much, MORAs can cause the patient's teeth to move so far out of proper position that orthodontics or facial reconstructive surgery is needed to correct the deformity.

Proponents of cranial osteopathy, craniosacral therapy, cranial therapy, and similar methods claim that the skull bones can be manipulated to relieve pain (especially TMJ pain) and remedy many other ailments. They also claim that a rhythm exists in the flow of the fluid that surrounds the brain and spinal cord and that diseases can be diagnosed by detecting aberrations in this rhythm and corrected by manipulating the skull. Proponents include dentists, physical therapists, osteopaths, and chiropractors. The theory underlying craniosacral therapy is erroneous because the bones of the skull are fused to each other, and cerebrospinal fluid does not have a palpable rhythm. In a recent test, three physical therapists who examined the same 12 patients diagnosed significantly different craniosacral rates.

Auriculotherapy is a variation of acupuncture based on the notion that the body and organs are represented on the surface of the ear. Proponents claim it is effective against facial pain and ailments throughout the body. Its practitioners twirl needles or administer small electrical currents at points on the ear that supposedly represent diseased organs. Courses on auriculotherapy are popular among holistic dentists. Complications from unsterile and broken needles have been reported.

A few dentists use a quack electrodiagnostic device that supposedly detects imbalances in the flow of vital energy through imaginary channels called meridians. These devices actually measure skin resistance to a low-voltage electric current, which the practitioners claim is related to electromagnetic energy imbalance. This procedure typically leads to multiple false diagnoses, unnecessary tooth removal, and/or the sale of useless and expensive products. The procedure is commonly referred to as electrodermal testing, galvanic testing, or electroacupuncture according to Voll (EAV). Some dentists who utilize such a device claim that each tooth is related to one or more of the body's internal organs.

Some dentists claim to specialize in the treatment of bad breath. Such dentists have no special expertise and are primarily interested in increasing their income by selling unproven products. One such product, Oxyfresh, has been sold through multilevel marketing with unsubstantiated claims that it eliminates mouth odors, cleans teeth, and conditions gums. The active ingredient is chlorine dioxide, which is also used as an algaecide in swimming pools.

A few hundred dentists claim that the mercury in silver-amalgam fillings is toxic and causes a wide range of health problems, including multiple sclerosis, arthritis, headaches, Parkinson's disease, and emotional stress. They recommend that mercury fillings be replaced with either gold or plastic ones and that vitamin supplements be taken to prevent trouble during the process. However, scientific testing has shown that the amount of mercury absorbed from fillings is only a small fraction of the average daily intake from food and is insignificant. In 1992 an extensive review by the U.S. Public Health Service concluded that it was inappropriate to recommend restricting the use of dental amalgam. The American Dental Association Council on Ethics, Bylaws, and Judicial Affairs considers the unnecessary removal of silver-amalgam fillings "improper and unethical."

The most outspoken advocate of mercury-amalgam toxicity has been Hal A. Huggins, D.D.S., of Colorado Springs, Colorado, who describes himself as one of Page's students. Huggins promoted balancing body chemistry so vigorously that in 1975 the American Dental Association Council on Dental Research denounced the diet that he recommended. Another Price follower is George A. Meinig, D.D.S., whose book *Root Canal Cover-up Exposed* was published in 1994.

In the mid-1980's the U.S. Food and Drug Administration forced Huggins to stop marketing mineral products with false claims that they would help the body rid itself of mercury. Huggins has also claimed that root canal therapy can make people susceptible to arthritis, multiple sclerosis, amyotrophic lateral sclerosis, and other autoimmune diseases. As with mercury-amalgam fillings, there is no objective evidence that teeth treated with root canal therapy have any adverse effect on the immune system or any other system or part of the body. Huggins's dental license was revoked in 1996. During the revocation proceedings the administrative law judge concluded: (a) Huggins had diagnosed mercury toxicity in all patients who consulted him in his office, even some without mercury fillings; (b) he had also recommended extraction of all teeth that had had root canal therapy; and (c) Huggins's treatments were "a sham, illusory and without scientific basis."

Huggins is among a small number of dentists who maintain that facial pain, heart disease, arthritis, and various other health problems are caused by infected cavitations, within the jaw bones, that are not detectable on x-ray examination or treatable with antibiotics. Advocates call this condition cavitational osteopathosis or neuralgia-inducing cavitational osteonecrosis (NICO) and claim they can cure the patient by locating and scraping out the affected tissues. They may also remove all root-canal-treated teeth and most of the vital teeth close to the area where they say an infection exists. There is no scientific evidence to support this assertion or the diagnostic and treatment methods based on it. Proponents of this dubious theory have formed the American Academy of Biological Dentistry.

Huggins's website states that, "Cavitations are hard to find. They require lots of skill, years of experience, and most of all, a vivid imagination to spot them on an X-ray film." Vivid imagination may well be the basic requirement of holistic dentistry.

Our advice is simple. Steer clear of dentists who practice holistic dentistry or biological dentistry or who use any of the dubious methods described in this chapter.

Chapter 13

Potential Risk for Lead Exposure in Dental Offices

In December 2000, the Washington State Health Department discovered white powder that was found to be lead oxide in boxes used to store dental intraoral radiograph film. The Washington State Health Department alerted state health departments throughout the United States. Subsequently, the Wisconsin Division of Public Health (WDPH) conducted an investigation of dental offices in the state. This report summarizes the investigation, which indicated that similar storage boxes are used in Wisconsin. The findings indicate that patients are at risk for exposure to a substantial amount of lead during a dental radiograph procedure if the office stores dental film in these boxes.

During January to March 2001, radiation safety inspectors in Wisconsin visited 240 (9%) of 2,748 dental offices with radiograph equipment. Of these, 43 (18%) stored radiograph film in table-top, lead-lined boxes. Of 11 dental offices in use for >20 years, four (36%) used this storage method.

The boxes were usually made of wood and shaped like a shoe box. All boxes contained a white powder residue. A bulk sample of the residue contained 77% lead identified as lead oxide. Visits to dental offices occurred before and after a mailing had been sent by WDPH to all dental offices with radiograph equipment warning about possible

Centers for Disease Control and Prevention, *Morbidity and Mortality Weekly Report*, October 12, 2001, 50(40);873–4. Available online at http://www.cdc.gov/mmwr; accessed May 2003.

lead exposure and recommending that lead-lined storage boxes be discarded. Many offices discarded the boxes before the inspection. In one office, after receiving the warning, paper was placed in the bottom of the box and film was placed on top of the paper. In another office, dental instruments had been placed in the box. Other offices used a vertical wall-mounted, lead-lined film dispensing box. Some of these boxes and the film in them also contained lead.

A mock dental radiograph procedure was performed during which wipes were placed on the tips of a dental hygienist's fingers whenever a patient's mouth was touched. Analysis of these wipe samples found 3,378μg [micrograms] lead that could have been transferred from the hygienist's fingers to a patient's mouth. Lead also could have been introduced directly from the film. Wipe samples of eight film packets from two dental offices that used the lead-lined storage boxes identified average lead levels of 3,352μg (range: 262μg to 34,000μg). During a typical radiographic procedure, usually conducted once per year, >4 separate views are taken. When children's teeth develop to the point where adjacent teeth touch (usually age 3 years), radiographs may be taken if the dentist suspects decay.

Because of the increased susceptibility of children and the developing fetus[1], lead exposure is particularly dangerous for children and for women who are or may soon become pregnant. The approximate half-life of lead in blood is 25 days[2]; as a result, the window for identifying lead exposure following dental radiographs is a few months. Health care providers who discover high blood lead levels of unexplained origin should consider this possible route of exposure.

Advances in dental radiograph technology have reduced scatter radiation—the reason for protective boxes—making lead-lined radiograph storage boxes unnecessary. Because lead oxide cannot be removed adequately, the film packets stored in lead-lined boxes and the film packets stored in them should be discarded.

References

1. Chisolm JJ, O'Hara DM. *Lead absorption in children.* Baltimore, Maryland: Urban & Schwarzenberg, 1982.

2. Hu H. Heavy metal poisoning. In: Fauci AS, ed. *Harrison's principles of internal medicine.* New York, New York: McGraw-Hill, 1998:2565–6.

Chapter 14

Dental Anxiety

Chapter Contents

Section 14.1

Calming the Anxious Child

Reprinted with permission from the American Academy of Pediatric Dentistry, www.aapd.org. © 2002.

How Does a Pediatric Dentist Help with Dental Anxiety?

Pediatric dentists have special training in helping anxious children feel secure during dental treatment. And pediatric dental offices are designed for children. Staff members choose to work in a pediatric dental practice because they like kids. So, most children are calm, comfortable, and confident in a pediatric dental office.

How Will a Pediatric Dentist Help My Child Feel Comfortable?

Pediatric dentists are trained in many methods to help children feel comfortable with dental treatment. For example, in the Tell-Show-Do technique, a pediatric dentist might name a dental instrument, demonstrate the instrument by using it to count your child's fingers, then apply the instrument in treatment.

The modeling technique pairs a timid child in dental treatment with a cooperative child of similar age. Coaching, distraction, and parent participation are other possibilities to give your child confidence in dentistry. But by far the most preferred technique is praise. Every child does something right during a dental visit, and pediatric dentists let children know that.

Should I Accompany My Child into Treatment?

Infants and some young children may feel more confident when parents stay close during treatment. With older children, doctor-child communication is often enhanced if parents remain in the reception room.

What If a Child Misbehaves during Treatment?

Occasionally a child's behavior during treatment requires assertive management to protect him or her from possible injury. Voice control (speaking calmly but firmly) usually takes care of it. Some children need gentle restraint of the arms or legs as well. Mild sedation, such as nitrous oxide/oxygen or a sedative, may benefit an anxious child. If a child is especially fearful or requires extensive treatment, other sedative techniques or general anesthesia may be recommended.

Section 14.2

Conquer Your Fear of the Dentist

"Dental Phobia, Dental Anxiety and Dental Fear Can Be Overcome," is reprinted with permission from www.saveyoursmile.com. © 2003 Dental Zone, Inc., dentalzone@aol.com.

Dental anxiety or fear of the dentist is a major stumbling block for many people. It usually prevents otherwise intelligent, rational people from optimizing and maintaining their dental health.

The key to good oral health is prevention—stopping problems before they arise. Unfortunately, people who suffer from dental anxiety often fail to visit the dentist for routine care. When they finally do go, often a small preventable problem has turned into a problem that will require major intervention.

In my years of successfully treating dental phobics, I have used a number of techniques. Some even involve the use of mild sedatives but most techniques involve face-to-face communication, answering the patient's questions, and a lot of listening.

Most dental phobics have had very negative experiences with either unskilled, uncaring, or incompetent dentists.

The most important step to overcoming dental anxiety is finding a good dentist. A good dentist is one who:

• is patient
• is highly competent

- endeavors to make each meeting pain free

- genuinely cares about you

- has the ability to nurture you through past traumas

Ask friends and family for dentists they recommend. Feel free to ask any potential dentist about his practice, practice philosophy, and the steps he or she takes to make dentistry pain free and anxiety free. Remember, do not be intimidated. You are the consumer and it is the dentist who should be selling you on his or her service.

It takes a true partnership between the patient and the dentist, a growing trust, and a growing relationship that cannot nor should not be pushed faster than the patient can accept.

In my practice, I have used this no-pressure approach with great success. Usually the first appointment is a get to know you visit where we take a complete medical and dental history and have a discussion with the patient.

I have found that by clearly explaining any planned procedures (what they are and why we plan to do them) and by answering all of the patient's questions, much of the anxiety can be eliminated. If all goes well, we may do an intraoral examination using a special camera that lets us see, on a monitor, the inside of the patient's mouth.

The second visit includes discussion on what is the most stressful thing about dentistry for the patient and ways we can reduce if not eliminate that stress. We perform an examination, take x-rays, and develop a treatment plan.

If the patient is ready for a cleaning of the teeth, we may proceed. The progress made in each visit is controlled by the patient and their readiness to continue. No pressure at all.

During future visits, we following through with the necessary procedures. I have dozens of patients who have been helped with this no-pressure approach. A person can also reduce their anxiety by bringing a friend or loved one along with them for support.

I often advise people not to schedule appointments during stressful times. Don't, for example, schedule an appointment before a major business meeting or in the middle of the day if you know you have several tasks to do after the appointment.

Also, during the procedure, I tell patients exactly what I am doing—when they are going to feel pressure and when they are going to feel coldness. I use all the techniques available to minimize pain. In the few cases where the patient will feel discomfort, I tell them. Surprisingly anxiety is reduced if a patient knows exactly what to expect. I cannot stress enough how important it is to find a dentist you can trust and who is willing to do what it takes to relieve your anxiety. Many dentists will use a technique known as guided imagery where they will tell you to think about pleasant experiences (such as sunbathing on a beach in the Bahamas) while the procedure is going on.

Some dentists may go over relaxation techniques with you. Others will play soothing music in the background or allow the patient to bring in a portable tape or CD player and headphones. Some dentists even have virtual reality goggles that the patient can wear during the procedure.

If your dentist is unwilling to discuss your anxiety or try things to help reduce your anxiety, it is time to get a new dentist.

Remember that an educated consumer is a less anxious consumer. Make sure your dentist explains each and every procedure you undergo. Good dentists usually have videos, pamphlets, or books explaining the procedures they perform. A good dentist will answer the questions you have thus lessening your anxiety.

With a good dentist-patient relationship and with good communication, dental anxiety can be overcome. You should feel comfortable discussing your anxieties with your dentist and should be confident that he or she will do everything possible to reduce your anxiety. If not, find a new dentist who is willing to do what it takes to overcome your anxiety.

This article was written by Dr. Eric Spieler. Dr. Spieler is a practicing physician in Philadelphia, Pennsylvania. To contact Dr. Spieler, E-mail him at DrSpieler@aol.com.

Chapter 15

Dental Visits and Exams

Chapter Contents

Section 15.1

Dental Visits and Teeth Cleaning

"Frequently Asked Questions—Dental Visits" is published by the Centers for Disease Control and Prevention, January 2001. Available online at www.cdc.gov/nohss/guideDV.htm; accessed May 2003.

Routine dental visits aid in the prevention, early detection and treatment of tooth decay, oral soft tissue disease, and periodontal diseases. All information collected at the dental checkup should be kept in a dental record for future reference. If you change dentists, a copy of your dental record (including radiographs) should be given to your new dentist.

How Often Should I Visit the Dentist?

Although annual (or more frequent) dental examinations are often recommended, there is little scientific evidence that this frequency is necessary for the maintenance of oral health in healthy children or adults. The frequency of routine dental visits should be based on individual need—some people will need to see the dentist more often than others. More frequent visits may be necessary for persons at increased risk for oral diseases due to age, pregnancy, tobacco and alcohol use, periodontal diseases, oral hygiene, and health conditions (e.g., diabetes, dry mouth, HIV infection). Your dentist or dental hygienist can help you determine how often you should have your teeth cleaned.

What Should a Complete Dental Examination Include?

A complete dental examination should include the following: (1) a soft tissue examination, (2) a screening and examination for periodontal diseases, and (3) a detailed charting of cavities, existing restorations (fillings and crowns), and other tooth conditions.

The purpose of the soft tissue examination is to detect pathological changes in the tissues that line the inside of the mouth. While the vast majority of pathology in the mouth is benign, precancerous and cancerous changes in the oral tissues may be found. It is best if detected at an early stage when it can be successfully treated. Tobacco and heavy alcohol use are major risk factors for oral cancer. A thorough soft tissue examination should include a visual inspection and finger exploration of the tongue, floor of the mouth (under the tongue), palate (roof of the mouth), salivary glands, insides of the cheek, and the back of the throat.

The tongue should be moved to allow for the inspection of its sides and base; the face, head, and neck should also be examined, and any enlarged lymph nodes identified.

In an examination for periodontal diseases, your dentist or hygienist should use a periodontal probe to measure the band of gum tissue that surrounds the tooth. The purpose of this examination is to detect gum disease at the early stages when prevention is most effective.

The third aspect of a complete dental examination is the inspection of every tooth surface for the presence of new decay and the status of existing restorations.

Dental radiographs (x-rays) may be part of your routine dental visit and will assist the dentist in locating disease that cannot be seen by the eye, such as cavities that develop between the teeth or bone loss that occurs beneath the gums.

When Should My Child First Visit the Dentist?

The American Academy of Pediatric Dentistry recommends an oral examination for all infants within 6 months of the eruption of the first tooth and no later than 12 months of age. An early examination will provide an opportunity for the parent or caregiver to receive anticipatory guidance regarding dental and oral development and oral health care. It will also help ensure that the infant's mouth is appropriately cleaned, that the infant has adequate fluoride exposure, and that the infant has no existing medical conditions or habits that could lead to oral disease.

Section 15.2

Frequently Asked Questions about Teeth Cleaning

"Frequently Asked Questions—Teeth Cleaning" is published by the Centers for Disease Control and Prevention, January 2001. Available online at www.cdc.gov/nohss/guideTC.htm; accessed May 2003.

When a dentist or dental hygienist cleans your teeth they remove soft (plaque) and hard (tartar, calculus, or stains) deposits from your teeth.

The primary purpose of having your teeth cleaned is to prevent or delay the progression of periodontal diseases. Professional dental care alone, however, is inadequate to prevent periodontal diseases. Smoking has been implicated in approximately 50% of periodontal disease cases in adults (Tomar 2000). Abstaining from tobacco use, maintaining good oral hygiene, and having your teeth cleaned professionally are the most effective ways to prevent periodontal diseases.

How Often Should I Get My Teeth Cleaned?

As with routine dental examinations, the frequency of professional teeth cleaning will depend on the health of your teeth and gums. Healthy children and adults should have their teeth cleaned at least once every 12-24 months. If you are at risk of periodontal diseases because of age, tobacco use, rate of accumulation of deposits, personal oral hygiene practices, or medical conditions such as diabetes or HIV infection, your teeth may need to be cleaned more often. Your dentist or dental hygienist can help you determine how often you should have your teeth cleaned.

Chapter 16

Why Some People Take Antibiotics before Visiting the Dentist

A relatively small but important group of individuals may need to be medicated before certain dental procedures are performed. Recommendations for premedication with antibiotics have changed as of September 1997. This article describes people that may be benefit from premedication and summarizes why premedication may be necessary. For specific recommendations, please personally visit your dentist or physician.

Who Needs Antibiotic Prophylaxis?

Individuals who are at risk for developing subacute bacterial endocarditis, an infection affecting the heart, should take antibiotics prior to certain dental procedures—especially procedures that produce gingival or mucosal bleeding. Bacterial endocarditis can develop in patients with certain underlying structural cardiac defects. The category of risk to which a patient belongs depends upon the condition present. The high risk category includes individuals with prosthetic heart valves, a history of endocarditis, complex cyanotic congenital heart disease, or surgically constructed systemic pulmonary shunts or conduits. The moderate risk category includes patients with congenital cardiac malformations (other than complex cyanotic disease), acquired valvular dysfunction (e.g., due to rheumatic fever), hypertropic

"Antibiotic Prophylaxis for Dental Treatment: An Overview," by Kimberly A. Loos, D.D.S. © 2003 Kimberly Loos. For additional information, visit www. smiledoc.com.

cardiomyopathy, mitral valve prolapse with valvular regurgitation and/or thickened leaflets, and certain types of heart murmurs. Individuals with isolated secundum atrial septal defects, surgical repair of atrial or ventricular septal defects, coronary bypass surgery, mitral valve prolapse without valvular regurgitation, innocent or physiological heart murmurs, previous Kawasaki disease or rheumatic fever without valvular dysfunction, and pacemakers do not necessarily need antibiotic prophylaxis.

The most controversial group of patients who might need antibiotic prophylaxis include individuals with total prosthetic joint replacements. Prophylaxis is recommended for some individuals with prosthetic joints because they may develop an infection at the site of the replaced joint. These individuals include patients who are immunocompromised or immunosuppressed such as those with rheumatoid arthritis, systemic lupus erythematosus, or disease-, drug-, or radiation-induced immunosuppression. Other at-risk patients with total joint replacements include those with insulin-dependent diabetes, previous prosthetic joint infections, malnourishment, and hemophilia. Patients that have had joint replacement surgery within the last two years should also consider antibiotic prophylaxis. Antibiotic prophylaxis is not recommended for patients with pins, plates, or screws.

Why Is Antibiotic Prophylaxis Necessary?

Certain dental procedures, including deep cleanings along the gum line, can cause bacteria normally present in the mouth to be released into the bloodstream. These bacteria can lodge in or near damaged areas of the heart causing endocarditis. Subacute bacterial endocarditis can be a life-threatening disease. Accordingly, prevention of endocarditis is very important. This infection can develop in persons with cardiac problems who develop a bacteremia or organisms likely to cause endocarditis. Some dental procedures involving the gum tissues can cause a bacteremia that rarely lasts longer than 15 minutes. The risk for bacteremia will be higher in a mouth with continuing inflammation; therefore, maintaining good oral hygiene is imperative. While there are currently no carefully controlled studies to prove antibiotic prophylaxis helps protect against endocarditis, *in vitro* bacteria studies, experimental animal models, and retrospective analysis of human antibiotic use provide the guidelines recommended for prevention of bacterial endocarditis.

Good dental health before and after surgery is important to reduce the incidence of bacteremias caused either by dental treatment or everyday occurrences. There is no scientific evidence which proves antibiotic prophylaxis is beneficial for preventing infection of total joint replacement, but it may prove beneficial for the small group of patients previously described in this article.

When Is Antibiotic Prophylaxis Needed?

Endocarditis prophylaxis and prophylaxis for those with total joint replacements is recommended before the following dental procedures are performed: tooth extraction, periodontal surgery, scaling and root planing, probing gingival pocket depths, a regular cleaning, implant surgery, root canal instrumentation or surgery beyond the apex of the root, and placement of orthodontic bands. Dental procedures for which antibiotic prophylaxis is not necessary include local anesthetic injections, fillings, crowns (unless bleeding is expected), suture removal, dental impressions and radiographs, fluoride treatments, orthodontic appliance adjustment, and shedding of primary teeth. Some of these procedures may require use of antibiotic prophylaxis depending upon the individual situation. Clinical judgment and physician consult is needed in some cases to establish the proper level of protection for the patient.

Which Antibiotic Is Recommended?

The regimen for prophylaxis for both endocarditis and prosthetic joints has changed. Previously, patients were required to take a certain amount of a specific antibiotic before and after their dental appointment. Now, patients are only required to take antibiotics prior to the dental procedure. The standard general prophylaxis is amoxicillin, 2.0 grams for adults and 50 mg/kg for children, taken one hour before the dental procedure. For those who are allergic to the penicillin family, another category, usually clindamycin, in varying dosages can be prescribed. For individuals who cannot take oral medications, an intramuscular (injection) or intravenous antibiotic (usually ampicillin or clindamycin) can be administered 30 minutes prior to initiating the dental procedure.

Chapter 17

Talk to Your Dentist
If You Use Herbal Medicines

Although many of the prescription and over-the-counter drugs used today are derived from plants, there is a big difference between the two. Conventional drugs, which must be approved for use by the Food and Drug Administration, are based on an active ingredient. Manufacturers find a chemical that provides a desired response when taken into the body, and then they synthesize that chemical. In other words, a conventional drug is based on a chemical that is made in a laboratory, even though it may have originally come from a plant.

Herbal or botanical medications are taken from the natural chemicals within a plant. Either the extract is taken in its original form, sometimes combined with other herbal extracts, or it is refined.

When an herbal medication is refined, the essential extract is taken out of the plant source, concentrated, and then added back to make the original herbal medication more potent.

Why Do I Need to Tell My Dentist If I Take Herbal Supplements?

Always tell your dentist about all medications and supplements you are taking and how much you take. From vitamins to echinacea,

"How Do Herbal Medications Differ from Conventional Drugs?" © 2003 Academy of General Dentistry. Reprinted with permission from the Academy of General Dentistry. For additional oral health topics, toll free access to a directory of members in your zip code area and other consumer services, see page 557 of this *Sourcebook* or contact the Academy of General Dentistry, 211 E. Chicago Avenue, Suite 900, Chicago, IL 60611, 312-440-4300, or visit their website at www.agd.org.

everything you put in your body causes a certain reaction, and some alternative medicines are very potent. That reaction can interfere with medications your dentist gives you or enhance them to cause a much stronger reaction. If your dentist doesn't know what drugs or supplements you have taken, he or she will not know how to protect you from possible substance interactions.

What Are Some Combinations I Should Avoid Taking?

Even the most common herbal and vitamin supplements can have serious side effects for some patients. Blood thinners, such as the popular *Ginkgo biloba* and even vitamin E can be dangerous when taken with aspirin, which also acts as a blood thinner. Because this may cause a situation in which some patients' blood will have difficulty clotting, serious surgical procedures should be avoided after taking such a combination of supplements.

Vitamins can be dangerous as well, if you aren't careful. Vitamin C, when taken in the thousands of grams as an intravenous cancer treatment, can cause problems and weaken the efficiency of anesthesia. On the other hand, if you are taking a calming supplement, such as Kava Kava or St. John's Wort, this can enhance the effects of the anesthesia your dentist gives you and cause problems.

Dandelion and bearberry are both herbal supplements that are said to work as a diuretic. These can interact with and over-enhance the effects of prescription diuretics, which can lead to dehydration, loss of potassium in the body, and even disruption of heart-rhythm.

What Will My Dentist Do When I Tell Him or Her?

It is important that your dentist has all the information, including your medical history, herbal medication, and conventional drugs you are taking. If your dentist knows that you are taking a medication that can interact with something he or she is planning on giving you, there are a variety of solutions from which to choose. Your dentist may have you stop taking the herbal medication until the treatment is over, or choose a different drug for treatment, if one is available. There are so many new alternative medications on the market today that a dentist may not know about all of them and their side effects. If your dentist is not familiar with the medication, he or she will make it his or her job to find out if a treatment is safe for your situation.

Many patients who take alternative medicines may not tell their dentist. They are afraid the dentist will not respect their decision to take an herbal medication and tell them to stop taking it. The truth is, as herbal medications become more popular, many dentists are beginning to use them in their practices. Your dentist might even have an alternative, herbal solution for you.

Where Can I Go for Information on Alternative Therapies?

The best person to ask is a licensed alternative MD. There are a few accredited schools in the United States that offer degrees in natural healing. Some of these schools can offer referrals to their graduates. For example, you can go to Bastyr University's referral page, http://www.bastyr.edu/contact/referral.asp, to look up a variety of practitioners.

Herbal remedies some dentists are using:

- Oil of calendula—For mouth wounds like cold sores.

- Plant-derived amica—Can be useful to patients after a tooth extraction or after oral surgery. It responds to minor trauma.

- Valerian—To calm nervous or anxious patients who are interested in an alternative to nitrous oxide.

- Aloe vera—Cold sores and fever blisters. The antibacterial and antiviral effects can shrink the lesion.

Part Three

Routine Dental Concerns

Chapter 18

Plaque: What It Is and How to Get Rid of It

People used to think that as you got older you naturally lost your teeth. We now know that's not true. By following easy steps for keeping your teeth and gums—healthy plus seeing your dentist regularly—you can have your teeth for a lifetime!

Plaque: What Is It?

Plaque is made up of invisible masses of harmful germs that live in the mouth and stick to the teeth.

- Some types of plaque cause tooth decay.
- Other types of plaque cause gum disease.

Red, puffy or bleeding gums can be the first signs of gum disease. If gum disease is not treated, the tissues holding the teeth in place are destroyed and the teeth are eventually lost.

Dental plaque is difficult to see unless it's stained, You can stain plaque by chewing red disclosing tablets, found at grocery stores and drugstores, or by using a cotton swab to smear green food coloring on your teeth. The red or green color left on the teeth will show you where there is still plaque—and where you have to brush again to remove it.

National Institute of Dental and Craniofacial Research (NIDCR), National Institutes of Health, NIH Publication Number 99-3245, July 1999. Available online at www.nidcr.nih.gov/health/pubs/plaque_brochure.pdf; accessed May 2003.

Stain and examine your teeth regularly to make sure you are removing all plaque.

Ask your dentist or dental hygienist if your plaque removal techniques are OK.

Floss

Use floss to remove germs and food particles between teeth. Rinse.

Ease the floss into place gently. Do not snap it into place—this could harm your gums.

Brush Teeth

Use any tooth brushing method that is comfortable, but do not scrub hard back and forth. Small circular motions and short back and forth motions work well. Rinse.

To prevent decay, it's what's on the toothbrush that counts. Use fluoride toothpaste. Fluoride is what protects teeth from decay.

Brush the tongue for a fresh feeling! Rinse again.

Remember: food residues, especially sweets, provide nutrients for the germs that cause tooth decay, as well as those that cause gum disease. That's why it is important to remove all food residues, as well as plaque, from teeth. Remove plaque at least once a day—twice a day is better. If you brush and floss once daily, do it before going to bed.

Another way of removing plaque between teeth is to use a dental pick—a thin plastic or wooden stick. These picks can be purchased at drug stores and grocery stores.

Chapter 19

Sealants

Chapter Contents

Section 19.1

Seal out Dental Decay

National Institute of Dental and Craniofacial Research (NIDCR), National
Oral Health Information Clearinghouse, NIH Publication Number 00-489,
January 2000. Available online at www.nidcr.nih.gov/health/pubs/sealants/
text.htm; accessed May 2003.

What Are Dental Sealants?

Sealants are thin, plastic coatings painted on the chewing surfaces
of the back teeth.

Sealants are put on in dentists' offices, clinics, and sometimes in
schools.

Getting sealants put on is simple and painless. Sealants are
painted on as a liquid and quickly harden to form a shield over the
tooth.

Sealants are clear or tinted. Tinted sealants are easier to see.

Are Sealants New?

No, sealants are not new. They have been around for a long time!
Research by NIDCR and others led to the development of sealants in
the early 1960s.

But many people still do not know what sealants are. In fact, fewer
than 20 percent of children in the United States have sealants!

How Long Do Sealants Last?

Sealants can last up to 10 years. But they need to be checked at
regular dental checkups to make sure they are not chipped or worn
away. The dentist can repair sealants by adding more sealant material.

How Much Do Sealants Cost?

Sealing one tooth usually costs less than filling one tooth.

Having sealants put on healthy teeth now will save you money in the long run by avoiding fillings, crowns, or caps used to fix decayed teeth.

But the most important reason for getting sealants is to avoid tooth decay. Healthy teeth can last a lifetime!

Does Insurance Pay for Sealants?

Many insurance companies pay for sealants. Check with your company for details.

Why Get Sealants?

By covering the chewing surfaces of the molars, sealants keep out the germs and food that cause decay.

What Causes Decay?

Germs in the mouth change the sugar in food to acid. The acid can eat a cavity in the tooth. The decay has to be cleaned out by drilling and then the tooth has to be filled.

Of course a healthy tooth is the best tooth. So it is important to prevent decay. That's why sealants are so important.

Why Do Back Teeth Decay So Easily?

The chewing surfaces of back teeth are rough and uneven because they have small pits and grooves. Food and germs can get stuck in the pits and stay there a long time because toothbrush bristles cannot brush them away.

Who Should Get Sealants?

Children should get sealants on their permanent molars as soon as the teeth come in—before decay attacks the teeth.

The first permanent molars—called 6-year molars—come in between the ages of 5 and 7.

The second permanent molars—12-year molars—come in when a child is between 11 and 14 years old.

The other teeth with pits and grooves—called premolars or bicuspids—right in front of the molars also may need to be sealed.

Teenagers and young adults without decay or fillings in their molars also may get sealants.

Should Sealants Also Be Put on Baby Teeth?

Your dentist might think it is a good idea, especially if your child's baby teeth have deep pits and grooves.

Baby teeth play an important role in holding the correct spacing for permanent teeth—so it is important to keep baby teeth healthy so they don't fall out early.

How Are Sealants Put on?

The tooth is cleaned.

The tooth is dried, and cotton or other material is put around the tooth so it stays dry.

A solution is put on the tooth surface that makes the tooth a little rough. (It is easier for the sealant to stick to a slightly rough tooth.)

The tooth is rinsed and dried. Then new cotton is put around the tooth so it stays dry.

The sealant is applied in liquid form and hardens in a few seconds.

What If a Small Cavity Is Accidentally Covered by a Sealant?

The decay will not spread because it is sealed off from its food and germ supply.

Besides Sealants, Are There Other Ways to Prevent Tooth Decay?

Yes. The best way you can help prevent tooth decay is to brush with a fluoride toothpaste and drink fluoridated water (water is fluoridated in about half the cities and towns of the United States). If your water is not fluoridated or if your teeth need more fluoride to stay healthy, your dentist can prescribe it in the form of a gel, mouth rinse, or tablet.

If you have a baby or a young child that needs fluoride and do not have fluoride in your water, your physician (pediatrician) or dentist can prescribe fluoride drops or tablets.

Fluoride is the best defense against tooth decay!

Remember:

- Sealants + Fluoride = Maximum Protection Against Cavities

- Sealants protect the chewing surfaces

- Fluoride protects the smooth surfaces

Fluoride:

- makes teeth more resistant to decay
- repairs tiny areas of decay before they become big cavities
- makes germs in the mouth less able to cause decay

Fluoride helps the smooth surfaces of the teeth the most. It is less effective on the chewing surfaces of the back teeth (molars).

Regular brushing—with fluoride toothpaste—and flossing also help prevent tooth decay.

Sealants and fluoride together can prevent almost all tooth decay.

How Can I Get More Information about Sealants?

For more information about sealants call your dentist, state or local dental society, or health department. Sometimes sealants are put on at school—check with your school or local health department to see if there is such a program in your area.

Section 19.2

Frequently Asked Questions about Dental Sealants

Centers for Disease Control and Prevention (CDC), January 2001. Available online at www.cdc.gov/nohss/guideDS.htm; accessed May 2003.

What Are Dental Sealants?

A dental sealant (also called a pit and fissure sealant) is a plastic, professionally applied material that is put on the chewing surfaces of back teeth to prevent cavities. Sealants provide a physical barrier so that cavity-causing bacteria cannot invade the pits and fissures on the chewing surfaces of teeth.

Why Should My Child Get Dental Sealants?

Since the early 1970's, childhood dental caries on smooth tooth surfaces (those without pits and fissures) has declined markedly because of widespread exposure to fluorides. By 1986-1987, approximately 90 percent of the decay in children's teeth occurred in tooth surfaces with pits and fissures, and almost two-thirds were found on the chewing surfaces alone.

Dental sealants have been shown to prevent decay on tooth surfaces with pits and fissures. Sealants have been approved for use for many years and are recommended by professional health associations and public health agencies.

When Should My Child Get Dental Sealants?

First permanent molars erupt into the mouth at about age 6 years. Placing sealants on these teeth shortly after they erupt protects them from developing caries in areas of the teeth where food and bacteria collect.

If sealants were applied routinely to susceptible tooth surfaces in conjunction with the appropriate use of fluoride, most tooth decay in children could be prevented.

Second permanent molars erupt into the mouth at about age 12 years. Pit and fissure surfaces of these teeth are as susceptible to dental caries as the first permanent molars of younger children. Therefore, young teens need to receive dental sealants shortly after the eruption of their second permanent molars.

Are Dental Sealants Just for Kids?

The potential to develop pit and fissure decay begins early in life, so children and teenagers are obvious candidates. But some adults at high risk of decay can benefit from sealants as well. Your dentist can tell you if you would benefit from dental sealants.

Do Dental Sealants Replace Fluoride?

No. Fluorides, such as those used in community water, toothpaste, gels, varnish, and mouth rinse also help to prevent decay. Fluoride works best on the smooth surfaces of teeth. The chewing surfaces on the back teeth, however, have tiny grooves where decay often begins. Sealants keep cavity-causing bacteria out of the grooves by covering them with a safe plastic coating. Sealants and fluorides work together to prevent tooth decay.

Chapter 20

X-Rays for Diagnosing Dental Problems

Chapter Contents

Section 20.1

X-Rays

"Frequently Asked Questions: X-Rays" reprinted with permission of the American Dental Association. © 2003 American Dental Association. For additional information, visit www.ada.org.

Table 20.1. Sources of Radiation and Estimated Exposure

Source	Estimated exposure (mSV)
Dental radiographs	
Bitewings (4 films)	0.038
Full-mouth series (about 19 films)	0.150
Medical radiographs	
Lower GI series	4.060
Upper GI series	2.440
Chest	0.080
Average radiation from outer space in Denver, CO (per year)	0.510
Average radiation in the U.S. from natural sources (per year)	3.000

Source: Adapted from Frederiksen NL. X-Rays: What is the Risk? *Texas Dental Journal.* 1995;112(2):68–72.

Note: A millisievert (mSV) is a unit of measure that allows for some comparison between radiation sources that expose the entire body (such as natural background radiation) and those that only expose a portion of the body (such as radiographs).

What Are the Benefits of a Dental X-Ray Examination?

Many diseases of the teeth and surrounding tissues cannot be seen when your dentist examines your mouth. An x-ray examination may reveal:

- small areas of decay between the teeth
- infections in the bone

- abscesses or cysts
- developmental abnormalities
- some types of tumors

Finding and treating dental problems at an early stage can save time, money, and unnecessary discomfort. It can detect damage to oral structures not visible during a regular exam. If you have a hidden tumor, radiographs may even help save your life.

How Do Dental X-Rays Compare to Other Sources of Radiation?

We are exposed to radiation every day from various sources, including outer space, minerals in the soil, and appliances in our homes (like smoke detectors and television screens).

Section 20.2

Protecting Yourself from X-Rays

"We Want You to Know about X-Rays: Get the Picture on Protection" is a brochure published by the U.S. Food and Drug Administration (FDA), Center for Devices and Radiological Health, November 3, 1999. Available online at www.fda.gov/cdrh/consumer/xraybrochure.html; accessed May 2003.

Will you be one of the 7 out of 10 Americans who will get a medical or dental x-ray picture this year? Most of the time that's fine because the x-ray will help your doctor find out what's wrong and decide how you should be treated The information from diagnostic x-rays can even save your life.

But sometimes x-rays are taken when they're not medically needed. And even when there is a good medical reason for an x-ray, if proper care is not taken, the patient can get more radiation than necessary. Like many things, x-rays may do harm as well as good. X-rays may add slightly to the chance of getting cancer in later life. And if the

X-RAY RECORD CARD

Name: _____

Health Ins.Co.: _____

Policy No.: _____

For additional cards, write to FDA, HFZ-220, 1350 Piccard Dr.,
Rockville, MD 20850

HELP REDUCE
X-RAY RISKS & COSTS

- Feel free to ask your doctor how an x-ray will help with the diagnosis and treatment.
- Don't refuse an x-ray if there's a clear need for it. Remember, the risk is small.
- Ask if a gonad shield can be used for yourself and for your children during x-rays of the abdomen.
- Tell the doctor or x-ray personnel if you are, or might be pregnant, before having an x-ray of the abdomen.
- Don't insist on an x-ray if the doctor explains there is no need for it.

DATE	TYPE OF EXAM	REFERRING PHYSICIAN	ADDRESS WHERE X-RAYS ARE KEPT

Figure 20.1. An x-ray record card may help you reduce your exposure to x-ray radiation.

sex organs are in or near the x-ray beam, changes could be produced in the reproductive cells. Those changes might be passed on and could cause harm in future children and grandchildren.

Because of the amount of radiation used in x-ray examinations is small, the chance that x-rays will cause these problems is very low. Still, it makes sense to avoid unnecessary risks, no matter how small. By avoiding x-rays that aren't medically needed, you avoid the risks, and you can also avoid unnecessary medical costs. You may now be asking, "How many x-ray exams are safe?" There's really no answer to this question. There is no number that is definitely safe, just as there is no number that is definitely dangerous. Every x-ray can involve some tiny risk. If the x-ray is needed to find out about a medical problem, then that small risk is certainly worth taking.

Here's what you can do:

- **Ask how it will help** to find out what's wrong. How will it help determine your treatment? Feel free to talk with your doctor; you have a right to understand why an x-ray is suggested.

- **Don't refuse an x-ray** if the doctor explains why it is medically needed. Remember, the risk of not having a needed x-ray is greater than the tiny risk from the radiation.

- **Don't insist on an x-ray.** Sometimes doctors give in to people who ask for an x-ray, even if it isn't medically needed.

- **Tell the doctor if you are or think you might be pregnant** before having an x-ray of your abdomen or lower back. Because the unborn baby is growing so quickly, it can be more easily affected by radiation than a grown-up. If you need an abdominal x-ray during your pregnancy, remember that the chance of harm to the unborn baby is very tiny. But be sure to talk with your doctor.

- **Keep up on new mammography information.** There is agreement that mammography (breast x-rays) is important in the fight against breast cancer. But scientific information is still growing on the proper role of mammography. Right now it is believed that women more likely to need mammography are those with symptoms, or those past menopause, or those with a personal or family history of breast cancer. Talk with your doctor about the value of breast x-rays in your particular case.

- **Ask if a gonad shield can be used** if you or your children are to have x-rays of the lower back, abdomen, or near the sex organs.

A lead shield over the sex organs can keep x-rays from reaching your reproductive cells, thereby protecting future generations. Gonad shielding should be considered if the patient might have children in the future. But remember, a shield can't always be used, particularly over the female ovaries, because it may hide what the doctor needs to see on the x-ray.

- **Keep an x-ray record card.** Copy the X-Ray Record Card in Figure 20.1 and keep it in your wallet. When an x-ray is taken, have the date, the type of exam, and where the x-ray is kept filled out on the card. Then, if another doctor suggests an x-ray of the same part of your body, you can tell him or her about the previous x-ray. Sometimes the doctor can use the previous x-ray instead of taking a new one. Or, if a new x-ray is needed, the previous one might help show any change in your medical problem. Keep a record card for everyone in your family.

Chapter 21

Tooth Pain

Symptom: Momentary Sensitivity to Hot or Cold Foods

Possible Problem: If the discomfort lasts only moments, sensitivity to hot and cold foods generally does not signal a problem. The sensitivity may be caused by a loose filling or by minimal gum recession, which exposes small areas of the root surface.

What to Do: Try using toothpastes made for sensitive teeth. Brush up and down with a soft brush; brushing sideways wears away exposed root surfaces. If this is unsuccessful, see your dentist.

Symptom: Sensitivity to Hot or Cold Foods after Dental Treatment

Possible Problem: Dental work may inflame the pulp, inside the tooth, causing temporary sensitivity.

What to Do: Wait four to six weeks. If the pain persists or worsens, see your dentist.

Symptom: Sharp Pain When Biting Down on Food

Possible Problem: There are several possible causes of this type of pain: decay, a loose filling, or a crack in the tooth. There may be damage to the pulp tissue inside the tooth.

"Tooth Pain Guide," Copyright © 2000 American Association of Endodontists. Reprinted by permission.

What to Do: See a dentist for evaluation. If the problem is a cracked tooth, your dentist may send you to an endodontist. Cracked tooth pain comes from damage to the inner soft tissue of the tooth, the pulp. Endodontists are dentists who specialize in pulp-related procedures. Endodontic treatment, also known as root canal treatment, can relieve that pain.

Symptom: Lingering Pain after Eating Hot or Cold Foods

Possible Problem: This probably means the pulp has been damaged by deep decay or physical trauma.

What to Do: See your endodontist to save the tooth with root canal treatment.

Symptom: Constant and Severe Pain and Pressure, Swelling of Gum, and Sensitivity to Touch

Possible Problem: A tooth may have become abscessed, causing the surrounding bone to become infected.

What to Do: See your endodontist for evaluation and treatment to relieve the pain and save the tooth. Take over-the-counter analgesics until you see the endodontist.

Symptom: Dull Ache and Pressure in Upper Teeth and Jaw

Possible Problem: The pain of a sinus headache is often felt in the face and teeth. Grinding of teeth, a condition known as bruxism, can also cause this type of ache.

What to Do: For sinus headache, try over-the-counter analgesics or sinus medicine. For bruxism, consult your dentist. If pain is severe and chronic, see your physician or endodontist for evaluation.

Symptom: Chronic Pain in Head, Neck, or Ear

Possible Problem: Sometimes pulp-damaged teeth cause pain in other parts of the head and neck, but other dental or medical problems may be responsible.

What to Do: See your endodontist for evaluation. If the problem is not related to the tooth, your endodontist will refer you to an appropriate dental specialist or a physician.

Chapter 22

Tooth Sensitivity

If you occasionally experience a sudden flash of pain or a mild tingly feeling when you bite into sweet or sour foods or drink hot or cold beverages, you may have sensitive teeth.

Pain from sensitive teeth is not always constant; it can come and go. Constant pain could be a sign of a more serious problem. It is still important, however, to discuss your symptoms with your dentist to determine the cause and proper treatment.

What Causes Sensitive Teeth?

In healthy teeth, porous tissue called dentin is protected by your gums and your teeth's hard enamel shell. Microscopic holes in the dentin, called tubules, connect back to the nerve triggering pain when irritated by certain foods and beverages. Dentin can be exposed by:

- Receding gums caused by improper brushing or gum disease
- Fractured or chipped teeth
- Clenching or grinding your teeth

Treatment

Depending on the diagnosis, your dentist may recommend one or more of the following treatments to relieve the symptoms of sensitive teeth:

"Sensitive Teeth" is reprinted with permission from HIVdent, www.hivdent.org. © 2000 HIVdent. Available online at www.hivdent.org/_peag/faq-sens.htm; accessed May 2003.

- A fluoride varnish, such as Duraphat, that can be applied by a dental professional

- A fluoride rinse or gel for sensitive teeth, prescribed by your dentist, for home use

- A soft-bristle or extra soft-bristle toothbrush to protect gums

- A special toothpaste for sensitive teeth that can either block access to the nerve or insulate the nerve itself. A sensitivity toothpaste usually eases pain in about two to four weeks.

Chapter 23

Cavities

Many of us remember sweating through the poking and prodding of the dentist. We prayed that he or she would not find cavities that would require the use of the dreaded dental drill. Armed with the right knowledge and proper home dental care, you can now rest at ease and fear cavities no more.

What Causes Cavities?

When it comes to cavities, bacteria are public enemy number one. Our mouths are full of bacteria that settle on our teeth in plaque, a goo of proteins, saliva, and food debris. Here bacteria devour food particles left on our teeth. These bacteria produce acid as a byproduct of their feasting. It is this acid which eats into the tooth enamel creating cavities.

The teeth have a moderate ability to repair tooth enamel by re-mineralizing the affected enamel with minerals from saliva. Unfortunately, the rate of destruction by acid exceeds this rate of repair. Normally, acids eating into tooth enamel is not painful. Left untreated, however, acid eats a hole through the enamel into the underlying dentin and pulp layers of the tooth. This does cause pain and left untreated the cavity will eventually destroy dentin, pulp and tooth nerve.

"How to Stop Cavities and Tooth Decay," reprinted with permission from www.saveyoursmile.com. © 2003 Dental Zone, Inc., dentalzone@aol.com.

What Can You Do to Reduce Your Chances of Getting Cavities?

Good oral hygiene significantly reduces your risk of getting cavities. Brushing removes bacteria as well as the food debris bacteria feed on. When brushing it is crucial to brush all tooth surfaces, which takes at least 2 to 3 minutes. Unfortunately, most people only brush for less than 45 seconds, missing a large percentage of their tooth surfaces.

Flossing every day is crucial to preventing cavities. Flossing reaches the nearly 35 percent of your mouth that your toothbrush cannot reach. In these areas, bacteria live happily pouring out cavity causing acid. Remember brushing without flossing is like taking a shower and only washing two thirds of your body. The remaining third still remains dirty!

In addition to practicing good oral hygiene, there are other things you can do to reduce your risk of getting cavities:

Watch What You Eat

Bacteria are particularly fond of foods containing sugars and carbohydrates. These foods provide bacteria with energy to grow, reproduce, and create enamel eating acid. A special favorite of bacteria are foods that tend to stick to teeth like peanut butter, caramel, and honey. When stuck to teeth these foods are not cleared by chewing and swallowing. Consequently they provide bacteria with a long-lasting food source from which to make acid.

When you eat meals or snacks containing large amounts of sugars, carbohydrates, or sticky foods that tend to get stuck to teeth, make sure to follow the meal with water to help wash off food particles remaining on teeth. If possible, brush your teeth immediately after the meal.

Watch the Timing of Snacks

The timing of your snacks is crucial to preventing cavities. The acid produced by bacteria is neutralized by saliva and cleared from the mouth. After the acid is cleared, minerals in saliva crystallize on the enamel to begin to repair areas damaged by the acid. Larger intervals between meals provide more opportunity for acid to be neutralized and more time for the acid damage to be repaired. Frequent snacks, however, provide for a constant acid attack and provide less time for tooth repair.

This explains why snacks eaten with a meal are better for teeth than snacks eaten between meals. A candy bar eaten with a meal, for example, is less likely to contribute to cavity formation than a candy bar eaten as a snack between meals.

This also explains why fewer larger-sized meals are better for teeth than more frequent smaller sized meals. Likewise, sipping on sugar-containing liquids through out the day is much more detrimental than drinking sugar-containing liquids with a meal.

Use Fluoride to Prevent Cavities

Fluoride is a wonder of modern dentistry. Fluoride incorporates itself into tooth enamel, strengthening the enamel and making it more resistant to acid attacks. Most adults receive adequate amounts of fluoride in their toothpastes. Children often receive adequate amounts in their drinking water. If your water is not fluoridated you may want to consult your pediatrician to see about providing fluoride supplements for your child.

Visit Your Dentist on a Regular Basis

Dental problems often remain silent creating pain only after significant damage has occurred. Dentists can identify many of these potentially devastating problems before they cause major damage. Additionally, dentists can detect places in your mouth that you miss when brushing. These areas are prime targets for cavity formation. In areas where cavities are just beginning to form, dentists can use high concentration fluoride treatments to prevent the need for the dental drills and fillings.

With proper oral hygiene and attention to what we eat and when we eat, cavities can be virtually eliminated.

Chapter 24

Cracked Teeth

Today, people are keeping their teeth longer thanks to advances in dental procedures. At the same time, people are also exposing their teeth to many more years of crack-inducing habits and stress. Although cracked teeth are becoming more and more common, these teeth can often be saved if treated promptly.

Cracked teeth exhibit a variety of symptoms. If your tooth is cracked, you might feel occasional pain when chewing, particularly between bites as you release the pressure on your teeth. You might also feel pain when you eat or drink something hot or cold. Cracks are difficult to diagnose because the pain comes and goes, and cracks rarely show up on x-rays. Because of this, you may see your dentist several times before the crack is diagnosed.

Why Does My Cracked Tooth Hurt?

A crack in a tooth usually affects the soft inner tissue of the tooth called the pulp. The pulp contains blood vessels and nerves. When it is damaged, it causes pain. That is why a cracked tooth hurts—the pulp is damaged. To relieve the pain and save your tooth, the pulp needs to be gently treated.

Why Have I Been Referred to an Endodontist?

Endodontists are dental specialists who diagnose and treat oral and facial pain. They specialize in root canal (endodontic) treatment, including any treatment for the inner soft tissues of the tooth. During dental school, all dentists are educated in treating the dental pulp. In addition to dental school, endodontists receive two or more years of advanced education in this kind of treatment. They study root canal techniques and procedures in greater depth, including the treatment of cracked teeth. For this reason, many dentists choose to refer their patients with cracked teeth to endodontists.

Why Does My Cracked Tooth Need to Be Treated?

As mentioned earlier, cracks in teeth often affect the inner tissue of the tooth, the pulp. The pulp contains blood vessels, nerves, and connective tissue. When a tooth is cracked, chewing can cause movement of the separate pieces of the tooth. This movement irritates the pulp and often causes pain. The tooth may also become sensitive to temperature extremes. In time, the pulp may become so irritated that your tooth may hurt by itself, even when you are not chewing or eating or drinking something hot or cold. When the pulp becomes irritated, it needs to be treated in order to save the tooth.

How Will My Cracked Tooth Be Treated?

The treatment of your cracked tooth depends on the type and severity of the crack. There are five common types of cracks.

Craze lines are tiny cracks that affect only the outer enamel of the tooth. They are common in all adult teeth and cause no pain. Craze lines need no treatment.

The second type of crack involves the cusp. The cusp is the pointed part of the chewing surface of your tooth. If a cusp becomes weakened, a fracture can result. Part of the cusp may break off or may need to be removed by your dentist. But this type of crack, a fractured cusp, rarely affects the pulp. Because the pulp is not affected, it is very unlikely that you would need root canal treatment. Your tooth can usually be restored by your dentist with a crown or other restoration.

If your crack is diagnosed as a cracked tooth, then the crack probably extends from the chewing surface of the tooth vertically towards the root. Sometimes it extends below the gum line and into the root. A cracked tooth is not separated into two distinct segments, but the soft inner tissue of the tooth is usually damaged anyway. If this happens, you will probably need root canal treatment to remove the damaged tissues and save the tooth. It is particularly important to diagnose this type of crack early. In its earlier stages, a cracked tooth can still be saved.

If you have a split tooth, on the other hand, it can never be saved intact. A split tooth is often the result of an untreated cracked tooth that splits into two distinct segments. With endodontic (root canal) treatment, however, a portion of the tooth can sometimes be saved.

Vertical root fractures are cracks that begin in the root and extend toward the chewing surface. They show very few signs and symptoms and therefore may go unnoticed for some time. You may discover that you have a vertical root fracture when the bone and gum surrounding the root become inflamed and infected. Treatment usually involves extraction of the tooth, but sometimes endodontic surgery can save a portion of the tooth.

After Treatment for a Cracked Tooth, Will My Tooth Completely Heal?

Unlike a broken bone, the fracture in a cracked tooth will never completely heal. In fact, even after treatment, it is possible that a crack may continue to worsen and separate, resulting in the loss of the tooth.

Despite the possibility for the tooth to worsen, the treatment you receive is important. It will relieve your pain and reduce the chances that the crack will worsen. Most cracked teeth continue to function for years after treatment. Your dentist or endodontist will be able to tell you more about your particular diagnosis and treatment recommendations.

What Can I Do to Prevent My Teeth from Cracking?

While cracked teeth are not completely preventable, you can take some steps to make your teeth less susceptible to cracks.

- Don't chew on hard objects such as ice, unpopped popcorn kernels, or pens.

- Don't clench or grind your teeth.

- If you clench or grind your teeth while you sleep, talk to your dentist about getting a retainer or other mouth guard to protect your teeth.

• Wear a mouth guard or a mask when playing contact sports.

And if you experience symptoms of a cracked tooth, see your dentist immediately. If detected early, a cracked tooth can often be saved.

Chapter 25

Dental Fillings

Chapter Contents

Section 25.1

How Dental Restoration Materials Compare

© 2002 Quackwatch, Inc. Reprinted with permission. Tables 25.1 and 25.2 are reprinted with permission of the American Dental Association. © 2003 American Dental Association. For additional information, visit www.ada.org.

Dental restorations can be classified into two types. Direct restorations are done by inserting filling material directly into the tooth. Indirect restorations are fabricated outside of the mouth.

In recent years, there has been a marked increase in the development of esthetic materials made of ceramic and plastic. These mimic the appearance of natural teeth and are more esthetically pleasing where they will be visible. But the strength and durability of traditional materials still make them useful, particularly in the back of the mouth where they must withstand the extreme forces that result from chewing. The traditional materials include gold, base metal alloys, and dental amalgam.

Amalgam, produced by mixing mercury and other metals, is still the most commonly used filling material. Some people have expressed concern about amalgam because of its alleged mercury content. In fact, amalgam is composed mostly of complex compounds where the mercury is bound chemically to the other ingredients. Although mercury by itself is classified as a toxic material, the mercury in amalgam is chemically bound to other metals to make it stable and therefore safe for use in dental applications. In fact, amalgam is the most thoroughly studied and tested restorative material now used. Compared to the rest, it is durable, easy to use, and inexpensive. The safety and effectiveness of amalgam have been reviewed by major U.S. and international scientific and health bodies, including the American Dental Association; the National Institutes of Health; the U.S. Public Health Service; the Centers for Disease Control and Prevention; the Food and Drug Administration; and the World Health Organization. All have concluded that amalgam is a safe and effective material for restoring teeth.

The charts below are reproduced with the kind permission of the American Dental Association, which developed them to help dentists

Table 25.1. Comparison of Direct Restorative Dental Materials (continued on next page)

Factors	Amalgam	Composites (Direct and Indirect)	Glass Ionomers	Resin-Ionomers
General description	A mixture of mercury and silver alloy powder that forms a hard solid metal filling. Self-hardening at mouth temperature.	A mixture of submicron glass filler and acrylic that forms a solid tooth-colored restoration. Self- or light-hardening at mouth temperature.	Self-hardening mixture of fluoride containing glass powder and organic acid that forms a solid tooth-colored restoration able to release fluoride.	Self or light-hardening mixture of sub-micron glass filler with fluoride-containing glass powder and acrylic resin that forms a solid tooth-colored restoration able to release fluoride.
Principal uses	Dental fillings and heavily loaded back tooth restorations.	Esthetic dental fillings and veneers.	Small non-load bearing fillings, cavity liners, and cements for crowns and bridges.	Small non-load bearing fillings, cavity liners, and cements for crowns and bridges.
Leakage and recurrent decay	Leakage is moderate, but recurrent decay is no more prevalent than other materials.	Leakage low when properly bonded to underlying tooth; recurrent decay depends on maintenance of the tooth-material bond.	Leakage is generally low; recurrent decay is comparable to other direct materials, fluoride release may be beneficial for patients at high risk for decay.	Leakage is low when properly bonded to the underlying tooth; recurrent decay is comparable to other direct materials, fluoride release may be beneficial for patients at high risk for decay.
Overall durability	Good to excellent in large load-bearing restorations.	Good in small-to-moderate size restorations.	Moderate to good in non-load-bearing restorations; poor in load-bearing.	Moderate to good in non-load-bearing restorations; poor in load-bearing.

187

Table 25.1. Comparison of Direct Restorative Dental Materials (continued)

Factors	Amalgam	Composites (Direct and Indirect)	Glass Ionomers	Resin-Ionomers
Cavity preparation considerations	Requires removal of tooth structure for adequate retention and thickness of the filling.	Adhesive bonding permits removing less tooth structure.	Adhesive bonding permits removing less tooth structure.	Adhesive bonding permits removing less tooth structure.
Clinical considerations	Tolerant to a wide range of clinical placement conditions, moderately tolerant to the presence of moisture during placement.	Must be placed in a well-controlled field of operation; very little tolerance to presence of moisture during placement.		
Resistance to wear	Highly resistant to wear.	Moderately resistant, but less so than amalgam.	High wear when placed on chewing surfaces.	
Resistance to fracture	Brittle, subject to chipping on filling edges, but good bulk strength in larger high-load restorations.	Moderate resistance to fracture in high-load restorations.	Low resistance to fracture.	Low to moderate resistance to fracture.
Biocompatibility	Well-tolerated with rare occurrences of allergenic response.			

Post-placement sensitivity	Early sensitivity to hot and cold possible.	Occurrence of sensitivity highly dependent on ability to adequately bond the restoration to the under-lying tooth.	Low.	Occurrence of sensitivity highly dependent on ability to adequately bond the restoration to the under-lying tooth.
Esthetics	Silver or gray metallic color does not mimic tooth color.	Mimics natural tooth color and translucency, but can be subject to staining and discoloration over time.	Mimics natural tooth color, but lacks natural translucency of enamel.	Mimics natural tooth color, but lacks natural translucency of enamel.
Relative cost to patient	Generally lower; actual cost of fillings depends on their size.	Moderate; actual cost of fillings depends on their size and technique.	Moderate; actual cost of fillings depends on their size and technique.	Moderate; actual cost of fillings depends on their size and technique.
Average number of visits to complete	One.	One for direct fillings; 2+ for indirect inlays, veneers, and crowns.	One.	One.

Table 25.2. Comparison of Indirect Restorative Dental Materials

Factors	All-porcelain (Ceramic)	Porcelain Fused to Metal	Gold Alloys (High-noble)	Base Metal Alloys (Non-noble)
General description	Porcelain, ceramic, or glass-like fillings and crowns.	Porcelain is fused to an underlying metal structure to provide strength to a filling, crown, or bridge.	Alloy of gold, copper, and other metals resulting in a strong, effective filling, crown, or bridge.	Alloys of non-noble metals with silver appearance resulting in high strength crowns and bridges.
Principal uses	Inlays, onlays, crowns, and aesthetic veneers.	Crowns and fixed bridges.	Inlays, onlays, crowns, and fixed bridges.	Crowns, fixed bridges, and partial dentures.
Leakage and recurrent decay	Sealing ability depends on materials, underlying tooth structure, and procedure used for placement.	The commonly used methods used for placement provide a good seal against leakage. The incidence of recurrent decay is similar to other restorative procedures.		
Durability	Brittle material; may fracture under heavy biting loads. Strength depends greatly on quality of bond to underlying tooth structure.	Very strong and durable.	High corrosion resistance prevents tarnishing; high strength and toughness resist fracture and wear.	
Cavity preparation considerations	Because strength depends on adequate porcelain thickness, it requires more aggressive tooth reduction during preparation.	Including both porcelain and metal creates a stronger restoration than porcelain alone; moderately aggressive tooth reduction is required.	The relative high strength of metals in thin sections requires the least amount of healthy tooth structure removal.	
Clinical considerations	These are multiple step procedures requiring highly accurate clinical and laboratory processing. Most restorations require multiple appointments and laboratory fabrication.			

Attribute	Porcelain (all-ceramic)	Porcelain-fused-to-metal	Gold alloys	Base-metal alloys
Resistance to wear	Highly resistant to wear, but porcelain can rapidly wear opposing teeth if its surface becomes rough.	Highly resistant to wear, but porcelain can rapidly wear opposing teeth if its surface becomes rough.	Resistant to wear and gentle to opposing teeth.	Resistant to wear and gentle to opposing teeth.
Resistance to fracture	Prone to fracture when placed under tension or on impact.	Porcelain is prone to impact fracture; the metal has high strength.	Highly resistant to fracture.	Highly resistant to fracture.
Biocompatibility	Well tolerated.	Well tolerated, but some patients may show allergenic sensitivity to base metals.	Well tolerated.	Well tolerated, but some patients may show allergenic sensitivity to base metals.
Post-placement sensitivity	Low thermal conductivity reduces the likelihood of discomfort from hot and cold.	*Sensitivity, if present, is usually not material specific.*	High thermal conductivity may result in early post-placement discomfort from hot and cold.	High thermal conductivity may result in early post-placement discomfort from hot and cold.
Esthetics	Color and translucency mimic natural tooth appearance.	Porcelain can mimic natural tooth appearance, but metal limits translucency.	Metal colors do not mimic natural teeth.	Metal colors do not mimic natural teeth.
Relative cost to patient	Higher; requires at least two office visits and laboratory services.	Higher; requires at least two office visits and laboratory services.	Higher; requires at least two office visits and laboratory services.	Higher; requires at least two office visits and laboratory services.
Average number of visits to complete	Minimum of two; matching esthetics of teeth may require more visits.	Minimum of two; matching esthetics of teeth may require more visits.	Minimum of two.	Minimum of two.

Note: The information in these tables is provided to help dentists discuss the attributes of commonly used dental restorative materials with their patients. The charts are a simple overview of the subject based on the current dental literature. It is not intended to be comprehensive. The attributes of a particular restorative material will vary from case to case depending on a number of factors.

Source: Reprinted with permission of the American Dental Association. © 2003 American Dental Association. For additional information, visit www.ada.org.

explain the relative advantages and disadvantages of the materials used in fillings, crowns, bridges, and inlays. They provide a simple overview of the subject based on the current dental literature and are not intended to be comprehensive. The attributes of a particular restorative material can vary from case to case depending on a number of factors.

Section 25.2

Tooth-Colored Fillings

Reprinted with permission from the American Academy of Pediatric Dentistry, www.aapd.org © 2002.

What Are Tooth-Colored Fillings?

Tooth-colored fillings are made from durable plastics called composite resins. Similar in color and texture to natural teeth, the fillings are less noticeable and much more attractive than other types of fillings.

What Are the Advantages of Tooth-Colored Fillings?

Because composite resins are tooth-colored, they look more natural than other filling materials. Your child can smile, talk, and eat with confidence. In addition, tooth-colored fillings are compatible with dental sealants. A tooth can be filled and sealed at the same time to prevent further decay.

What Are the Disadvantages?

First, tooth-colored fillings are not for every tooth. They work best in small restorations and low-stress areas. For example, your pediatric dentist may not recommend a tooth-colored filling for a large cavity or for the chewing surface of a back tooth. Second, tooth-colored fillings may cost a bit more than silver fillings because they take longer to place.

How Do I Decide If Tooth-Colored Fillings Are Right for My Child?

Talk to your pediatric dentist. Together you will decide what type of filling is best for your child.

How Do I Care for a Tooth-Colored Filling?

Take care of a tooth-colored filling the same way you take care of a silver filling: Brush, floss, and visit your dentist. Any filling will last longer with good oral hygiene. Your pediatric dentist will regularly check the fillings for color change, leakage, or unusual wear and inform you of the need for repair or replacement.

Section 25.3

All about Amalgam Fillings

"NCAHF Position Paper on Amalgam Fillings," © 2002 National Coalition Against Health Fraud. Reprinted with permission.

This chapter was written in response to claims that the mercury content of amalgam fillings causes toxic amounts of mercury to enter the body. Advocates of this belief are seeking to ban amalgam use and to force dentists and dental organizations to compensate all persons who claim that amalgam has damaged their health. The National Council Against Health Fraud believes that amalgam fillings are safe, that anti-amalgam activities endanger public welfare, and that so-called mercury-free dentistry is substandard practice. NCAHF is a nonprofit consumer protection organization that promotes rational health care.

Background History

Dental amalgam has been widely used for over 150 years. It is made by mixing approximately equal parts of elemental liquid mercury (43 to 54 percent) and an alloy powder (57 to 46 percent) composed of silver, tin, copper, and sometimes smaller amounts of zinc, palladium, or indium.[1] Although some forms of mercury are hazardous, the mercury in amalgam is chemically bound to the other metals to make it stable and therefore safe for use in dental applications.

The difference between bound and unbound chemicals can be illustrated by a simple comparison. Elemental hydrogen is an explosive gas. Elemental oxygen is a gas that supports combustion. When combined, however, they form water, which has neither of these effects. Saying that amalgam will poison you is like saying that drinking water will make you explode and burst into flames.

Amalgam is the most thoroughly studied and tested filling material now used. Compared to other restorative materials, it is durable, easy to use, and inexpensive. The American Dental Association, Consumers Union, the U.S. Food and Drug Administration, the U.S. Public Health Service, the World Health Organization, and many other prominent organizations have concluded that amalgam is safe and effective for restoring teeth.[2-6] It is safe to assume that if a better material is developed, the dental profession will adopt and use it.

Amalgam Safety

The amount of mercury released from installed amalgam and absorbed by the body is minuscule. Mercury is found in the earth's crust and is ubiquitous in the environment. Thus, even without amalgam fillings, everyone has small but measurable blood and urine levels. Amalgam fillings may raise these levels slightly, but this has no practical or clinical significance.

The legal limit of safe mercury exposure for industrial workers is 50 micrograms per cubic meter of air for 8 hours per day and 50 weeks per year. Regular exposure at this level will produce urine mercury levels of about 135 micrograms per liter. These levels are much higher than those of the general public but produce no symptoms and are considered safe.

Most people with fillings have less than 5 micrograms per liter of urine. Nearly all practicing dentists have levels below 10 micrograms per liter, even though they are exposed to mercury vapor when placing or removing amalgam filings and typically have amalgams in their own teeth. Thus, even with that exposure, the maximum levels found in dentists are only slightly higher than those of their patients and are far below the levels known to affect health, even in a minor way.[7-12]

No illness has ever been associated with amalgam use in patients, except for rare instances of allergies. Moreover, there is insufficient evidence to assure that components of other restorative materials have fewer potential health effects than dental amalgam, including allergic reactions.

Improper Claims

Despite the above facts, some dentists and other health professionals advise people to avoid amalgam and to have their amalgam fillings replaced with other materials. Dentists who oppose the use of amalgam may refer to their approach as holistic dentistry, biological dentistry, or mercury-free dentistry.

Offbeat practitioners often diagnose amalgam toxicity or amalgam illness in patients who suffer from multiple common symptoms. One study found that people with symptoms they related to amalgam fillings did not have mercury blood and urine mercury levels that were significant or higher than those of a control group.[12] Several studies have found that many symptoms attributed to amalgam restorations are psychosomatic in nature and have been exacerbated greatly by information from the media or from a dentist.[13-17] False diagnoses of mercury toxicity are also made by many of the physicians who offer chelation therapy, a series of intravenous infusions that costs thousands of dollars.

The leading anti-amalgamist has been Hal Huggins, D.D.S., of Colorado Springs, Colorado. Huggins claims that sensitive individuals can develop emotional problems (depression, anxiety, irritability), neurological disorders (facial twitches, muscle spasms, epilepsy, multiple sclerosis), cardiovascular problems (unexplained rapid heart rate, unidentified chest pains), collagen diseases (arthritis, scleroderma, lupus erythematosus), allergies, digestive problems (ulcers, regional ileitis), and immunologic disorders (which he claims include leukemia, Hodgkin's disease, and mononucleosis). He recommends replacing amalgam with other materials and taking vitamins and other supplements to prevent trouble after amalgam removal.[18] There is no scientific evidence that amalgam fillings cause or contribute to the development of these diseases.

Huggins's dental license was revoked in 1996. During the revocation proceedings, the administrative law judge concluded:

- Huggins had diagnosed mercury toxicity in all patients who consulted him in his office, even some without mercury fillings.

- He had also recommended extraction of all teeth that had had root canal therapy.

- Huggins's treatments were "a sham, illusory and without scientific basis."[19]

- A practitioner who does not wish to use amalgam can still practice ethically by giving appropriate advice and referring patients elsewhere when amalgam is the best choice. But advertising a practice as mercury-free is unethical because it falsely implies that amalgam fillings are dangerous and that mercury-free methods are superior.

Dubious Tests

The advice from anti-amalgam practitioners is typically accompanied by one or more tests that are either misinterpreted or completely bogus.

Breath Testing

Breath testing involves probing the mouth with a vacuum device after the patient chews gum vigorously for several minutes. The procedure causes tiny amounts of mercury to be released from amalgam fillings and deposited on a gold foil within the device. Because people only chew during a small part of the day, the resultant readings are much higher than the average amounts released per 24 hours. In addition, the amounts deposited on the foil are artificially high because most mercury vapor is exhaled rather than absorbed by the body and the device remeasures the same air several times, which inflates the reading. The readouts of the device are also raised by the presence of traces of foods, bacterial gases, and other substances commonly found within the mouth.

Urine Testing

Because mercury is ubiquitous, the body reaches a steady state in which tiny amounts are absorbed and excreted. Thus, mercury is commonly found in people's urine. Mercury can also be found in the blood, because this is the major medium for transporting materials around the body. Large-scale studies have shown that the general population has urine-mercury levels below 10 micrograms/liter. Industrial workers, and dentists, who have regular exposure to mercury vapor also have low values. Urine testing, which is a fairly reliable indicator of chronic exposure, is best performed on a 24-hour urine specimen. Urine mercury levels can be temporarily raised by administering a chelating agent such as DMSA [dimercaptosuccinic acid] or DMPS [dimercapto-1-propane-sulphonic acid], which collects the small amounts of mercury from the body, concentrates them, and then forces them to be excreted. In other words, mercury that normally recirculates within the body is now bound and excreted. The urine level under such circumstances is artificially raised above the steady-state level. The use of a chelating agent before testing should be considered fraudulent.

Blood Testing

Mercury is excreted by the kidneys, which filter the blood. The mercury levels of blood are lower than those of urine and therefore more difficult to detect. Even at high levels of mercury exposure, industrial workers show blood concentrations in the parts-per-billion range, typically less than 5 parts per billion. In this range, the amounts are too small to identify the type of mercury or its source. Urine mercury testing gives a more meaningful picture of exposure and is also more accurate because the mercury is more concentrated.

Skin Testing

Some anti-amalgamists administer a patch test with a dilute solution of corrosive mercury salts that cause the skin to redden and possibly swell.[20] The reaction is misinterpreted as a sign of mercury allergy or toxicity.

Stool Testing

Fecal mercury levels are not an accurate indicator of mercury exposure. The amount found in stool reflects the amount eaten and not absorbed plus anything excreted in the stool. At best, a stool test might indicate that mercury entered the gastrointestinal tract, but it could not provide an accurate measurement of either exposure or what was absorbed into the body.

Hair Analysis

Hair analysis is performed by sending a sample of hair to a commercial hair analysis laboratory, which issues a computerized report indicating the number of micrograms found and whether that amount should be considered harmful. This procedure is not valid. Hair contains trace amounts of mercury from food, water, and air, regardless of whether the person has amalgam fillings. Because hair can absorb mercury from external sources, amount of mercury it contains does not necessarily reflect the amount within the body. In addition, hair mercury testing cannot be standardized because hair thickness, density, shape, surface area, and growth rate vary from person to person. The laboratory used most for hair analysis is Doctor's Data of Chicago, which reports toxic mineral levels as high when the amounts are near the top of their reference range.[21] This merely means that the specimen contained more than most other hair specimens handled by the lab. It does not mean that the level is abnormal or that the level within the patient's body is dangerous. Thus even if hair analysis were valid, the reporting process is not.

Electrodermal Testing

Some practitioners use quack diagnostic devices that are said to detect electromagnetic imbalances. One wire from the device goes to a brass cylinder that the patient holds in one hand. A second wire is connected to a probe, which the operator touches to various points inside the mouth. This completes a low-voltage circuit, and the device registers the flow of current, which the operator misinterprets as abnormal.

Physical Harm

Inappropriate removal of amalgam fillings is usually followed by replacement with a more costly material. But removing good fillings is not merely a waste of money. In some cases, it results in significant damage or loss of the tooth. To remove an intact filling, it is necessary to drill into the tooth around the outer edges of the amalgam. If the filling is large or deep, the tooth can be significantly weakened and the heat from the drilling process can injure the relatively delicate tissues of the pulp beneath the filling. To this risks must be added the general risks of anesthesia and other types of mechanical injury that are uncommon but are inexcusable when a procedure is unnecessary.

In 1985, a $100,000 settlement was awarded to a 55-year-old California woman whose dentist removed her amalgam fillings. Based on testing with a phony electrodiagnostic device, the dentist had claimed that six of her fillings were a liability to her large intestine.[22] In removing the fillings, the dentist caused severe nerve damage necessitating root canal therapy for two teeth and extraction of two others.

Regulatory Action

The American Dental Association Council on Ethics, Bylaws, and Judicial Affairs has concluded that "removal of amalgam restorations from the non-allergic patient for the alleged purpose of removing toxic substances from the body, when such treatment is performed at the recommendation or suggestion of the dentist, is improper and unethical."[23] The policy, initiated in 1986, was triggered in part by the case of an Iowa dentist who had extracted all 28 teeth of a patient with multiple sclerosis. The dentist received a 9-month license suspension followed by 51 months of probation.

Dentists who attempt to diagnose or treat heavy metal toxicity, or who test patients for heavy metals by any means, are not practicing dentistry. These activities fall outside the scope of dental licensure. Any dentist who believes a patient requires diagnosis or treatment for any medical condition outside of the scope of dentistry is obliged to make a referral to a physician or other health professional as appropriate. Failure to make such a referral should be considered negligence.

Selection of a material should be based only on its known clinical properties and performance for the particular placement situation, coupled with the needs of a patient. A dentist who excludes any material from possible selection for a given restoration on the sole basis of personal opinion or unsupported conjecture cannot be providing optimal services for all of his/her patients.

Such a dentist may be denying a patient the benefits of a material that is most suitable for that patient's needs. Such denial should be considered unprofessional conduct.

No dentist is required to use amalgam. However, dentists who make false claims about amalgam safety create unnecessary patient anxiety, and undermine confidence in the profession. Such behavior should be considered unprofessional conduct. Consumers Union (CU) has concluded: dentists who purport to treat health problems by ripping out fillings are putting their own economic interests ahead of their patients' welfare. The false diagnosis of mercury-amalgam toxicity has such harmful potential and shows such poor judgment on the part of the practitioner that CU believes dentists who engage in this practice should have their license revoked.[24]

Legal and Political Action

Class-action suits have been filed in Maryland and California claiming that patients have been harmed by amalgam fillings and that the American Dental Association (ADA) and state dental associations have engaged in unfair and deceptive trade practices as well as fraud and conspiracy to defraud by not informing patients that amalgam fillings contain mercury . The ADA has countered that the suits are part of a "coordinated attempt by some to have judges decide matters of scientific debate, and stifles discussion within the scientific community, most of whose members simply do not agree with their views."[25] In a news report, an ADA official referred to a California suit as "an egregious abuse of the legal system."[26] NCAHF concurs with this assessment.

U.S. Representative Diane Watson (D-CA) has introduced a bill to prohibit interstate commerce of mercury intended for use in dental fillings by 2007. She does not appear to understand that the properties of chemical combinations can differ greatly from those of the individual ingredients that form them. Calling Watson "scientifically unsophisticated," *Time* magazine science writer Leon Jaroff has urged Watson to get over her "amalgam hang-up" and "learn not to be taken in by quacks."[27] NCAHF hopes that she will do so.

Recommendations

To Consumers

- There is no logical reason to worry about the safety of amalgam fillings.

- Anyone told that a urine mercury level produced after taking DMPS represents a toxic state is being misled.

- Avoid health professionals who advise you that amalgam fillings cause disease or should be removed as a preventive measure.

- Report any such advice to the practitioner's state licensing board.

To Dental Organizations

- Issue clear and forceful guidelines indicating that unnecessary amalgam removal is unethical and unprofessional and that the diagnosis of mercury toxicity is outside the proper scope of dentistry.

- Issue a position statement about dubious mercury testing

To Dental Licensing Boards

- Practice standards should be based solely on scientifically gathered objective evidence.

- Classify as unprofessional conduct any advice that amalgam fillings are dangerous and therefore should be avoided or removed.

- Ban the use of hair analysis and chelating agents by dentists.

- Ban any advertising of mercury-free dentistry, which falsely implies that amalgam fillings are dangerous and should therefore be avoided or removed.

To Legislators

- Do not be misled by false claims that amalgam is dangerous.

- Do not support special laws that would restrict or discourage amalgam use.

References

1. Dental amalgam use and benefits. U.S. Centers for Disease Control Resource Library Fact Sheet, December 2001.

2. ADA Council on Scientific Affairs. Dental amalgam: Update on safety concerns. *JADA* 1998;129:494–501.

3. The mercury in your mouth. *Consumer Reports* 1991;56:316–319.

4. Benson JS and others. Dental Amalgam: A Scientific Review and Recommended Public Health Strategy for Research, Education and Regulation. Washington, D, US Public Health Service, 1993.

5. Consumer Update: Dental amalgams. FDA Center for Devices and Radiological Health, Feb 11, 2002.

6. World Health Organization. Consensus Statement on Dental Amalgam. Mjor IA, Pakhomov GN. Dental Amalgam and Alternative Direct Restorative Materials. Geneva: World Health Organization, 1999.

7. Mackert JR. Dental amalgam and mercury. *JADA* 1991;122:54–61.

8. Olsson S, Bergman M. Daily dose calculations from measurements of intra-oral mercury vapor. *J Dent Res* 1992;71:414–423.

9. Mackert JR. Factors affecting estimation of dental amalgam exposure from measurements of mercury vapor in levels in intraoral and expired air. *J Dent Res* 1987;66:1175–1180.

10. Mackert JR Jr, Berglund A. Mercury exposure from dental amalgam fillings: absorbed dose and the potential for adverse health effects. *Crit Rev Oral Biol Med* 1997;8:410–436.

11. Berglund A. Molin M. Mercury vapor release from dental amalgam in patients with symptoms allegedly caused by amalgam fillings. *Eur J Oral Sci* 1996;104:56–63.

12. Dodes J. The amalgam controversy: An evidence-based analysis. *JADA* 2002;132:348–356.

13. Herrstrom P, Hogstedt B. Clinical study of oral galvanism: No evidence of toxic mercury exposure but anxiety disorder an important background factor. *Scand J Dent Res* 1993;101:232–237.

14. Lindberg NE, Lindberg E, Larsson G. Psychological factors in the etiology of amalgam illness. *Acta Odontol Scand* 1994;52: 219–228.

15. A multidisciplinary clinical study of patients suffering from illness associated with mercury release from dental restorations: Psychiatric aspects. *Acta Psychiatr Scandinavia* 1997; 96:475–482.

16. Malt UF, Nerdrum P, Oppedal B, et al. Physical and mental problems attributed to dental amalgam fillings: a descriptive study of 99 self-referred patients compared to 272 controls. *Psychosom Med* 1997;59:32–41.

17. Bailer J, Rist F, Rudolf A, at el. Adverse health effects related to mercury exposure from dental amalgam fillings: toxicological or psychological causes? *Psychol Med* 2001;31:255–263.

18. Huggins HE, Huggins SA. It's All in Your Head. Self-published, Colorado Springs, Colorado, 1985.

19. Connick N. Before the State Board of Dental Examiners, State Board of Colorado. Case No. 95-04. In the matter of the disciplinary proceedings regarding the license to practice dentistry

in the State of Colorado of Hal A. Huggins, D.D.S., License No. 3057. Feb 29, 1996.

20. Fisher AA. The misuse of the patch test to determine "hypersensitivity" to mercury amalgam dental fillings. *Cutis* 1985; 35:109, 112, 117.

21. Druyan ME and others. Determination of reference ranges for elements in human scalp hair. *Trace Elem Res* 1998;62: 183–197.

22. *Sherry v Doe*. California Sonoma County Superior Court, No. 134740, March 1, 1985.

23. Dental amalgam and other restorative materials. Advisory opinion 5.A.1, American Dental Association Principles of Ethics and Code of Professional Conduct, revised April 2002.

24. Barrett S and the editors of *Consumer Reports*. Health Schemes, Scams, and Frauds. New York: Consumer Reports Books, 1990.

25. Berry J. ADA pledges vigorous defense' against Maryland amalgam suit. *ADA News* March 4, 2002.

26. Another amalgam suit filed in California. ADA news release, March 21, 2002.

27. Jaroff, L. There's nothing dangerous about 'silver' fillings: But some in Congress continue to insist there is. http://www.time. com. May 8, 2002.

Section 25.4

Consumer Update: Dental Amalgams

U.S. Food and Drug Administration (FDA), Center for Devices and Radiological Health; December 2002. Available online at www.fda.gov/ cdrh/consumer/amalgams.html; accessed May 2003.

The U.S. Food and Drug Administration and other organizations of the U.S. Public Health Service (USPHS) continue to investigate the safety of amalgams used in dental restorations (fillings). However, no valid scientific evidence has shown that amalgams cause harm to patients with dental restorations, except in the rare case of allergy.

The safety of dental amalgams has been reviewed extensively over the past ten years, both nationally and internationally. In 1994, an international conference of health officials concluded there is no scientific evidence that dental amalgam presents a significant health hazard to the general population, although a small number of patients had mild, temporary allergic reactions. The World Health Organization (WHO), in its Consensus Statement on Dental Amalgam reached a similar conclusion. They wrote: "Amalgam restorations are safe and cost-effective ...Components in dental restorative materials, including amalgam, may, in rare instances, result in local side-effects or allergic reactions. The risk of adverse side-effects is very low for all types of restorative materials, including amalgam and all resin-based materials." Similar conclusions were reached by the USPHS, the European Commission, the National Board of Health and Welfare in Sweden, the New Zealand Ministry of Health, Health Canada, and the province of Quebec.

In January 1993, the USPHS published a broad scientific report about the safety and use of dental amalgam and other materials commonly used to fill dental cavities. USPHS reaffirmed these conclusions in 1995 and 1997.

Since then, the National Institutes of Health (NIH), the Centers for Disease Control and Prevention (CDC), and the Food and Drug Administration (FDA) have continued to study the issue. The National Institute of Dental & Craniofacial Research at NIH has also provided money to study the safety of dental amalgams and to develop non-mercury alternatives. This effort includes research and clinical studies of dental amalgam use in children.

These studies are ongoing and will require several years of follow up in order to detect any subtle and long-range health effects.

Also, USPHS scientists analyzed approximately 175 peer-reviewed studies submitted in support of three citizen petitions received by FDA after the 1993 report. The USPHS concluded that data in these studies did not support claims that individuals with dental amalgam restorations will experience problems, including neurologic, renal, or developmental effects, except for rare allergic or hypersensitivity reactions.

Although there is international agreement that the scientific data do not confirm the presence of a significant health hazard, several countries restrict the use of dental amalgams or have recommended limitations on their use. For example, Health Canada recommended that dental amalgam be avoided in people allergic to mercury or with impaired kidney function; if possible, to avoid its placement or removal in the teeth of pregnant women; and to consider the use of alternatives in the primary teeth of children. Some manufacturers now include these contraindications (against using) in their labeling of dental amalgams sold in those countries. If a manufacturer wishes to make a similar labeling change in its dental amalgam sold in the United States, FDA will require the manufacturer to submit a new marketing application with data supporting the change.

FDA is examining its regulation of dental amalgam alloy and pre-encapsulated dental amalgam. To reduce possible allergic reactions from restorative materials, FDA is proposing in labeling guidance that the product's labeling list the ingredients in descending order of weight by percentage and include lot numbers, appropriate warnings and precautions, handling instructions, and expiration dating. The labeling guidance will be most useful with new restorative materials.

While research, regulatory changes, and educational efforts are underway, the use of dental amalgams in the United States is declining. Pediatric dentists, in particular, are using resin (plastic) FDA cleared tooth-colored materials that are bonded to the tooth. They may release fluoride and are mercury-free. Other reasons for the decline in amalgam use include increasing use of sealants and community fluoridation, an expanding selection of fluoride-containing dental products, improved oral hygiene practices, and greater access to dental care. With the improvement of alternative restorative materials over the past few years, dentists increased their use of these products.

The USPHS will continue to gather data about possible risks of dental amalgams and other restorative products and to pursue new methods of dental treatment and oral health. As an important part of this plan, USPHS will continue working with the dental profession to bring about changes in the delivery of oral healthcare based on valid scientific research.

Section 25.5

Dental Amalgam: Myths vs. Facts

Reprinted with permission of the American Dental Association. © 2003 American Dental Association. For additional information, visit www.ada.org.

The following information from the American Dental Association corrects much of the misinformation about silver-colored fillings known as amalgam.

Myth: Dental amalgam causes numerous health problems.

Fact: Not true. You should feel very secure that the many organizations responsible for protecting the public's health have said time and time again that amalgam fillings are safe. Those organizations include the World Health Organization, United States Public Health Service, the National Institutes of Health, and the Food and Drug Administration.

Myth: There are better materials for treating cavities, but the ADA continues to promote use of dental amalgam because it receives money from amalgam manufacturers through its Seal of Acceptance program.

Fact: Be assured that the ADA does not profit from amalgam, nor does it promote the material. The cost of maintaining the ADA Seal program is financed primarily through ADA member dentist dues.

What the ADA does promote is having patients make informed decisions about their dental care in consultation with their dentist. The choice of a particular filling material is determined in partnership by the dentist and patient, and based upon a variety of considerations, including size and location of the cavity, patient history, cosmetic concerns, and cost.

Myth: *The ADA justifies amalgam use by saying the filling has been around for 150 years.*

Fact: When making treatment recommendations, dentists rely on the best-available science and their own clinical experience. Because amalgam has been around so long, the dental profession and scientific community have learned a great deal about its durability, reliability, and safety. Just like aspirin, amalgam has withstood the test of time and is still a valued option for patients.

Myth: *Removal of amalgam cures some diseases.*

Fact: It is unconscionable to lead people to believe that their serious illnesses may improve by undergoing unnecessary dental treatment. In fact, leading medical experts and health organizations have negated such statements and conclusions. For example:

- "There is no scientific evidence to connect the development of MS or other neurological diseases with dental fillings containing mercury."—National Multiple Sclerosis Society

- "According to the best available scientific evidence there is no relationship between silver dental fillings and Alzheimer's."—Alzheimer's Association

- "There is no scientific evidence of any measurable clinical toxic effects [of dental amalgam]."—American Academy of Pediatrics

Myth: *Dental amalgam fillings release mercury vapors that are harmful to the body.*

Fact: Minute amounts of mercury vapor (between 1–3 micrograms [1 microgram is equal to 35.2 billionths of an ounce] per day) may be released from amalgam under the pressure of chewing or grinding, but there is no scientific evidence that such low-level exposure is harmful. In fact, dental materials experts say one would have to have almost 500 amalgam fillings to even see the subtlest symptoms in the most sensitive person.

Myth: Dentists cannot tell their patients that amalgam contains mercury.

Fact: Actually, the ADA encourages dentists to discuss the full range of filling options with their patients so together they can decide what is the most appropriate treatment.

Chapter 26

The Use of Lasers in Dentistry

Laser use in dentistry was suggested approximately 35 years ago as a means of using energy generated by light to remove or modify soft and hard tissues in the oral cavity. Laser is an acronym for "Light Amplification by Stimulated Emission of Radiation." The radiation involved in generating laser light is nonionizing and does not produce the same effects attributed to x-radiation. The Food and Drug Administration has approved the use of various lasers as devices to remove diseased gingival tissues and for other soft tissue applications, the removal of dental caries, as an aid in placing tooth-colored restorations, and as an adjunct in root canal procedures, such as pulpotomies. This chapter concentrates on root canals.

Lasers emit light energy that can interact with biologic tissues, such as tooth enamel, dentin, gingiva, or dental pulp. The interaction is the effect of the particular properties of laser light including: 1) monochromaticity, where the light is all the same color (same wavelength); 2) coherence, where the waves of light are all in phase; and 3) collimation, where the light rays are parallel to each other and do not diverge. Applying this light energy results in the modification or removal of tissue. In root canal treatment, the dental pulp is removed and the walls of the root canal system are enlarged by melting and resolidifying the dentin. Once the preparation is completed, the root canal is obturated, and the laser is used to soften and mold the obturating material

---

to the prepared root canal system. These procedures are accomplished by the interactions between the laser light and the tooth substances enamel and dentin. These interactions are thermal (increased temperature), chemical (breaking of tissue chemical bonds), and acoustic (generation of temporary stress waves that can lead to fracture of enamel and/or dentin or cavitation of tissue).

Root canal treatment is currently performed using a combination of hand and rotary instruments to remove the soft tissue, clean the root canal space, and shape the space to receive the obturating material, usually gutta-percha. This biocompatible material is then placed with an adhesive cement using special hand instruments to ensure complete sealing of the root canals. These procedures are performed by endodontists, dental specialists who limit their practices to endodontics, with an exceptionally high success rate on the majority of teeth.

Laser energy, when added to root canal procedures, presents advantages and disadvantages. Currently, root canal procedures clean the canal space. Studies using extracted teeth inoculated with bacteria have shown that lasers can reduce the quantity of microorganisms. The walls of the prepared canal space contain tubular openings that harbor organisms, and the preparation itself causes formation of a layer of debris (smear layer) composed of organisms and tooth substances. Laser energy can remove the smear layer as well as dentin from the canal wall and will melt and resolidify the dentin to close the tubular openings. The laser also may aid in welding tooth-like materials (not as yet produced) to the resolidified walls, resulting in denser root canal packing.

The advantages of using the laser, however, are balanced by several disadvantages. Root canal spaces are rarely straight and more often are curved in at least two dimensions. Root canal instruments used to clean the space throughout its length can be curved to follow the curvatures in a tooth root. Laser probes can clean an area in a root canal space that is straight as long as the probe is in contact with the dentinal wall. The probes are made of glass and cannot be curved to follow the natural curvatures of the tooth root. When in contact with the dentinal wall, laser probes are capable of cleaning an area in the root canal space that is straight.

Further, the interactions involved between laser energy and the tissue cause rises in temperature. These increased temperatures can char the canal space, damaging it to the point that the tooth may be lost. The increased temperatures also may extend to the outer surfaces of the tooth, damaging the soft tissue that connects the tooth to the surrounding bone. If the temperature is high enough, the bone surrounding the tooth may also be damaged, adversely affecting the entire area, which can result in ankylosis [stiffness in the joint].

While the FDA has approved one laser (diode) as an adjunct for removal of pulp tissue in a pulpotomy procedure, more research is required to develop laser energy for use in endodontics so that it is equal, if not superior, to present treatment modalities. Until that research is complete, patients should ask about the use of lasers in root canal treatment, especially in light of the high success rate of non-laser procedures carried out by those trained to perform them.

Chapter 27

Pain Management in Dental Care

Chapter Contents

Section 27.1

Conscious Sedation

Reprinted with permission from the American Academy of Pediatric
Dentistry, www.aapd.org. © 2002.

What Is Conscious Sedation?

Conscious sedation is a management technique that uses medications to assist the child to cope with fear and anxiety and cooperate with dental treatment. Medications and dosages should be selected that are unlikely to cause loss of consciousness in the patient.

Who Should Be Sedated?

Children who have a level of anxiety that prevents good coping skills or are very young and do not understand how to cope in a cooperative fashion for the delivery of dental care should be sedated. Conscious sedation is often helpful for some children who have special needs.

Why Utilize Conscious Sedation?

Conscious sedation aids in allowing a child to cope better with dental treatment. This can help prevent injury to the child from patient movement and promote a better environment for providing dental care.

What Medications Are Used?

Many different medications can be used for conscious sedation. Your pediatric dentist will discuss different options for your child.

Is Sedation Safe?

Sedation is safe when administered by a trained pediatric dentist who follows the sedation guidelines of the American Academy of Pediatric

Dentistry. Your pediatric dentist will discuss sedation options and patient monitoring for the protection of your child.

What Special Instructions Should I Follow before the Sedation Appointment?

In order to alleviate potential anxiety in your child, your pediatric dentist may recommend minimal discussion of the dental appointment with your child. Should your child become ill, contact your pediatric dentist to see if it is necessary to postpone the appointment. It is very important to follow the directions of your pediatric dentist regarding fasting from fluids and foods prior to the sedation appointment.

What Special Instructions Should I Follow after the Sedation Appointment?

Your pediatric dentist will not discharge your child until the child is alert and ready to go. Children who have been sedated are usually requested to remain at home for the rest of the day with adult supervision. Your pediatric dentist will discuss specific post-sedation instructions with you, including appropriate diet, physical activity, and requested supervision.

Section 27.2

Anesthesia

Reprinted with permission of the American Dental Association. © 2003 American Dental Association. For additional information, visit www.ada.org.

Advances in dental techniques and medications can greatly reduce—even eliminate—discomfort during dental treatment, and your dentist and the ADA [American Dental Association] want you to know about them. Here are some of the options available to help alleviate anxiety or pain that may be associated with dental care.

Analgesics

Non-narcotic analgesics are the most commonly used drugs for relief of toothache or pain following dental treatment. This category includes aspirin, acetaminophen, and non-steroidal anti-inflammatory drugs such as ibuprofen.

Narcotic analgesics, such as those containing codeine, act on the central nervous system to relieve pain. They are used for more severe pain.

Local Anesthesia

Topical anesthetics are applied to mouth tissues with a swab to prevent pain on the surface level. Your dentist may use a topical anesthetic to numb an area in preparation for administering an injectable local anesthetic. Topical anesthetics also may be used to soothe painful mouth sores.

Injectable local anesthetics, such as Novocain, prevent pain in a specific area of your mouth during treatment by blocking the nerves that sense or transmit pain and numbing mouth tissues. They cause the temporary numbness often referred to as a fat-lip feeling. Injectable anesthetics may be used in such procedures as filling cavities, preparing teeth for crowns, or treating gum disease.

Sedation and General Anesthesia

Anti-anxiety agents, such as nitrous oxide, or sedatives may help you relax during dental visits and often may be used along with local anesthetics. Dentists also can use these agents to induce conscious sedation, in which the patient achieves a relaxed state during treatment but can respond to speech or touch. Sedatives can be administered before, during, or after dental procedures by mouth, inhalation, or injection.

More complex treatments may require drugs that can induce deep sedation, causing a loss of feeling and reducing consciousness in order to relieve both pain and anxiety. On occasion, patients undergo general anesthesia, in which drugs cause a temporary loss of consciousness. Deep sedation and general anesthesia may be recommended in certain procedures for children or others who have severe anxiety or who have difficulty controlling their movements.

The ADA provides guidelines to help dentists administer pain controllers in the safest manner possible. Dentists use the pain and anxiety control techniques mentioned above to treat tens of millions of patients safely every year. Even so, taking any medication involves a certain amount of risk. That's why the ADA urges you to take an active role in your oral health care. This includes knowing your health status and telling your dentist about any illnesses or health conditions, whether you are taking any medications (prescription or nonprescription), and whether you've ever had any problems such as allergic reactions to any medications. It also includes understanding the risks and benefits involved in dental treatment, so that you and your dentist can make the best decisions about the treatment that is right for you.

Understanding the range of choices that are available to relieve anxiety and discomfort makes you a well-informed dental consumer. If you have questions or concerns about your oral health care, don't hesitate to talk to your dentist. If you still have concerns, consider getting a second opinion. Working together, you and your dentist can choose the appropriate steps to make your dental visit as safe and comfortable as possible and to help you keep a healthy smile.

Section 27.3

Safety Suggestions Regarding Anesthesia in the Dental Office

"When Having Anesthesia in the Office Setting: SOBA Safety Suggestions," © 2000 Society for Office Based Anesthesia. Reprinted with permission. For additional information, visit www.soba.org.

Things you should know before you have anesthesia for an office-based surgery.

- Is this a true conscious sedation? (Which means I will be lightly sedated, still respond to verbal commands, and be able to breathe normally without heavy snoring.)

- Is this a deep sedation technique? (I will not respond to verbal commands and I may need some airway support, i.e., chin lift, mechanical airways.)

- Will I be given general anesthesia? (I will be completely asleep, the intravenous medications may be supplemented with an inhalation anesthetic, and a type of artificial airway will probably be used, i.e., oral airway or intratracheal [breathing tube].)

When you receive general anesthesia or deep sedation (which can quickly change to general anesthesia), your anesthesia care should be provided by a specialist in anesthesia, i.e., physician or dentist anesthesiologist or CRNA.

When you receive only conscious sedation (local anesthesia may also be used), it may be appropriate to have this care provided by your surgeon and an appropriately trained assistant (preferably an RN) whose only responsibility is to monitor you. Questions to ask:

- Who will monitor me during the procedure?

- Will this person have any other responsibilities besides the anesthetic? (The answer should be no.)

- How much training and experience with this type of anesthetic does he/she have?

218

- What type of monitors will be used? (During conscious sedation, your blood pressure, oxygen saturation, heart rate, and respirations should be continuously monitored. Additional monitors are needed if a deep sedation or general anesthesia is planned.)

Ask a few more questions:

- How many drugs will be used during this procedure? (When two or three drugs are used together, it increases the likelihood that your sedation may become deep sedation rather than conscious sedation.)
- If there were a problem, where would I be transferred? Have you ever had to do a transfer before?
- Who in the office is CPR certified?
- How can I reach the anesthesia provider after hours?

Section 27.4

Painless Drilling

"Dental More Gentle with Painless Drillings and Matching Fillings," by Paula Kurtzweil, *FDA Consumer*, U.S. Food and Drug Administration, May 1999.

Kids today have it so good—computers in the classroom, Nickelodeon on cable TV, popcorn in the microwave. They also have it good because they rarely get dental cavities. And, for those who do develop tooth decay, newer dental devices the Food and Drug Administration has cleared in the past two to five years are less painful than the traditional dentist's drill.

Public health measures, such as fluoridation of drinking water and consumer education on proper dental hygiene, have helped bring about a decline in cavities in the past 50 years. Today, half of all American children under 12 have never had a cavity. For adults, these preventive measures, along with new filling materials, are enabling many of them to keep their own teeth for the rest of their lives.

"There's really no reason in this country today that [people] can't maintain their own teeth for their entire life," says Kimberly Harms, D.D.S., a dentist in Farmington, Minnesota.

Digging out the Decay

The only way to treat tooth decay, technically known as dental caries, is by cutting away the decaying portion of the tooth, a procedure that is done almost 170 million times a year. Until about five years ago, the only way to do that was with the standard handpiece, commonly known as the dental drill, a device that dates to the 1700s. Modern high-speed handpieces revolutionized dentistry when they were introduced in the 1960s.

Today, dentists have two other options—the erbium:YAG laser and the microair abrasion unit. FDA cleared the erbium:YAG laser for marketing for use on adults in May 1997 and for use on children in October 1998. Though the clearances were the first of their kind for treating hard tissue in the mouth, the laser actually was introduced into dentistry in 1995, when FDA cleared a laser device for gum surgery.

As of March 1999, two companies market the laser for dental decay: Premier Laser Systems Inc., of Irvine, California, and BioLase, of San Clemente, California.

The erbium:YAG laser essentially vaporizes decayed tooth tissue. A stream of laser light that passes through a fiber connected to a pencil-like handpiece is directed to the decay. The laser handpiece looks like the standard handpiece and, like the standard handpiece, must be used in a controlled manner so that it doesn't slip and damage healthy tissue.

"The laser is a cutting instrument," says Susan Runner, D.D.S., branch chief of dental devices in FDA's Center for Devices and Radiological Health. "And like any cutting instrument, dentists have to be careful any time they use it. The laser has many of the same risks as the drill."

Another similarity between the dental drill and the laser is that both use water and air to cool the tooth and clean the surface during removal of decay. While dentists and patients may wear eye protection during conventional treatment to protect against the spray of water and particles, they must wear goggles during the laser procedure to protect their eyes from straying laser light.

The laser has several benefits over the handpiece: Because laser treatment is usually painless, there is no need for anesthesia—or anesthetic injections—in many patients, and dentists do not have to wait until their patients' mouths are numb to begin treatment. Also, the laser eliminates the vibrating sensations of the high-speed handpiece.

Also, compared with the standard handpiece, the laser can work with better precision, saving more of the healthy tooth. And when the laser procedure is done, patients do not have to wait for the numbness and puffiness related to the use of anesthesia to fade.

For many patients, especially those particularly fearful of the dental drill, the laser has drawn rave reviews. "My patients love it," says Edward Romano, a dentist in Morristown, N.J., who has used the laser since 1997. "They say: 'I can't believe it's so comfortable, that dentistry has come this far.'"

However, the laser is not without its own shortcomings. For one, it can't be used on teeth with fillings already in place. According to Runner, there is the risk of damage to the tooth because the filling heats up. Romano says silver fillings also damage the laser tip. Also, studies show that the laser procedure takes longer than the conventional method.

"The laser is really ideal for virgin teeth—for new decay," Runner says. "Dental lasers is a growing field, but they can't do everything. There's still a need for the standard handpiece."

Another potential pitfall is expense. In December, Premier Laser Systems was citing a list price of about $45,000 for its Centauri laser. That includes training for the dentist. The standard high-speed handpiece typically sells for around $600.

Premier Laser estimates, however, that while the typical laser procedure costs about $13 more on average than the same drill procedure, the cost reductions of not using anesthesia and having more time to spend with other patients could actually save dentists about $70,000 over three years.

Still, some dentists say they are putting off buying a laser for treating cavities, at least for the near future. "Our position [in my dental practice] is that the laser looks promising," Harms says. "But we're not using it yet. We're waiting for long-term studies and newer tools."

The other alternative to the traditional high-speed handpiece is the air abrasion handpiece. Air abrasion involves the use of a high-pressured instrument similar to a tiny sandblaster. A stream of tiny aluminum oxide particles cuts away the decay. There is no heat and no vibration, and often, it can be used without anesthesia. It also can be used to remove some fillings, although it is not yet cleared for removing amalgams (silver-colored fillings).

Harms, who uses air abrasion, says the technique is ideal for small cavities and fillings in children, but she notes, "It doesn't replace the drill."

Fillings

Once decay is removed, a filling is placed inside the cut-out area to retain the tooth's shape and function, including chewing. Today, a variety of filling materials is available.

One of the oldest and now most commonly used is amalgam, a metal alloy of silver, tin, copper, and sometimes indium, palladium and zinc that is mixed with about an equal amount of mercury. FDA regulates amalgam alloy as a medical device.

According to a November 1998 article in the *Journal of the American Dental Association*, dentists continue to use amalgam primarily because it is inexpensive and durable and withstands the tremendous forces of chewing. A 1993 U.S. Public Health Service report on dental amalgam said that amalgam typically lasts from 8 to 12 years. Only gold alloy and metal-ceramic crowns last longer—up to 18 years.

Amalgam has drawn controversy in the past 10 years because its critics contend that the mercury emits minute amounts of vapor, causing a variety of health problems ranging from multiple sclerosis and arthritis to mental disorders. However, several investigations by the federal government and others have not borne this out, and the use of amalgam is supported by FDA, the National Institute on Dental and Craniofacial Research, the American Dental Association, and other professional organizations.

In a scientific literature review published in the November 1998 *Journal of the American Dental Association*, professors of dentistry in the United States and China found that research has not yet shown that mercury vapors escaping amalgams are "in concentrations high enough to produce any detectable effect on the body." The authors concluded that, contrary to some dentists' current practice, "dentists cannot ethically tell patients that amalgam is a health hazard and that removal of restorations will benefit their health."

While amalgam remains the most commonly used dental filling, its use does appear to be declining. According to the dental association's journal article, the use of amalgam for filling back teeth has dropped from 85 percent in 1988 to 58 percent in 1997. "The use of amalgam will likely continue to diminish, and it will eventually disappear from the scene," the journal article said.

One reason for the decline is the introduction of new materials that afford similar durability and strength as amalgam and, unlike the silver-colored fillings, can be made to match the color of a patient's teeth. "The aesthetics' side of it is very important to many patients," Runner says. However, using these materials—composites, glass ionomers, and metal-ceramic crowns—can cost a patient from 1.5 times to 8 times the cost of an amalgam restoration.

Prevention of Decay

Of course, much of the pain and expense of treating cavities can be eliminated through preventive measures.

Many of these measures, says Dennis Mangan, Ph.D., chief of the Infectious Diseases Branch of the extramural division of the National Institute on Dental and Craniofacial Research, are aimed at interrupting the decay process—for example, eliminating the sugars that serve as a source of food for bacteria in the mouth, eliminating the bacteria that feed on the sugars, strengthening the tooth's enamel to make it harder for acids to attack. Or, Mangan says, "It can be some combination of all of them."

Some of the most successful preventive measures involve fluoride, a mineral that occurs naturally in many foods and water. Fluoride helps prevent decay by making the tooth more resistant to acid attacks. It also has been found to reverse early decay where acid has broken through the enamel by remineralizing the affected area.

To function effectively as an anti-decay substance, fluoride should not only be applied to the teeth but ingested, as well. The most important way in which fluoride is ingested is through fluoridated public drinking water. Dental experts cite water fluoridation, which began 50 years ago, as the main reason for the decline in cavities in children since World War II.

In areas with inadequate or no water fluoridation, children between 6 months and 16 years may need fluoride supplements. A dentist can prescribe the correct dose.

Fluoride can be applied directly to teeth with the use of fluoridated toothpastes and mouth rinses. Less-concentrated rinses are available over-the-counter, while stronger concentrations require a dentist's prescription.

Consumers need to be sure that children don't use fluoride products without supervision because excess ingestion of fluoride can cause defects in the tooth's enamel that range from barely noticeable white specks or streaks to cosmetically objectionable brown discoloration. The defects, known as fluorosis, occur while the teeth are forming, usually in children under 6 years. Although tooth staining from fluorosis cannot be removed with normal hygiene, a dentist may be able to lighten or remove these stains with professional-strength abrasives or bleaches.

Although excess fluoride intake can be toxic, most reported adverse reactions involve vomiting, diarrhea, and eye irritation. Because fluoride is a drug, FDA requires toothpaste manufacturers to include on the labels of fluoride toothpastes a warning that the products should be kept out of the reach of children under 6. In addition, because FDA requires all over-the-counter oral drugs to bear an accidental-ingestion warning, toothpaste labels also must carry a warning that instructs consumers to contact a professional or a Poison Control Center if more than the normal amount used for brushing is swallowed. This labeling requirement took effect April 1997.

Another highly effective way to prevent cavities is sealants. Plastic material that is usually applied to the chewing surfaces of the permanent back teeth, sealants bond into the depressions and grooves of the chewing surfaces, acting as a barrier to plaque and acid.

According to the American Dental Association (ADA), sealants are "virtually 100-percent effective at preventing tooth decay." They can be used on the permanent teeth of both children and adults.

Though sealants are considered to be most beneficial to children, a 1996 study published in ADA's journal found that only 20 percent of school-aged children have dental sealants on their permanent molars. Cost-wise, sealants average about half the cost of a filling, according to the American Academy of Pediatric Dentistry.

Another reason for the decline in dental caries can be attributed to public education aimed at encouraging consumers to follow good oral health practices at home and see a dentist regularly, beginning as early as age 1.

"Most patients now know [they should] see a dentist regularly," says Cleveland dentist Matthew Mecini, D.D.S., citing statistics that show that 50 to 55 percent of adults actually follow that advice. "We [the dental community] are doing a better job of educating the public on the need for regular dental care."

What's Ahead

Efforts to reduce cavities don't end there. One of the most promising preventives on the horizon is a vaccine-like product against decay. In April 1998, British scientists reported that they had developed a plant-based treatment, which, when applied to the teeth, effectively prevented *Streptococcus* bacteria, the main bacteria involved in tooth decay in humans, from growing in the mouth for up to four months.

In the United States, researchers funded by the National Institute of Dental and Craniofacial Research are studying a similar preventive, known as plantibodies. Using genetic engineering techniques, scientists transfer a gene for antibodies specific for streptococci to the tobacco plant, which produces large quantities of these antibodies. Antibodies purified from the tobacco plant are then applied to the teeth with a goal of preventing streptococci from adhering to the teeth.

"The concept is good," Mangan says, but notes that the high cost of genetic engineering and the bother of applying the substance on a routine schedule may make the product somewhat impractical.

Other research, he says, focuses on a vaccine that boosts children's immune systems to prevent decay. The intent of this experimental product is to stimulate the body's own production of antibodies to prevent streptococci from adhering to the teeth.

While these experimental products promise an even brighter dental outlook for future generations, kids today can look forward to a life of dental care that even their parents never envisioned.

"If you can reduce the anxiety that often accompanies dental treatment," FDA's Runner says, "that's a very positive step, especially for children. That's where a lot of these devices have the most potential—in children."

How Decay Occurs

For most people, the first sign of a cavity is pain, but the actual start of tooth decay begins much earlier, with the accumulation of minute amounts of a sticky film, called plaque, on the tooth's surface.

Plaque contains bacteria, which feed on carbohydrates in the mouth. As a result of their feeding frenzy, the bacteria produce acids, which can attack the tooth enamel—the outermost layer of the tooth. If the plaque isn't removed, it continues to build, creating more acid that continues to damage the tooth enamel. There usually is no pain until the acids eat through to the tooth's underlying dentin and pulp layers, where the nerves are located. This decay, technically known as dental caries, is the point at which treatment is needed to prevent further tooth damage and loss.

Cavities usually form:

- in depressions and grooves of chewing surfaces
- between teeth

- on the root surfaces of people whose gums have receded.

Dental decay usually occurs in the back teeth, where it is more difficult to remove food debris and plaque. There are two notable exceptions: early childhood decay in bottle-fed babies and root decay in older adults.

Baby-bottle decay usually occurs in the upper front teeth as a result of continuous feeding on sweet liquids, including milk, formula, and fruit juice. Nighttime use of a bottle is the most dangerous because the sugars sit on the baby's teeth for an extended time. Tooth loss can result, causing spacing and development problems when the permanent teeth erupt.

"It's very nasty," says Cleveland dentist Matthew Mecini, D.D.S. "You don't see it too often, but when you do, it's severe. The amount of damage that can be done to children's teeth in a short time is amazing."

Root decay occurs on the exposed root surfaces of older adults whose gums have receded as a result of gum disease. Many types of medicines older people typically use decrease saliva production, which can aggravate the problem. Saliva is important in preventing tooth decay because it can wash away food particles and bacteria and help neutralize acids formed by bacteria in the mouth.

The first sign of a cavity forming may be a white spot that in time may turn brown. Most patients, however, remain unaware of the decay until it is well advanced. Common signs that people notice include sensitivity of the tooth when exposed to hot or cold and brief pain after eating a sugar-containing food.

The dentist can diagnose decay with x-rays or by probing the tooth with a sharp instrument. Decayed enamel or dentin will feel soft.

Paula Kurtzweil is a member of FDA's public affairs staff.

Chapter 28

Periodontal (Gum) Disease

Chapter Contents

Section 28.1

Receding Gums

From "Receding Gums," © 2001 California Dental Association. Reprinted with Permission. For more information, visit the website of the California Dental Association at www.cda.org. As a public service, the California Dental Association also maintains a consumer information website at www.smilecalifornia.org.

At first, receding gums may not sound like such a disastrous affliction, but when one considers the possible causes and consequences of the condition, it suddenly becomes much more than a vanity issue.

In many cases, receding gums are caused by periodontal disease also known as gum disease. Three out of four adults have some form of it. And, in most cases, it doesn't cause any pain and therefore goes unnoticed.

Most common in adults, gum disease starts when plaque, containing bacteria, builds up on the teeth and gums. When the plaque is not removed daily, it produces toxins that irritate the gums. Eventually these toxins destroy the gum tissues, causing them to separate from the tooth (recede) and form spaces called pockets. The pockets hold more bacteria, which only compounds the problem.

In the early stages (gingivitis), marked by red or swollen gums that bleed easily, gum disease is reversible and can be detected by your dentist during regular checkups. As the disease progresses (periodontitis), it can destroy the bone and soft tissues that support the teeth. Teeth can become loose, fall out, or have to be removed by a dentist. In fact, periodontitis is the culprit in 70 percent of tooth loss in adults over 40.

The good news is that gum disease is easily prevented through brushing and flossing daily, eating a balanced diet, and visiting the dentist regularly for professional cleanings. Following this simple regimen, adults can look forward to keeping their natural teeth throughout their lives.

Section 28.2

Periodontal Diseases

Reprinted with permission from The American Academy of Periodontology. Figure 28.1 © American Academy of Periodontology.

What Are Periodontal Diseases?

The American Academy of Periodontology [AAP] defines inflammatory periodontal diseases, also known as gum disease, as chronic bacterial infections that inflame the supporting tissues of the teeth and destroy attachment fibers (periodontal ligaments) and supporting bone that hold teeth into the mouth. Periodontal diseases can affect one tooth or many teeth, and begins when the bacteria in plaque (the sticky, colorless film that constantly forms on your teeth) causes the gums to become inflamed. It usually progresses, leading to the loss of bone and periodontal ligament adjacent to the gums.

Common Forms of Periodontal Diseases

Gingivitis

Gingivitis is the mildest form of periodontal diseases. Development of gingivitis requires the presence of plaque bacteria, which are thought to induce pathological changes in the tissues by both direct and indirect means. The initial lesion appears as an acute inflammatory response with characteristic infiltration of neutrophils (type of white blood cell produced in bone marrow). Gums become red, swell, and bleed easily with brushing or flossing. There is usually little or no discomfort at this stage, and the condition is reversible with professional cleaning and good oral home care.

Chronic Periodontitis

Chronic periodontitis is an infectious disease resulting in inflammation within the supporting tissues of the teeth and progressive attachment and bone loss. It is clinically differentiated from gingivitis by the

229

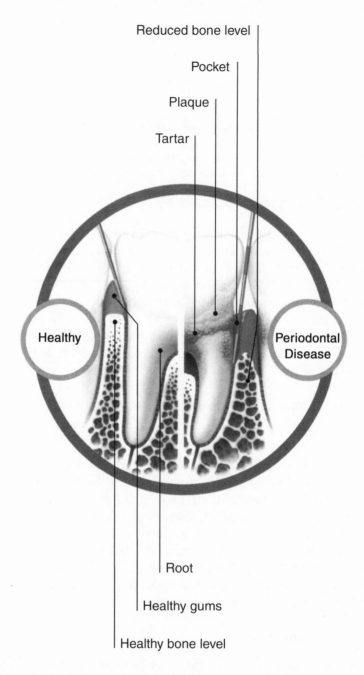

Reduced bone level

Pocket

Plaque

Tartar

Healthy

Periodontal Disease

Root

Healthy gums

Healthy bone level

Figure 28.1. Healthy gums versus periodontal disease. © American Academy of Periodontology.

loss of the connective tissue attachment to the teeth in the presence of gingival inflammation.

Chronic periodontitis is characterized by pocket formation and/or receding gums, and is recognized as the most frequently occurring form of periodontitis. It is most prevalent in adults, but can occur at any age.

The primary clinical features of periodontitis include clinical attachment loss (CAL), alveolar bone loss (BL), periodontal pocketing, and gingival inflammation. In addition, enlargement or recession of the gingival tissue; bleeding of the gingiva following application of pressure; and increased mobility, drifting, and/or tooth exfoliation may occur.

Additionally, chronic periodontitis can be further characterized by extent and severity. As a general guide, extent can be categorized as localized if ≤ 30 percent of the pocket sites (the areas between the teeth and gums that are examined for periodontitis) are affected and generalized if > 30 percent of the sites are affected. Severity can be described for the entire dentition or for individual teeth and sites. Attachment loss reflects the effect of a more common clinical measurement for periodontal disease called pocket depth: slight = 4-5 mm [millimeters], moderate = 5-6 mm, and severe = 7 mm or greater.

Aggressive Periodontitis

Aggressive periodontitis is a form of periodontitis that occurs in patients who are otherwise in good oral health. Common features include rapid attachment loss and bone destruction. Secondary features that are generally, but not universally, present are:

- Amounts of microbial deposits are inconsistent with the severity of periodontal tissue destruction

- Elevated proportions of specific bacteria, such as *Actinobacillus actinomycetemcomitans* and, in some populations, *Porphyromonas gingivalis*

- Phagocyte (cells that defend the body against infections) abnormalities

- Hyper-responsive macrophage phenotype, including elevated levels of prostaglandin E_2 and the gene interleukin-1 beta

There are two forms of aggressive periodontitis (localized and generalized). In addition to features common to all forms of aggressive periodontitis, the below features differentiate localized from generalized:

Localized Aggressive Periodontitis

• Circumpubertal onset

• Robust serum antibody response to infecting agents

• Localized first molar/incisor presentation with interproximal (in between teeth) attachment loss on at least two permanent teeth, one of which is a first molar, and involving no more than two teeth other than first molars and incisors

Generalized Aggressive Periodontitis

• Usually affecting persons under 30 years of age, but patients may be older

• Poor serum antibody response to infecting agents

• Pronounced episodic nature of the destruction of attachment and alveolar bone

• Generalized interproximal attachment loss affecting at least three permanent teeth other than first molars and incisors

Periodontitis as a Manifestation of Systemic Diseases

This type of periodontitis is associated with one of several systemic diseases, such as diabetes.

Necrotizing Periodontal Diseases

An infection characterized by necrosis (death of tissue by disease) of gingival tissues, periodontal ligament, and alveolar bone. These lesions are most commonly observed in individuals with systemic conditions including, but not limited to, HIV infection, malnutrition, and immunosuppression.

Symptoms of Periodontal Disease

Periodontal diseases are often silent, meaning symptoms may not appear until an advanced stage of the disease. Some people may have periodontal disease and not have any of these symptoms. Therefore, the only way to detect the disease is through a periodontal evaluation.

Signs and symptoms of periodontal diseases established by the American Academy of Periodontology include:

- Red, swollen, or tender gums

- Bleeding while brushing or flossing

- Gums that pull away from the teeth

- Loose or separating teeth

- Pus between the gum and the tooth

- Persistent bad breath

- A change in the way your teeth fit together when you bite

- A change in the fit of partial dentures

Diagnosing Periodontal Diseases

Assessing periodontal health is based primarily on traditional clinical and radiographic (X-ray) assessment. Periodontists (dentists who specialize in the prevention, diagnosis, and treatment of tissues surrounding the teeth) depend heavily on factors such as: 1) presence or absence of clinically detectable inflammation; 2) extent and pattern of clinical attachment loss; 3) patient's age at onset; 4) rate of progression; and 5) presence or absence of miscellaneous signs and symptoms, including pain and amount of observable plaque and calculus.

During a periodontal examination, a periodontist will ask patients about their medical and dental history. He/she will inspect gums for color and firmness and check the teeth for looseness and the way they fit together when biting. X-rays may be taken to evaluate the bone supporting the teeth. In cases of aggressive or advanced disease, the periodontist may order microbiologic testing to determine the level of periodontal pathogens.

More specifically, the following procedures may be performed and findings noted on the patient's chart during a clinical examination:

- Visual evaluation inside and outside of the mouth to detect non-periodontal oral diseases or conditions.

- Periodontal probing. During a periodontal probing, the periodontist will gently place a small measuring instrument (periodontal probe) in the pocket between the teeth and gums to measure pocket depths, recession, and attachment level; and to evaluate the subgingival area (area below the gum line) for findings such as bleeding, suppuration (pus), furcation (bone loss) status, and the detection of endodontic-periodontal lesions.

- Dental examination, including caries (dental decay) assessment, proximal contact relationships, the status of dental restorations and prosthetic appliances (crowns, bridges, dental implants, fixed retainers, etc.) and other tooth or implant problems.

- Determination of the degree tooth and implant looseness.

- Occlusal (bite) examination.

- Review and interpretation of a satisfactory number of updated, diagnostic-quality x-rays. In addition, other diagnostic imaging might be needed for implant therapy.

- Evaluation of potential relationships between periodontal health and overall health.

- Assessment of suitability to receive dental implants as needed.

The primary clinical importance of periodontal pockets is that they are a major habitat for putative periodontal pathogens. Deep pockets are a source of concern because the sites are difficult for the patient and dentist to clean, and they could increase the risk for the progression of periodontal diseases. Deep periodontal pockets do not necessarily mean that specific site will lose additional attachment in the future, but untreated periodontal disease is progressive and leads to tooth loss.

The probing depth in healthy gum attachments is 1-3 mm. Areas of damage from periodontal destruction reflect loss of increased gum attachment. Probing depths of 4-5 mm indicates slight periodontal disease, 5-6 mm suggests moderate, and 7 mm or greater could reveal severe periodontal disease.

These are the numbers patients may hear their periodontists call out during a periodontal exam.

Causes of Periodontal Diseases

The American Academy of Periodontology confirms the main cause of inflammatory periodontal diseases is periodontal pathogens in bacterial plaque, a sticky colorless film that constantly forms on the teeth. The mouth is full of several hundred types of bacteria of which approximately a dozen are considered periodontal pathogens (e.g.,

Porphyromonas gingivalis, Prevotella intermedia, Actinobacillus actinomycetemcomitans). Periodontal pathogens are Gram-negative and anaerobic (don't require oxygen to live); therefore, these bacteria thrive in deep defects or pockets below the gum line.

If plaque is not removed, it can turn into a hard substance called calculus in less than two days (calculus is so hard it can only be removed by a professional cleaning). Toxins produced by bacterial plaque irritate the gums and stimulate a chronic inflammatory response in which the tissues and bone that support the teeth are broken down and damaged. Gums separate from the teeth, forming deepening pockets that become infected with pathogens causing the disease to progress. As the disease progresses, the pockets deepen further and more gum tissue attachment and bone are lost. Often, this destructive process has very mild symptoms. Eventually, teeth can become loose and may have to be removed. Other factors that contribute to an increased susceptibility and/or severity of periodontal diseases include: smoking/tobacco use; genetics; hormonal changes; stress; medications; clenching or grinding your teeth; diabetes; poor nutrition; and systemic diseases.

Preventing Periodontal Diseases

The best way to prevent periodontal diseases and tooth decay is to remove the bacterial plaque by thorough brushing and flossing and by regular dental visits that include a periodontal evaluation. Typically, periodontists recommend that patients with good periodontal health have their teeth cleaned every 6 months. For the majority of the population, this routine, plus good personal oral hygiene including daily brushing and flossing, appears to be sufficient to maintaining healthy gums.

Brushing

It's important for the patient to begin with the right equipment. A soft-bristled toothbrush allows the brush bristles to get between the teeth better. If the bristles on the toothbrush are bent or frayed, the brush should be replaced with a new one.

To clean the surfaces of the teeth, the toothbrush should be positioned at a 45-degree angle where the gums and teeth meet. The patient should gently move the brush in a circular motion for several short, gentle strokes, and apply light pressure to get the bristles between the teeth.

To clean the biting surfaces of the teeth, the patient should use short, gentle strokes. Since the toothbrush can clean only one or two teeth at a time, the position of the brush can be changed as often as necessary to reach and clean all tooth surfaces.

Flossing

Since periodontal diseases occur primarily between the teeth where a toothbrush cannot reach, flossing daily will break up the bacterial colonies between teeth that can cause diseases.

To floss, it's best to begin with a piece of waxed or unwaxed floss about 18 inches long. The floss can be lightly wrapped around the middle finger of one hand. The remaining floss can be wrapped around the rest of the patient's middle finger of the opposite hand.

To floss the upper teeth, hold the floss tightly between the thumb and forefinger of each hand (no more than one-half inch apart) and gently insert it between the teeth, using a back-and-forth motion. The fingers controlling the floss should be no more than one-half inch apart. It's important not to force the floss or snap it into place. The floss should be guided to the gum line by curving the floss into a C-shape against one tooth. The floss can slide into the space between the gum and the tooth until the patient feels light resistance.

Using both hands, the patient can move the floss up and down each of the two sides of the teeth that face each other. As the floss becomes frayed or soiled, a turn from one middle finger to the other will bring up a fresh section.

To clean between the bottom teeth, the floss can be guided using the forefingers of both hands. Don't forget the backside of the last tooth on both sides, upper and lower.

After flossing, the patient can rinse vigorously with water to remove the plaque and food particles. During the first week of flossing, the patient's gums may bleed or be sore. As the plaque is removed daily, gums will heal and the bleeding should stop. If the bleeding does not stop within seven to ten days, the periodontist should be notified.

Who Gets Periodontal Diseases?

Even though good oral hygiene and regular dental visits go a long way toward prevention, periodontal diseases are still widespread. Research shows that nearly one in three U.S. adults aged 30 to 54 have some form of periodontal disease or a more advanced stage of the disease, as do a startling 50 percent of adults aged 55 to 90.

Tobacco Users

Smoking may contribute to the severity of more than half of the cases of periodontal diseases among adults in the United States, according to a study published in the *Journal of Periodontology* (*JOP*). In fact, researchers found that current smokers are about four times more likely than people who have never smoked to have advanced periodontitis.

The study also found that smoking increases the risk for periodontal treatment complications and/or failure. It reduces the delivery of oxygen and nutrients to gingival tissue and impairs the body's defense mechanisms, making a person more susceptible to infections like periodontitis.

Many chemicals found in tobacco, such as nicotine and tar, may have harmful effects on the periodontal tissues. One study even found that current smokers had more plaque and periodontal destruction than former or never smokers.

As a result, tobacco users are likely to have calculus form on their teeth, have deeper pockets between the teeth and gums, and lose more of the bone and tissue that support the teeth. Loss of bone and tissue may potentially cause tooth loss.

Research also shows that smokers lose more teeth than nonsmokers. According to data from the Centers for Disease Control and Prevention, only about 20 percent of people over age 65 who have never smoked are toothless, while 41.3 percent of daily smokers over age 65 are toothless.

Smokeless tobacco users aren't out of harm's way either. In fact, smokeless tobacco users are also at a greater risk of having more severe and rapidly progressing periodontitis, as well as receding gums. When gums recede to the point where the tooth roots are exposed, teeth may become susceptible to root cavities or sensitive to cold and touch—not to mention the fact that the chances of developing oral cancer also increases with smokeless tobacco use.

Oral health will begin to improve once the tobacco user quits. According to the *JOP* study, 11 years after quitting, former smokers' likelihood of having periodontitis was not significantly different from those who had never smoked.

Families and Periodontal Diseases

Research provides further evidence that genetics plays a major role in the onset and severity of periodontal diseases. A study, published in the *Journal of Periodontology* (*JOP*), concluded that approximately half of the variance in periodontal diseases in the population can be attributed to genetic differences.

Patients can be tested for genetic links to periodontal diseases with a simple swab of saliva from the inside of the cheek. Identification of people at high risk for periodontal diseases, before they even display signs and symptoms, may provide new avenues for prevention and treatment.

For patients who are genetically susceptible to periodontal diseases, closer and more intensive preventive measures may be required to maintain the same level of oral health.

Periodontal diseases may also be passed from parents to children and between people in relationships, according to a study in the *JOP*.

Researchers suggest bacteria that cause periodontal diseases pass via saliva. This means that the common contact of saliva in families puts children and couples at risk for contracting the periodontal diseases of another family member.

Based on this research, the American Academy of Periodontology (AAP) recognizes that treatment of periodontal diseases may involve entire families. If one family member has periodontitis, the AAP recommends that all family members see a dental professional for a periodontal screening.

Periodontitis: A Risk Factor for Systemic Diseases

Recent research has revealed that some forms of periodontal diseases may represent a far more serious threat to the health of millions of Americans than previously realized.

These studies found that periodontal infections might contribute to the development of heart disease, increase the risk of premature, underweight babies and pose a serious threat to people whose health is already compromised due to diabetes and respiratory diseases.

Heart Disease

Research suggests more advanced forms of periodontal diseases may increase the risk of heart disease. For example, recent studies suggest that people with periodontitis may have nearly twice the risk of having a fatal heart attack as those without periodontitis.

While more research is needed to confirm how periodontal bacteria may affect your heart, one possibility is that periodontal bacteria enter the blood through inflamed gums and cause small blood clots that contribute to clogged arteries. Another possibility is that inflammation caused by periodontitis may contribute to the buildup of fatty deposits inside the heart arteries.

Since periodontitis is a bacterial infection of the gums, bone and periodontal ligament, the bacteria can enter the bloodstream and travel to major organs and begin new infections. It can also exacerbate certain existing heart conditions. Patients at risk for infective endocarditis may require antibiotics prior to dental procedures. The periodontist and cardiologist will determine if a heart condition requires use of antibiotics prior to dental procedures.

Preterm Underweight Births

Pregnant women who have periodontitis may be up to seven times more likely to have a baby that is born too early and too small.

While more research is needed to confirm how advanced forms of periodontal diseases may affect pregnancy outcomes, one theory is that they may trigger increased levels of biological fluids that induce labor. Furthermore, data suggest that women whose periodontal condition worsens during pregnancy are at significant risk of having a premature baby.

An ongoing study of more than 2,000 pregnant women shows that the more of the mouth affected with certain forms of periodontal diseases (meaning they affect at least 30 percent), the more likely a woman is to deliver a premature baby. The study was presented at the AAP's Specialty Conference on Periodontal Medicine in Washington, D.C.

All infections are cause for concern among pregnant women because they pose a risk to the health of the baby. Therefore, the American Academy of Periodontology recommends that women considering pregnancy have a periodontal evaluation.

Diabetes and Periodontal Diseases

For years we've known that people with diabetes are more likely to have periodontal diseases than people without diabetes. In fact, the link is well documented. Studies have found periodontal diseases to be more prevalent in diabetic individuals. This is probably because people with diabetes are more susceptible to contracting infections. In fact, they lose more teeth than non-diabetic people do.

While it has been established that people with diabetes are more prone to developing periodontal disease, new research suggests that severe forms of periodontal diseases might be a risk factor for diabetes.

Severe forms of periodontal diseases can cause bacteria to enter the bloodstream and activate immune cells. These activated cells produce inflammatory biological signals (cytokines) that have a destructive effect throughout the entire body. In the pancreas, the cells responsible for insulin production can be damaged or destroyed by chronically elevated levels of cytokines that have been found in some systemic diseases. Once this happens, it may induce type 2 diabetes, even in otherwise healthy individuals with no other risk factors for the disease.

Respiratory and Periodontal Disease

Bacterial respiratory infections are thought to be acquired through inhalation of fine droplets from the mouth and throat into the lungs. These droplets contain germs that can breed and multiply within the lungs. Research suggests that bacteria found in the throat as well as bacteria found in the mouth can be drawn into the lower respiratory tract, which causes infections or worsens existing lung conditions.

Now research confirms findings that periodontitis may increase a person's risk for the respiratory disorder chronic obstructive pulmonary disease (COPD), the sixth leading cause of mortality in the United States.

This study analyzed data from a national survey, which examined patients with periodontal diseases defined by mean periodontal attachment loss (MAL) of greater than 3 millimeters. Patients with periodontal diseases were found to have nearly a one-and-a-half times greater risk of COPD. A distinct trend also was noted with lung function, which seems to diminish with increased periodontal attachment loss. This suggests that periodontitis activity may promote the progression of COPD.

Economic, Psychological, and Social Burden

A silent epidemic of oral diseases is affecting vulnerable citizens— poor children, the elderly, and many members of racial and ethnic minority groups. These diseases are progressive, cumulative, and become more complex over time. They can affect the ability to eat, how people look, and the way they communicate. In addition, oral diseases can affect economic productivity and compromise the ability to work at home, at school, or on the job.

According to the U.S. Surgeon General's first report on oral health, expenditures for dental services in the United States alone made up 4.7 percent of the nation's general health expenditures in 1998—$53.8 billion out of $1.1 trillion.

The social impact of oral diseases in children is substantial. About 37 percent of children have not had a dental visit before starting school, and more than 51 million school hours are lost each year to dental-related illness. When children don't see dental professionals, they miss the opportunity to have problems caught early before they escalate into larger, more expensive problems to treat. Parents also miss the opportunity to learn how to promote good oral habits in their children.

Additionally, over one third of the U.S. population (100 million people) has no access to community water fluoridation, which prevents tooth decay. A little less than two thirds of adults report having visited a dentist in the past 12 months. And employed adults lose more than 164 million hours of work each year due to dental diseases or dental visits.

Periodontal Treatment

Periodontists are dentists who specialize in the prevention, diagnosis, and treatment of tissues surrounding the teeth and in the placement of dental implants. They receive extensive training in these areas, including three additional years of education beyond dental school. Periodontists are familiar with the latest techniques for diagnosing and treating periodontal diseases. In addition, they can perform cosmetic periodontal procedures and dental implants to help patients achieve the smiles they desire. Periodontics is one of nine dental specialties recognized by the American Dental Association.

Periodontists are like physicians of the mouth. Similar to infectious disease experts and geneticists, they look at microbiological aspects of periodontal diseases as well as how genetics may influence disease progression and/or treatment. Just as organ transplant experts, who are looking at home tissue engineering may one day be used to grow organs, periodontists are examining how this same body of research can help them regrow supporting tooth structures and even teeth. And, like an orthopedic surgeon who today is able to place implants and improve the quality of life for patients who have failing hips and knees, periodontists can offer patients dental implants as a tooth replacement option over crowns, bridges, or dentures.

Often, general practitioner dentists and other dental specialists refer their patients to a periodontist when periodontal diseases are present. However, many patients don't know that they can go directly to a periodontist or refer a family member or friend if they detect symptoms of the disease and/or are seeking solutions to functional and esthetic concerns caused by periodontal diseases.

241

Periodontal Examination

All patients should receive a comprehensive periodontal examination. During this exam, the periodontist discusses with the patient the chief complaint, reviews medical and dental histories, and performs a clinical examination and radiographic (x-ray) analysis. In some cases, microbiological, genetic, biochemical, or other diagnostic tests may be performed.

Surgical Procedures

Pocket Depth Reduction

Bone and gum tissue should fit snugly around the teeth like a turtleneck around the neck. Periodontal diseases destroy these supporting tissues and pockets form around the teeth.

Over time, these pockets become deeper, providing a larger space for bacteria to live. As bacteria develop around the teeth, they can accumulate and advance under the gum tissue. These deep pockets collect even more bacteria, resulting in further bone and tissue loss. Eventually, too much bone is lost, and the teeth need to be extracted.

As explained in an earlier section, periodontists measure pocket depths with an instrument called a periodontal probe to determine if there is any breakdown in soft tissue or pocket development between the teeth and gums. Pocket depth reduction procedures are performed when patients have pockets that are too deep to clean with daily at-home oral hygiene and a professional care routine. During this procedure, periodontists fold back the gum tissue and remove the disease-causing bacteria before securing the tissue into place. In some cases, irregular surfaces of the damaged bone are smoothed to limit areas where disease-causing bacteria can hide (also known as osseous surgery). This allows the gum tissue to better reattach to healthy bone.

Reducing pocket depth and eliminating existing bacteria are important to prevent damage caused by the progression of periodontal diseases and to maintain a healthy smile. Eliminating bacteria alone may not be sufficient to prevent disease recurrence.

Regeneration

When periodontal diseases destroy too much of the bone and tissue that support the teeth, regenerative procedures may be recommended to reverse some of the damage by regenerating lost bone and tissue.

During regenerative procedures, periodontists fold back the gum tissue and remove the disease-causing bacteria. Membranes (filters), bone grafts, or tissue-stimulating proteins may also be used to stimulate the body's natural ability to regenerate bone and tissue. Regenerated tissues can increase support for the teeth; thus increasing their stability and long-term outlook.

Soft Tissue Grafts

Exposed tooth roots are the result of gum recession. They can make the teeth appear too long or cause patients to cringe because they are sensitive to hot and cold. Exposed roots are also more sensitive to decay.

Once the factors that contributed to the recession are controlled, a soft tissue graft procedure can repair the defect and help to prevent additional recession and bone loss. During this procedure, periodontists take gum tissue from the palate or another donor source to cover the exposed root. Soft tissue grafts can be done for one tooth or several teeth.

Functional Crown Lengthening

Crown lengthening recontours the gum tissue and often the underlying bone surrounding one or more teeth so that an adequate amount of healthy tooth is exposed. This procedure is often used as part of a treatment plan for a tooth that is to be fitted with a crown. It provides the necessary space between the supporting bone and crown, preventing the new crown from damaging gum tissues and bone. In some cases, if a tooth is badly worn, decayed, or fractured below the gum line, crown lengthening adjusts the gum and bone levels to gain access to more of the tooth so it can be restored.

Dental Implants

A dental implant is an artificial tooth root placed into the jaw to hold a replacement tooth or bridge in place. While high-tech in nature, dental implants are actually more tooth saving than traditional bridgework, since implants do not rely on neighboring teeth for support.

Implants, which look like screws or cylinders, are placed into the jaw. Over two to six months, the implants and bone are allowed to bond together to form anchors (osseointegration). During this time, a temporary tooth replacement option can be worn over the implant sites.

Often, a second step of the procedure is necessary to uncover the implants and attach extensions. These small metal posts, called abutments, complete the foundation on which the new teeth will be placed. The gums will be allowed to heal for a couple of weeks following this procedure.

These are some implant systems (one-stage) that do not require this second step. These systems use an implant that already has the extension piece attached.

Dental implants can be used to replace a single tooth, several teeth, or an entire mouthful of teeth.

Dental implants are intimately connected with the gum tissues and underlying bone in the mouth. Since periodontists are the dental experts who specialize in precisely these areas, they are ideal members of the dental implant team. Not only do periodontists have experience working with other dental professionals, they also have the special knowledge, training, and facilities needed to help patients have teeth that look and feel natural.

Sinus Augmentation

The upper back jaw has traditionally been one of the most difficult areas to successfully place dental implants due to insufficient bone quantity and quality and the close proximity to the sinus. Patients who have lost bone in that area due to periodontal diseases and/or tooth loss may be left without enough bone to place implants.

Sinus augmentation can help correct this problem by raising the sinus floor and developing bone for the placement of dental implants. Several techniques can be used to raise the sinus and allow for new bone to form. In one common technique, an incision is made to expose the bone. Then a small circle is cut into the bone. This bony piece is lifted into the sinus cavity, much like a trap door, and the space underneath is filled with bone graft material. As with standard regenerative procedures, membranes (filters), bone grafts or tissue-stimulating proteins may be used to stimulate the body's natural ability to regenerate bone and tissue.

Finally, the incision is closed and healing takes place. Depending on the patient's individual needs, the bone usually will be allowed to develop for about four to 12 months before implants can be placed. After the implants are placed, an additional healing period is required. In some cases, the implant can be placed at the same time the sinus is augmented.

Ridge Modification

Deformities in the upper or lower jaw can leave patients with inadequate bone in which to place dental implants. Wearing dentures, developmental defects, injury, or trauma can cause this defect. Not only does this deformity cause problems in placing the implant, it can also cause an unattractive indentation in the jaw line near the missing teeth that may be difficult to clean and maintain.

To correct the problem, the gum is lifted away from the ridge to expose the bony defect. The defect is then filled with bone or bone substitute to build up the ridge. As with standard regenerative procedures and sinus augmentation, membranes (filters), bone grafts, or tissue-stimulating proteins may be used to stimulate the body's natural ability regenerate bone and tissue.

Finally, the incision is closed and healing takes place. Depending on the patient's individual needs, the bone usually will be allowed to develop for about four to 12 months before implants can be placed. In some cases, the implant can be placed at the same time the ridge is modified.

Non-Surgical Procedures

Scaling and Root Planing

Mechanical methods of subgingival debridement accomplished by thorough scaling and root planing (a careful cleaning of the root surfaces to remove plaque and calculus [tartar] from deep periodontal pockets and to smooth the tooth root to remove bacterial toxins), accompanied by oral hygiene procedures, have served as the gold standard of periodontal therapy for decades.

Clinical trials have consistently demonstrated that scaling and root planing reduces gingival inflammation, reduces probing depth, and results in a gain of clinical attachment in most patients and sites with adult periodontitis. Furthermore, available evidence supports that scaling and root planing results in a shift of the subgingival microbiota from one associated with disease toward one associated with health. Thus, mechanical therapy is usually the first mode of treatment recommended for most periodontal infections. Following adequate time to evaluate healing response, the patient must be reevaluated to determine if further mechanical, adjunctive pharmacological, and/or surgical treatment is indicated.

Antimicrobials

The reported effects of locally delivered sustained release antimicrobials on subgingival microbiota have been mixed. In some cases, the effect was minimal or nondetectable, resulting in a return to baseline bacterial levels within a short period of time. Other studies have shown suppression of the disease-associated microbiota, some for extended periods of time.

Furthermore, the indications for systemic antibiotics include their possible adjunctive use in the management of microbially induced periodontal diseases as well as in patients who are put at risk because of bacteremia. In addition to the medical contraindications for the use of systemic antibiotics, they are not indicated for the treatment of chronic gingivitis.

Host-Modulating Drugs

Current research on host-modulating drugs indicates potential therapeutic value in the management of the patient with periodontal diseases. This could be a promising new area in periodontal treatment.

Surgical versus Non-Surgical Procedures

Some studies suggest that scaling and root planing with antimicrobial support might be substituted for periodontal surgery, and that it is a more cost-effective, user-friendly means of periodontal treatment. However, other recent studies have concluded that surgery may provide a better long-term outcome with less need for adjunctive treatments than non-surgical therapy. The American Academy of Periodontology is concerned that these studies have initiated debate that is confusing for practitioners and patients and may thwart thoughtful discussion and better understanding of the key issue: what is the most effective means to keep periodontal diseases at bay for each individual patient?

AAP treatment guidelines have always stressed that periodontal health should be achieved in the least invasive and most cost-effective manner. This is often accomplished through non-surgical periodontal treatment, including scaling and root planing followed by adjunctive therapy such as systemic and local delivery antimicrobials and host modulation, as needed and on a case-by-case basis.

Most periodontists would agree that after scaling and root planing, many patients do not require any further active treatment, including surgical therapy. However, the majority of patients will require ongoing maintenance therapy to sustain health. Non-surgical treatment does have its limitations, and when it does not achieve periodontal health, surgery might be indicated to restore periodontal anatomy damaged by periodontal diseases and to facilitate oral hygiene practices.

Some studies propose that patients receive antibiotics at the time of scaling and root planing. This blanket use of antibiotics is not necessary for most patients because they usually respond well to non-surgical treatment without antibiotics. Blanket antibiotic use disregards the Centers for Disease Control and Prevention recommendations for appropriate antibiotic use for healthcare providers. As healthcare providers, it is important for all dentists to consider antibiotic usage guidelines in treatment planning, so that the effectiveness of their use is preserved for patients who do not initially respond to therapy; and to avoid contributing to one of the world's most pressing health problems, namely, antibiotic resistance.

The AAP continually monitors emerging research to identify therapies that further its members' understanding of cost-effective, minimally invasive procedures in the treatment of periodontal diseases. Unfortunately, when the overly simplistic dispute over non-surgical versus surgical procedures arises, it often misleads patients and the dental community into thinking it's an either-or debate. In fact, the procedures are complementary, with each having their place in treatment, and each having their limitations.

Periodontal Maintenance Procedures

Periodontal maintenance procedures (PMP) are specialized treatment for patients who have already been diagnosed with and treated for periodontal diseases. PMP is different from traditional six-month cleanings by a patient's general dentist, which help to protect the health of the teeth.

During PMP visits, periodontists update the patient's medical and dental histories to note any factors that may influence periodontal health and treatment effectiveness. A thorough periodontal evaluation is also performed, including a comprehensive periodontal probing; an oral cancer screening of the inner and outer oral tissues; and x-rays to evaluate the teeth and bone supporting the teeth, if necessary. Harmful bacterial plaque and calculus are then removed from above and below the gum line. If appropriate, a detailed, non-surgical treatment is used to smooth root surfaces that may be particularly infected (root planing). Finally, the patient's at-home oral hygiene routine will be reviewed and modification suggestions tailored for the condition.

If new or recurrent periodontal diseases are identified during a PMP visit, then additional periodontal treatment may be recommended.

Laser Treatment

Advertisements have recommended the use of lasers in many of the above-listed treatments, suggesting that it is "revolutionary and pain-free." The use of lasers for any periodontal treatment should be evaluated in light of FDA-accepted functions and currently available evidence. At the time of this writing, no evidence has been published in peer-reviewed literature indicating that lasers alter the level of periodontal pathogens in periodontal pockets. Additionally, no evidence exists that the use of lasers in gingival curettage as adjunctive therapy to scaling and root planing is superior to scaling and root planing alone.

The AAP feels that further research on the potential use of laser energy in periodontal therapy is necessary, and that the scientific literature should be followed to evaluate treatments that may benefit patients.

References

1. The American Academy of Periodontology. 1999 International Workshop for a Classification of Periodontal Diseases and Conditions. *Annals of Periodontology* 1999; 4:1:2–3.

2. The American Academy of Periodontology. The Pathogenesis of Periodontal Diseases (position paper). *J. Periodontol*; April 1999; 70;457–470.

3. Flemming, Thomas F. Periodontitis. *J. Periodontol* 1999; 4:1:32–37.

4. The American Academy of Periodontology. Consensus Report: Chronic Periodontitis. *Annals of Periodontology* 1999:4;38.

5. The American Academy of Periodontology. Consensus Report: Aggressive Periodontitis. *Annals of Periodontology* 1999:4;53.

6. The American Academy of Periodontology. Consensus Report: Necrotizing Periodontal Diseases. *Annals of Periodontology* 1999:4;78.

7. The American Academy of Periodontology. Diagnosis of Periodontal Diseases (position paper) April 1995; 1–13.

8. Armitage Gary. Periodontal Diseases: Diagnosis. *Annals of Periodontology* 1996:1:1:37–215.

9. Zambon Joseph. Periodontal Diseases: Microbial Factors. *Annals of Periodontology* 1996:1:1:879–925.

10. Oral Health in America: A Report of the Surgeon General. Rockville, MD: U.S. Department of Health and Human Services, National Institute of Dental and Craniofacial Research, National Institutes of Health, 2000; NIH Publication No. 00-4713; 1–308.

11. Soder B, Nedlich U, Jin Jian L. Longitudinal effect of nonsurgical treatment and systemic metronidazole for one week in smokers and nonsmokers with refractory periodontitis: A 5-year study. *J Periodontol* 1999;70:761–771.

12. The American Academy of Periodontology. Tobacco use and the periodontal patient. *J Periodontol* 1999; 70:1419–1427.

13. Centers from Disease Control and Prevention, National Center for Chronic Prevention and Health Promotion, Division of Oral Health. Total tooth loss among persons Aged ≤ 65 Years—Selected States, 1995-1997 *Morbidity and Mortality Weekly Report* 1999;48:10:206–210.

14. Albandar JM, Brunelle JA, Kingman A. Destructive periodontal disease in adults 30 years of age and older in the United States, 1988-1994. *J Periodontol* 1999;1:13–29.

15. Irfan U, Dawson D, Bissada N. Assessment of familial patterns of microbial infection in periodontitis. *J Periodontol* 1999;70:1406–1418.

16. The American Academy of Periodontology. Periodontal disease as a potential risk factor for systemic diseases. *J Periodontol* 1998;69:841–850.

17. Jeffcoat M. Geurs N, Reddy M, Goldenberg R, Hauth J. Current evidence regarding periodontal disease as a risk factor in preterm birth. *Annals Periodontol* 2001;6:183–188.

18. The epidemiological and clinical aspects of periodontal disease in diabetics. *Annals of Periodontol* 1998;3:1:2–12.

19. Proceedings of the Periodontal-Systemic Connection: A State-of-the-Science Symposium. *Annals of Periodontol* 2001;6:127–128.

20. Scannapieco F, Ho A. Potential associations between chronic respiratory disease and periodontal disease: Analysis of National Health and Nutrition examination survey III. *J Periodontol* 2001;72:50–56.

21. The American Academy of Periodontology. Guidelines for periodontal therapy. *J Periodontol* 2001;72:1624–1628.

22. The American Academy of Periodontology. Consensus Report Non-Surgical Pocket Therapy: Mechanical, Pharmacotherapeutics, and Dental Occlusion. *Annals of Periodontology* 1996; 1:1:581–587.

Section 28.3

Fighting Gum Disease: How to Keep Your Teeth

By Carol Lewis, *FDA Consumer*, U.S. Food and Drug Administration (FDA), May 2002.

More than 75 percent of Americans over 35 have some form of gum disease. In its earliest stage, your gums might swell and bleed easily. At its worst, you might lose your teeth. The bottom line? If you want to keep your teeth, you must take care of your gums.

The mouth is a busy place, with millions of bacteria constantly on the move. While some bacteria are harmless, others can attack the teeth and gums. Harmful bacteria are contained in a colorless sticky film called plaque, the cause of gum disease. If not removed, plaque builds up on the teeth and ultimately irritates the gums and causes bleeding. Left unchecked, bone and connective tissue are destroyed, and teeth often become loose and may have to be removed.

A recent poll of 1,000 people over 35 done by Harris Interactive Inc. found that 60 percent of adults surveyed knew little, if anything, about gum disease, the symptoms, available treatments, and—most importantly—the consequences. And 39 percent do not visit a dentist regularly. Yet, gum disease is the leading cause of adult tooth loss.

Moreover, a Surgeon General's report issued in May 2000 labeled Americans' bad oral health a "silent epidemic" and called for a national effort to improve oral health among all Americans.

The good news is that in most people gum disease is preventable. Attention to everyday oral hygiene (brushing and flossing), coupled with professional cleanings twice a year, could be all that's needed to prevent gum disease—and actually reverse the early stage—and help you keep your teeth for a lifetime.

In addition, several products have been approved by the Food and Drug Administration specifically to diagnose and treat gum disease, and even regenerate lost bone. These products may help improve the effectiveness of the professional care you receive.

What Is Gum Disease?

In the broadest sense, the term gum disease—or periodontal disease—describes bacterial growth and production of factors that gradually destroy the tissue surrounding and supporting the teeth. Periodontal means around the tooth.

Gum disease begins with plaque, which is always forming on your teeth, without you even knowing it. When it accumulates to excessive levels, it can harden into a substance called tartar (calculus) in as little as 24 hours. Tartar is so tightly bound to teeth that it can be removed only during a professional cleaning.

Gingivitis and periodontitis are the two main stages of gum disease. Each stage is characterized by what a dentist sees and feels in your mouth, and by what's happening under your gum line. Although gingivitis usually precedes periodontitis, it's important to know that not all gingivitis progresses to periodontitis.

In the early stage of gingivitis, the gums can become red and swollen and bleed easily, often during tooth brushing. Bleeding, although not always a symptom of gingivitis, is a signal that your mouth is unhealthy and needs attention. The gums may be irritated, but the teeth are still firmly planted in their sockets.

No bone or other tissue damage has occurred at this stage. Although dental disease in America remains a serious public health concern, recent developments indicate that the situation is far from hopeless. Frederick N. Hyman, D.D.S., a dental officer in the FDA's dermatologic and dental drug products division, says that because people seem to be paying more attention to oral hygiene as part of personal grooming, the payoff is "a decline in gingivitis over recent years." Hyman adds that "gingivitis can be reversed in nearly all cases when proper plaque control is practiced," consisting, in part, of daily brushing and flossing.

When gingivitis is left untreated, it can advance to periodontitis. At this point, the inner layer of the gum and bone pull away from the teeth (recede) and form pockets. These small spaces between teeth and gums may collect debris and can become infected. The body's immune system fights the bacteria as the plaque spreads and grows below the gum line. Bacterial toxins and the body's enzymes fighting the infection actually start to break down the bone and connective tissue that hold teeth in place. As the disease progresses, the pockets deepen and more gum tissue and bone are destroyed.

At this point, because there is no longer an anchor for the teeth, they become progressively looser, and the ultimate outcome is tooth loss.

Signs and Symptoms

Periodontal disease may progress painlessly, producing few obvious signs, even in the late stages of the disease. Then one day, on a visit to your dentist, you might be told that you have chronic gum disease and that you may be at increased risk of losing your teeth.

Although the symptoms of periodontal disease often are subtle, the condition is not entirely without warning signs. Certain symptoms may point to some form of the disease. They include:

- gums that bleed during and after tooth brushing
- red, swollen, or tender gums
- persistent bad breath or bad taste in the mouth
- receding gums
- formation of deep pockets between teeth and gums
- loose or shifting teeth
- changes in the way teeth fit together on biting or in the fit of partial dentures.

Even if you don't notice any symptoms, you may still have some degree of gum disease. Some people have gum disease only around certain teeth, such as those in the back of the mouth, which they cannot see. Only a dentist or a periodontist—a dentist who specializes in gum disease—can recognize and determine the progression of gum disease.

The American Academy of Periodontology (AAP) says that up to 30 percent of the U.S. population may be genetically susceptible to gum disease. And, despite aggressive oral care habits, people who are genetically predisposed may be up to six times more likely to develop some form of gum disease. Genetic testing to identify these people can help by encouraging early treatment that may help them keep their teeth for a lifetime.

Diagnosis

During a periodontal exam, your gums are checked for bleeding, swelling, and firmness. The teeth are checked for movement and sensitivity. Your bite is assessed. Full-mouth X-rays can help detect breakdown of bone surrounding your teeth.

Periodontal probing determines how severe your disease is. A probe is like a tiny ruler that is gently inserted into pockets around teeth. The deeper the pocket, the more severe the disease.

In healthy gums, the pockets measure less than 3 millimeters—about one-eighth of an inch—and no bone loss appears on x-rays. Gums are tight against the teeth and have pink tips. Pockets that measure 3 millimeters to 5 millimeters indicate signs of disease. Tartar may be progressing below the gum line and some bone loss could be evident. Pockets that are 5 millimeters or deeper indicate a serious condition that usually includes receding gums and a greater degree of bone loss.

Following the evaluation, your dentist or periodontist will recommend treatment options. Methods used to treat gum disease vary and are based on the stage of the disease.

Treatment

The goal of periodontal treatment is to control any infection that exists and to halt progression of the disease. Treatment options involve home care that includes healthy eating and proper brushing and flossing, non-surgical therapy that controls the growth of harmful bacteria and, in more advanced cases of disease, surgery to restore supportive tissues.

Although brushing and flossing are equally important, brushing eliminates only the plaque from the surfaces of the teeth that the brush can reach. Flossing, on the other hand, removes plaque from in between the teeth and under the gum line.

Both should be used as part of a regular at-home, self-care treatment plan. Some dentists also recommend specialized toothbrushes, such as those that are motorized and have smaller heads, which may be a more effective method of removing plaque than a standard toothbrush.

John J. Golski, D.D.S., a Frederick, Maryland, periodontist, says that the rationale behind flossing is not "just to get the food out." From the periodontal standpoint, Golski says, "You're flossing to remove plaque—the real culprit behind gum disease," adding that proper brushing and flossing techniques are critical.

During a typical checkup your dentist or dental hygienist will remove the plaque and tartar from above and below the gum line of all your teeth. If you have some signs of gingivitis, your dentist may recommend that you return for future cleanings more often than twice a year. Your dentist may also recommend that you use a toothpaste or mouth rinse that is FDA-approved for fighting gingivitis.

In addition to containing fluoride to fight cavities, Colgate Total®—the only toothpaste approved by the FDA for helping to prevent gingivitis—also contains triclosan, a mild antimicrobial that has been clinically proven to reduce plaque and gingivitis if used regularly. A chlorhexidine-containing rinse, also approved to fight plaque and gingivitis, is available only with a prescription.

If your dentist determines that you have some bone loss or that the gums have receded from the teeth, the standard treatment is an intensive deep-cleaning, non-surgical method called scaling and root planing (SRP). Scaling scrapes the plaque and tartar from above and below the gum line. Root planing smoothes rough spots on the tooth root where germs collect and helps remove bacteria that can contribute to the disease. This smooth, clean surface helps allow the gums to reattach to the teeth.

A relatively new drug in the arsenal against serious gum disease called Periostat® (doxycycline hyclate) was approved by the FDA in 1998 to be used in combination with SRP. While SRP primarily eliminates bacteria, Periostat®, which is taken orally, suppresses the action of collagenase, an enzyme that causes destruction of the teeth and gums.

Periodontal procedures such as SRP, and even surgery, are most often done in the office. The time spent, the degree of discomfort, and healing times vary. All depend on the type and extent of the procedure and the person's overall health.

Local anesthesia to numb the treatment area usually is given before some treatments. If necessary, medication is given to help you relax. Incisions may be closed with stitches designed to dissolve and may be covered with a protective dressing.

Susan Runner, D.D.S., chief of the Dental Devices Branch in the FDA's Center for Devices and Radiological Health, says that devices have been approved both for diagnosing gum diseases and promoting regeneration of periodontal tissue.

"Periodontal membranes, along with bone-filling material, are used in treatment of the condition to help repair damage resulting from periodontal disease," Runner says. "Tissue engineering devices mimic the biological characteristics of the wound-healing process, and may help stimulate bone cells to grow."

Opinions about which treatment methods to use vary in the periodontal field. For some people, certain procedures may be safer, more effective, and more comfortable than others may be. Which treatment your dentist or periodontist chooses will most likely depend on how far your disease has progressed, how you may have responded to earlier treatments, or your overall health.

"Generally, we all have the same goals, but the methods for getting to them may be different," says Golski. "One size doesn't fit all." Professional treatment can promote reattachment of healthy gums to teeth, reduce swelling, the depth of pockets, and the risk of infection, and stop further damage.

"But in the end," Golski says, "nothing will work without a compliant patient."

Antibiotic Treatments

Antibiotic treatments can be used either in combination with surgery and other therapies, or alone, to reduce or temporarily eliminate the bacteria associated with periodontal disease.

However, doctors, dentists, and public health officials are becoming more concerned that overuse of these antibiotics can increase the risk of bacterial resistance to these drugs. When germs become resistant to antibiotics, the drugs lose the ability to fight infection.

"The resistance we're worried about," explains Robert Genco, D.D.S., Ph.D., chairman of the oral biology department at The State University of New York at Buffalo, "is in association with antibiotics in the traditional use; those at higher levels in the blood that kill bacteria."

Jerry Gordon, D.M.D., of Bensalem, Pennsylvania, shares Genco's concerns. "There is a role for antibiotics in periodontal disease," Gordon says, "but you have to be very selective in your use."

Each time a person takes penicillin or another antibiotic for a bacterial infection, the drug may kill most of the bacteria. But a few germs may survive by mutating or acquiring resistance genes from other bacteria. These surviving genes can multiply quickly, creating drug-resistant strains. The presence of these strains may mean that the person's next infection will not respond to another dose of the same antibiotic. And this overuse would be detrimental to people if they develop a life-threatening illness for which antibiotics would no longer be helpful.

John V. Kelsey, D.D.S., dental team leader in the FDA's dermatologic and dental drug products division, says, "The widespread use of systemic antibiotics is generating resistant organisms, and that's a problem." And that fact, he says, "has prompted the industry to develop new strategies that would reduce the risk of resistance developing."

Table 28.1. FDA-Approved Products for Gum Disease (continued on next page)

A number of products are available to control infection and reduce inflammation.

Name	What It Is	Why It's Used	How It's Used
Colgate Total® (triclosan and fluoride toothpaste)	Over-the-counter toothpaste containing the antibacterial triclosan	The antibacterial ingredient reduces plaque and resulting gingivitis. The fluoride protects against cavities.	Used like a regular toothpaste
Peridex® or generic (chlorhexidine mouth rinse)	Prescription mouth rinse containing an anti-microbial called chlorhexidine	To control bacteria, resulting in less plaque and gingivitis	Used like a regular mouthwash
PerioChip®	A tiny piece of gelatin filled with chlorhexidine	To control bacteria and reduce the size of periodontal pockets	Chip is placed in the pockets after root planing, where the medicine is slowly released over time.
Atridox™	A gel that contains the antibiotic doxycycline	To control bacteria and reduce the size of periodontal pockets	Placed in pockets after scaling and root planing. Antibiotic is released slowly over a period of about seven days.

For example, three relatively new drugs—Atridox™ (doxycycline hyclate), PerioChip® (chlorhexidine gluconate), and Arestin™ (minocycline)—are antibiotics that were approved in sustained-release doses to be applied into the periodontal pocket. Local application of antibiotics to the gum surface may not affect the entire body, as do oral antibiotics.

Oral Health and Overall Health

According to the Centers for Disease Control and Prevention (CDC), researchers have uncovered potential links between periodontal disease and other serious health conditions. In people with healthy

Table 28.1. FDA-Approved Products for Gum Disease (continued from previous page)

A number of products are available to control infection and reduce inflammation.

Name	What It Is	Why It's Used	How It's Used
Actisite®	Thread-like fiber that contains the antibiotic tetracycline	To control bacteria and reduce the size of periodontal pockets	These fibers are placed in the pockets. The medicine is released slowly over 10 days. The fibers are then removed.
Arestin™ microspheres	Tiny round particles that contain the antibiotic minocycline	To control bacteria and reduce the size of periodontal pockets	Microspheres placed into pockets after scaling and root planing. Particles release minocycline slowly over time.
Periostat®	A low dose of the medication doxycycline that keeps destructive enzymes in check	To hold back the body's enzyme response—if not controlled, certain enzymes can break down bone and connective tissue.	This medication is in pill form. It is used in combination with scaling and root planing.

immune systems, the influx of oral bacteria into the bloodstream is usually harmless. But under certain circumstances, the CDC says, the microorganisms that live in the human mouth can cause problems elsewhere in the body "if normal protective barriers in the mouth are breached."

If you have diabetes, for example, you are at higher risk of developing infections such as periodontal disease. These infections can impair the body's ability to process or use insulin, which may cause your diabetes to be more difficult to manage. Diabetes is not only a risk factor for periodontal disease, but periodontal disease may make diabetes worse.

However, the CDC cautions that there is not enough evidence to conclude that oral infections actually cause or contribute to cardiovascular disease, diabetes, and other serious health problems. More research is underway to determine whether the associations are causal or coincidental.

Other Common Measures for Treating Gum Disease

- Curettage—a scraping away of the diseased gum tissue in the infected pocket, which permits the infected area to heal.

- Flap surgery—involves lifting back the gums and removing the tartar. The gums are then sewn back in place so that the tissue fits snugly around the tooth. This method also reduces the pocket and areas where bacteria grow.

- Bone grafts—used to replace bone destroyed by periodontitis. Tiny fragments of your own bone, synthetic bone, or donated bone are placed where bone was lost. These grafts serve as a platform for the regrowth of bone, which restores stability to teeth.

- Soft tissue grafts—reinforce thin gums or fill in places where gums have receded. Grafted tissue, most often taken from the roof of the mouth, is stitched in place over the affected area.

- Guided tissue regeneration—stimulates bone and gum tissue growth. Done in combination with flap surgery, a small piece of mesh-like fabric is inserted between the bone and gum tissue. This keeps the gum tissue from growing into the area where the bone should be, allowing the bone and connective tissue to regrow to better support the teeth.

- Bone (osseous) surgery—smoothes shallow craters in the bone due to moderate and advanced bone loss. Following flap surgery, the bone around the tooth is reshaped to decrease the craters. This makes it harder for bacteria to collect and grow.

- Medications in pill form—are used to help kill the germs that cause periodontitis or suppress the destruction of the tooth's attachment to the bone. There are also antibiotic gels, fibers, or chips applied directly to the infected pocket. In some cases, a dentist will prescribe a special anti-germ mouth rinse containing a chemical called chlorhexidine to help control plaque and gingivitis. These are the only mouth rinses approved for treating periodontal disease.

Other Potential Factors That Contribute to Gum Disease

While plaque is the primary cause of periodontal disease, the American Academy of Periodontology (AAP) says that other factors are thought to increase the risk, severity, and speed of gum disease development. These can include:

- Tobacco use—one of the most significant risk factors associated with the development of periodontitis. People who smoke are seven times more likely to get periodontitis than nonsmokers, and smoking can lower the chances of success of some treatments.

- Hormonal changes—may make gums more sensitive and make it easier for gingivitis to develop.

- Stress—may make it difficult for the body's immune system to fight off infection.

- Medications—can affect oral health because they lessen the flow of saliva, which has a protective effect on teeth and gums. Some drugs, such as the anticonvulsant medication diphenylhydantoin and the anti-angina drug nifedipine, can cause abnormal growth of gum tissue.

- Poor nutrition—may make it difficult for the immune system to fight off infection, especially if the diet is low in important nutrients. Additionally, the bacteria that cause periodontal disease thrive in acidic environments. Eating sugars and other foods that increase the acidity in the mouth increases bacterial counts.

- Illnesses—may affect the condition of your gums. This includes diseases such as cancer or AIDS that interfere with the immune system.

- Clenching and grinding teeth—may put excess force on the supporting tissues of the teeth and could speed up the rate at which these tissues are destroyed.

Chapter 29

Dental Emergencies

Chapter Contents

Section 29.1

Saving a Knocked-Out Tooth

Approximately one to three million permanent teeth are accidentally knocked out each year. Both adults and children are at risk.

With proper emergency action, a tooth that has been entirely knocked out of its socket often can be successfully replanted and last for years. Because of this, it is important to be prepared and know what to do if this happens to you or someone with you. The key is to act quickly, yet calmly, and follow these simple steps.

1. Pick up the tooth by the crown (the chewing surface) not the root. The tooth should be handled carefully—touch only the crown—to minimize injury to the root.

2. Clean tooth with water. If dirty, gently rinse the tooth with water, remembering not to handle the root surface.

   • Do not use soap or chemicals.

   • Do not scrub the tooth.

   • Do not dry the tooth.

   • Do not wrap it in a tissue or cloth.

3. Reposition tooth in socket immediately, if possible. The sooner the tooth is replaced, the greater the likelihood it will survive. To reinsert, carefully push the tooth into the socket with fingers, or position above the socket and close mouth slowly. Hold the tooth in place with fingers or by gently biting down on it.

4. Keep tooth moist at all times. The tooth must not be left outside the mouth to dry. If it cannot be replaced on the socket, put it in one of the following:

   • Emergency tooth preservation kit

   • Milk

   • Mouth (next to cheek)

- If none of these is practical, use water (with pinch of salt if possible).

5. See a dentist as soon as possible. Bring the tooth to a dentist or endodontist as soon as possible—ideally within 30 minutes. However, it is possible to save the tooth even if it has been outside the mouth for an hour or more.

Section 29.2

Facial Injuries

Reprinted with permission from the American Association of Oral and Maxillofacial Surgeons. © 1999. For additional information, visit www.aaoms.org.

There are people specially trained to deal with injuries to the mouth, face, and jaw: oral and maxillofacial surgeons.

Their training and experience uniquely qualify them to deal with these types of injuries. These can include a wide range of injuries, from facial cuts and lacerations to more serious problems, like broken teeth and fractured facial bones.

The Serious Side of Facial Injury

One of the most common types of serious injury to the face occurs when bones are broken. Fractures can involve the lower jaw, upper jaw, palate, cheekbones, eye socket, and combinations of these bones. These injuries can affect sight and the ability to breathe, speak, and swallow. Treatment often requires hospitalization.

Specialized Treatment

The principles of treatment for facial fractures are the same as for a broken arm or leg. The parts of the bone must be lined up (reduced) and held in position long enough to permit them time to heal. This may require six or more weeks depending on the patient's age and the fracture's complexity.

When fractures are extensive, multiple incisions to expose the bones and a combination of wiring or plating techniques may be needed. The repositioning technique used by the oral and maxillofacial surgeon depends upon the location and severity of the fracture. In the case of a break of the upper or lower jaw, metal braces may be fastened to the teeth and rubber bands or wires used to hold the jaws together. Patients with few or no teeth may need dentures or specially constructed splints to align and secure the fracture.

What's more, many individuals who sustain facial fractures have other medical problems and the oral and maxillofacial surgeon is trained to coordinate his or her treatment with that of other doctors.

During the healing period, when jaws are wired shut, the oral and maxillofacial surgeon prescribes a nutritional diet.

This helps the injury heal as quickly as possible by keeping the patient in good health. After discharge from the hospital, the doctor gives the patient instructions for dealing with continued facial and oral care.

Don't Treat Any Facial Injury Lightly

Of course, not all facial injuries are extensive. The thing you should remember, though, is that they are all complex. Even in the case of a moderately cut lip, the expertise of the oral and maxillofacial surgeon is indispensable. If sutures are needed, placement must be precise to bring about the desired cosmetic result.

So a good rule of thumb is that you shouldn't take any facial injury lightly. Not only that, but facial injuries are in a critical area of the body. After all, the functions of breathing, eating, speaking, and seeing are located there.

Prevention—The Best Policy

Because avoiding injury is always best, the oral and maxillofacial surgeon is a staunch advocate of the use of automobile seat belts. For the same reason, the use of protective mouth guards and appropriate masks and helmets for athletes is recommended. The oral and maxillofacial surgeon maintains a constant vigilance, warning the public of hidden everyday hazards to their health.

Now, as always, your oral and maxillofacial surgeon's concern is not just with oral health, but extends to the total health of the individual.

Section 29.3

Mouth Protectors

Reprinted with permission from the American Academy of Pediatric
Dentistry, www.aapd.org. © 2002.

What Are Athletic Mouth Protectors?

Athletic mouth protectors, or mouth guards, are made of soft plastic. They are adapted to fit comfortably to the shape of the upper teeth.

Why Are Mouth Guards Important?

Mouth guards hold top priority as sports equipment. They protect not just the teeth, but the lips, cheeks, and tongue. They help protect children from such head and neck injuries as concussions and jaw fractures. Increasingly, organized sports are requiring mouth guards to prevent injury to their athletes. Research shows that most oral injuries occur when athletes are not wearing mouth protection.

When Should My Child Wear a Mouth Guard?

Whenever he or she is in an activity with a risk of falls or of head contact with other players or equipment. This includes football, baseball, basketball, soccer, hockey, skateboarding, even gymnastics. We usually think of football and hockey as the most dangerous to the teeth, but nearly half of sports-related mouth injuries occur in basketball and baseball.

How Do I Choose a Mouth Guard for My Child?

Any mouth guard works better than no mouth guard. So, choose a mouth guard that your child can wear comfortably. If a mouth guard feels bulky or interferes with speech, it will be left in the locker room.

You can select from several options in mouth guards. First, preformed or boil-to-fit mouth guards are found in sports stores. Different types and brands vary in terms of comfort, protection, and cost.

265

Second, customized mouth guards are provided through your pediatric dentist. They cost a bit more, but are more comfortable and more effective in preventing injuries. Your pediatric dentist can advise you on what type of mouth guard is best for your child.

Section 29.4

Sports Safety

Reprinted with permission from the American Association of Oral and Maxillofacial Surgeons. © 1999. For additional information, visit www.aaoms.org.

Despite the new innovations in mouth and face guard technology, many athletes still subject themselves to needless sports-related injuries to the mouth and face.

Members of the American Association of Oral and Maxillofacial Surgeons would like to see helmets, face masks, and mouth guards—every kind of safety gear that reduces the risk of injury—become standard pieces of athletic equipment.

Guard against Injuries

Oral and maxillofacial surgeons are the specialists called in to treat the broken jaws, splint the loosened teeth, and replant the knocked-out tooth. Every day they treat the painful results of needless sports-related injuries. That's why oral and maxillofacial surgeons support the mandatory use of safety equipment. As always, prevention is the best policy.

Protection Is the Best Protection

Elaborate protective equipment is available for sports that involve contact and present a greater probability of injury. Among these sports are:

- **Football.** Helmets with face guards and mouth guards should be worn. Many of the helmets manufactured for younger players have plastic face guards that can be bent back into the face and cause injury. These should be replaced by carbon steel wire guards.

- **Baseball.** A catcher should always wear a mask. Batting helmets with a clear molded plastic face guard are now available; these can also be worn while fielding.

- **Ice Hockey.** Many ice hockey players are beginning to wear cage-like face guards attached to the helmet. These are superior to the hard plastic face masks worn by some goalies as the face guard and the helmet take the pressure of a blow instead of the face. For extra protection both face and mouth guards—including external mouth guards made of hard plastic and secured with straps—can be worn.

- **Wrestling.** More and more high school athletic associations require wrestlers to wear head gear. A strap with a chin cup holds the gear in place and helps to steady the jaw. Recently, face masks have been developed for wrestlers who have suffered facial injuries. Mouth guards should also be worn by wrestlers.

- **Boxing.** Mouth guards are mandatory in this sport. A new pacifier-like mouth guard for pugilists has been designed with a thicker front, including air holes to aid breathing.

- **Lacrosse.** Hard plastic helmets resembling baseball batting helmets, with wire cage face masks, are manufactured for this sport.

- **Field Hockey.** Oral and maxillofacial surgeons recommend that athletes participating in this sport wear mouth guards. Goalies can receive extra protection by wearing Lacrosse helmets.

- **Soccer.** Soccer players should wear mouth guards for protection. Oral and maxillofacial surgeons advise goalies to also wear helmets.

By encouraging athletes to wear mouth guards and other protective equipment, oral surgeons hope to help change the face of sports.

In the event that a facial or mouth injury occurs that requires a trip to the emergency room, the injured athlete, his parent, or coach should be sure to ask that an oral and maxillofacial surgeon is called for consultation. With their background and training, oral and maxillofacial surgeons are the specialists most qualified to deal with these types of injuries. In some cases, they may even detect a hidden injury that might otherwise go unnoticed.

Changing the Face of Sports

From their experience with athletes—ranging from NFL All-Pros to Olympians to the kid playing sandlot ball—oral and maxillofacial surgeons recommend that athletes participating in such sports as basketball, soccer, water polo, handball, rugby, karate, judo, gymnastics, and horseback riding, be fitted with mouth guards.

New synthetic materials and advances in engineering and design have resulted in mouth guards that are sturdier yet lightweight enough to allow ease of breathing. Mouth guards can vary from very inexpensive boil and bite models to custom-fabricated guards made by dentists, which can be adapted to the sport and are generally more comfortable.

A mouth protector should be evaluated from the standpoint of retention, comfort, ability to speak and breathe, tear resistance, and protection provided to the teeth, gums, and lips.

There are five criteria to use when being fitted for a mouth protector. The device should cover the upper and/or lower teeth and gums; be fitted so that it does not misalign the jaw and throw off the bite; be light; be strong; and be easy to clean.

Part Four

Surgical, Orthodontic, and Other Specialized Procedures

Chapter 30

Root Canal Treatment

Chapter Contents

Section 30.1

About Root Canal Treatment

Nothing is as good as a natural tooth! And sometimes your natural tooth may need root canal (endodontic) treatment for it to remain a healthy part of your mouth.

Most patients report that having root canal (endodontic) treatment today is as unremarkable as having a cavity filled.

If you've been told you need root canal (endodontic) treatment, you can find the answers to your questions below.

Who Performs Endodontic Treatment?

All dentists, including your general dentist, received some training in endodontics while in dental school. Often general dentists refer patients needing root canal treatment to endodontists.

What Is an Endodontist?

Endodontists are dentists who specialize in treating the soft inner tissue of your tooth's roots. After they complete dental school, they attend another dental school program for two or three more years. This program is called an advanced specialty education program. They study only endodontic treatment and learn advanced techniques so they can give you the very best care.

Endodontists are specialists. In their offices, they perform only endodontic procedures, both routine and complex. They are also experienced at finding the cause of oral and facial pain that is difficult to diagnose.

Why Is There a Need for Endodontic Treatment?

Sometimes the pulp inside your tooth becomes inflamed or infected. This can be caused by deep decay, repeated dental procedures on the tooth, a crack or chip in the tooth, or a blow to the tooth.

What Are the Signs of Needing Endodontic Treatment?

Signs to look for include pain, prolonged sensitivity to heat or cold, discoloration of the tooth, and swelling and tenderness in the nearby gums. But sometimes, there are no symptoms.

How Does Endodontic Treatment Save the Tooth?

The endodontist removes the inflamed or infected pulp, carefully cleans and shapes the inside of the tooth, then fills and seals the space. Afterward, you return to your general dentist, who will place a crown or other restoration on the tooth to protect it and restore it to full function.

Will I Feel Pain during or after the Procedure?

While many patients may be in great pain before seeing an endodontist, most report that the pain is relieved by the endodontist and that they are comfortable during the procedure. For the first few days after treatment, the tooth may feel sensitive, especially if there was pain or infection before the procedure. This discomfort can be relieved with over-the-counter or prescription medications. The endodontist will tell you how to care for your tooth at home.

How Much Will the Procedure Cost?

The cost varies depending on how severe the problem is and which tooth is affected. Many dental insurance policies cover endodontic treatment. Generally, treatment and restoration of your natural tooth is the least expensive option. The only alternative is having the tooth extracted and replaced with a bridge, implant, or removable partial denture to restore chewing function and prevent adjacent teeth from shifting.

Will the Tooth Need Any Special Care or Additional Treatment?

You should not chew or bite on the treated tooth until you have had it restored by your general dentist because your tooth could fracture. Otherwise, just practice good oral hygiene—brushing, flossing, and regular checkups and cleanings. Endodontically treated teeth can last for many years, even a lifetime.

What Causes an Endodontically Treated Tooth to Need Additional Treatment?

New trauma, deep decay, or a loose, cracked, or broken filling can cause new infection in your tooth. In some cases, your endodontist may discover very narrow or curved canals that could not be treated during the initial procedure. Sometimes a treated tooth may need endodontic surgery to be saved.

What Is Endodontic Surgery?

The most common endodontic surgical procedure is an apicoectomy or root-end resection. It is used to relieve inflammation or infection in the bony area around the end of your tooth that continues after endodontic treatment. The endodontist opens the gum tissue and removes the infected tissue and may remove the very end of the root. A small filling may be placed to seal the root canal.

Endodontists use local anesthetics, like those used when you have a cavity filled. Most patients return to their normal activities the next day.

Section 30.2

Endodontic Surgery

Why Do I Need Endodontic Surgery?

Before understanding endodontic surgery, it is important to understand nonsurgical endodontic treatment. Nonsurgical endodontic treatment is more commonly known as root canal treatment. It is necessary when the soft inner tissue of the tooth, the pulp, becomes inflamed or infected. Endodontic treatment involves removal of the damaged pulp. The canals are then cleaned, filled, and sealed to preserve the tooth.

Sometimes endodontic treatment alone cannot save your tooth, and your dentist or endodontist may recommend endodontic surgery. Endodontic surgery includes any surgical procedures used to remove infection from your root canals and surrounding areas. Surgery can also be used in diagnosing problems that do not appear on your x-ray, such as root fractures, or in treating problems in the surrounding bone.

Who Performs Endodontic Surgery?

All dentists are trained in endodontic treatment. Because endodontic surgery can often be more challenging than routine treatment, many dentists refer patients needing surgery to endodontists. Endodontists are dental specialists who diagnose and treat oral pain. They specialize in endodontic (root canal) treatment, including any treatment for the inner tissues of the tooth. In addition to dental school, endodontists receive two or more years of advanced education. They study root canal techniques and procedures in greater depth, including the area of endodontic surgery.

What Is an Apicoectomy?

An apicoectomy is the most common endodontic surgical procedure. This procedure is used to remove infection or inflammation from the bony area around the end of your tooth. The endodontist starts by opening the gum tissue near the tooth. This allows him or her to see the underlying bone. Next, your endodontist will remove any inflamed or infected tissue. The very end of the root is also removed.

After the inflamed or infected tissue is removed, a small filling may be placed in the root end to seal the root canal. A few stitches are placed in the gum to help the tissue heal properly. Within a few months, the bone heals around the end of the root.

Are There Other Types of Endodontic Surgery?

There are several other types of surgery that are performed, depending upon the situation. Your endodontist will be happy to discuss the specific type of surgery that you might need.

Will Endodontic Surgery Hurt?

Your endodontist will provide you with local anesthetics that will make the procedure comfortable. You may feel some discomfort or experience slight swelling after the procedure, but this is normal for any surgical procedure. If necessary, your endodontist will recommend appropriate pain medication to alleviate your discomfort.

What Do I Do after the Surgery?

Your endodontist will give you specific postoperative instructions to follow. If you have questions or if you have pain that does not respond to medication, call your endodontist.

Can I Drive Myself Home?

Patients who have had endodontic surgery are usually able to drive themselves home. But it is a good idea to talk to your endodontist about this prior to your appointment to decide if other transportation arrangements will be necessary.

When Can I Return to My Normal Activities?

Most patients return to their normal daily activities one or two days after their surgery. Your endodontist will discuss your expected recovery time with you.

Does Insurance Cover Endodontic Surgery?

Many insurance plans do cover endodontic surgery. Each insurance plan is different, however. You should consult with your employer or insurance company prior to treatment.

What Are the Chances That the Surgery Will Be Successful?

Your dentist and endodontist have suggested endodontic surgery because they believe it is the best option for you. Your endodontist will discuss your chances for a successful surgery so you can make an informed decision. Keep in mind that there are no guarantees with any surgical procedure.

What Are the Alternatives If I Choose Not to Have Surgery?

Most often, the only alternative to surgery is extraction of the tooth. You must then replace the extracted tooth with an implant, bridge, or removable partial denture. These will restore chewing function and prevent adjacent teeth from shifting. Because these alternatives require surgery or dental procedures on adjacent healthy teeth, endodontic surgery is usually the most cost-effective option. No matter how effective modern tooth replacements are, nothing is as good as your natural tooth.

Section 30.3

Endodontic Retreatment

If you have a tooth that has had endodontic (root canal) treatment, it can last as long as your other natural teeth. In some cases, however, complete healing may not occur. There may be new problems months or even years after the initial treatment. When this happens, it is sometimes possible for your endodontist to perform the treatment again with more successful results. This process is called retreatment.

Who Performs Endodontic Retreatment?

All dentists are educated in endodontic treatment. Retreatment, however, can be more challenging than the initial treatment. For this reason, many dentists refer their patients in need of retreatment to endodontists.

What Is an Endodontist?

Endodontists are dental specialists who diagnose and treat oral and facial pain. They specialize in endodontic (root canal) treatment, including any treatment for the soft inner tissues of the tooth, the pulp. In addition to dental school, endodontists receive another two or more years of advanced education. They study root canal techniques and procedures in greater depth, including the area of retreatment.

Why Does My Tooth Need Retreatment?

Occasionally, healing may not occur as expected after an initial root canal procedure. This can happen for a variety of reasons—new decay, a broken or cracked crown, or canals that were not detected during the first procedure. By performing the procedure a second time, endodontists can often save your tooth.

What Happens during Endodontic Retreatment?

First, your endodontist will remove the restoration or crown and the filling materials inside your tooth to reclean the canals and take a closer look at the inside of your tooth. Examination of the inside of your tooth may determine what caused the first treatment to fail.

Next, your endodontist will fill and seal the canals with a rubbery material called gutta-percha, and then place a temporary filling in the tooth.

The entire root canal procedure may require just one or perhaps several trips to your endodontist's office. Talk to your endodontist for information on your retreatment.

After retreatment, your family dentist should place a new crown or other restoration on your tooth. Returning to your dentist is very important because the crown will restore your tooth and help protect it from more damage.

Is Retreatment the Best Treatment Option for Me?

The decision to retreat should be made by you, your dentist, and your endodontist. While retreated teeth can last a lifetime, there is no guarantee that treatment will be more successful the second time. The treatment option for any particular patient must be chosen on an individual basis.

How Much Will Retreatment Cost?

The cost of retreatment varies depending on the complexity of the procedure. It will probably cost more than the initial procedure, because your restoration and root filling materials must be removed before the second treatment can begin. Also, your endodontist may need to spend more time searching for problems that may have caused the initial treatment to fail.

The only alternatives to retreatment are having the tooth extracted or having it retreated surgically, if the root cannot be accessed through the crown. If the tooth is extracted, it must be replaced with a bridge, implant, or removable partial denture. This will restore chewing function and prevent adjacent teeth from shifting.

Generally, nonsurgical retreatment and restoration of your natural tooth is the least expensive option. Your dentist will be happy to discuss the various treatment options and their costs with you.

Chapter 31

Extractions and Restorations

Chapter Contents

Section 31.1

Tooth Extractions

From *Gale Encyclopedia of Medicine, 2ⁿᵈ Edition,* by Bethany Thivierge, 5, Gale Group, © 2002, Gale Group. Reprinted by permission of The Gale Group.

Definition

Tooth extraction is the removal of a tooth from its socket in the bone.

Purpose

Extraction is performed for positional, structural, or economic reasons. Teeth are often removed because they are impacted. Teeth become impacted when they are prevented from growing into their normal position in the mouth by gum tissue, bone, or other teeth. Impaction is a common reason for the extraction of wisdom teeth. Extraction is the only known method that will prevent further problems. Teeth may also be extracted to make more room in the mouth prior to straightening the remaining teeth (orthodontic treatment), or because they are so badly positioned that straightening is impossible. Extraction may be used to remove teeth that are so badly decayed or broken that they cannot be restored. In addition, patients sometimes choose extraction as a less expensive alternative to filling or placing a crown on a severely decayed tooth.

Precautions

In some situations, tooth extractions may need to be postponed temporarily. These situations include:

- Infection that has progressed from the tooth into the bone. Infections may make anesthesia difficult. They can be treated with antibiotics before the tooth is extracted.

- The patient's use of drugs that thin the blood (anticoagulants). These medications include warfarin (Coumadin) and aspirin.

The patient should stop using these medications for three days prior to extraction.

- Patients who have had any of the following procedures in the previous six months: heart valve replacement, open heart surgery, prosthetic joint replacement, or placement of a medical shunt. These patients may be given antibiotics to reduce the risk of bacterial infection.

Description

Tooth extraction can be performed with local anesthesia if the tooth is exposed and appears to be easily removable in one piece. An instrument called an elevator is used to loosen (luxate) the tooth, widen the space in the bone, and break the tiny elastic fibers that attach the tooth to the bone. Once the tooth is dislocated from the bone, it can be lifted and removed with forceps.

If the extraction is likely to be difficult, the dentist may refer the patient to an oral surgeon. Oral surgeons are specialists who are trained to give nitrous oxide, an intravenous sedative, or a general anesthetic to relieve pain. Extracting an impacted tooth or a tooth with curved roots typically requires cutting through gum tissue to expose the tooth. It may also require removing portions of bone to free the tooth. Some teeth must be cut and removed in sections. The extraction site may or may not require one or more stitches to close the cut (incision).

Preparation

Before an extraction, the dentist will take the patient's medical history, noting allergies and prescription medications. A dental history is also taken, with particular attention to previous extractions and reactions to anesthetics. The dentist may then prescribe antibiotics or recommend stopping certain medications prior to the extraction. The tooth is x-rayed to determine its full shape and position, especially if it is impacted.

If the patient is going to have deep anesthesia, he or she should wear loose clothing with sleeves that are easily rolled up to allow for an intravenous line. The patient should not eat or drink anything for at least six hours before the procedure. Arrangements should be made for a friend or relative to drive the patient home after the surgery.

Aftercare

An important aspect of aftercare is encouraging a clot to form at the extraction site. The patient should put pressure on the area by biting gently on a roll or wad of gauze for several hours after surgery. Once the clot is formed, it should not be disturbed. The patient should not rinse, spit, drink with a straw, or smoke for at least 24 hours after the extraction and preferably longer. Vigorous exercise should not be done for the first three to five days.

For the first two days after the procedure, the patient should drink liquids without using a straw, and eat soft foods. Any chewing must be done on the side away from the extraction site. Hard or sticky foods should be avoided. The mouth may be gently cleaned with a toothbrush, but the extraction area should not be scrubbed.

Wrapped ice packs can be applied to reduce facial swelling. Swelling is a normal part of the healing process. It is most noticeable in the first 48 to 72 hours. As the swelling subsides, the patient may experience muscle stiffness. Moist heat and gentle exercise will restore jaw movement. The dentist may prescribe medications to relieve the postoperative pain.

Risks

Potential complications of tooth extraction include postoperative infection, temporary numbness from nerve irritation, jaw fracture, and jaw joint pain. An additional complication is called dry socket. When a blood clot does not properly form in the empty tooth socket, the bone beneath the socket is painfully exposed to air and food, and the extraction site heals more slowly.

Normal Results

After an extraction, the wound usually closes in about two weeks. It takes three to six months for the bone and soft tissue to be restructured. Complications such as infection or dry socket may prolong the healing time.

Key Terms

Dry socket: A painful condition following tooth extraction in which a blood clot does not properly fill the empty socket. Dry socket leaves the underlying bone exposed to air and food.

Extraction site: The empty tooth socket following removal of the tooth.

Impacted tooth: A tooth that is growing against another tooth, bone, or soft tissue.

Luxate: To loosen or dislocate the tooth from the socket.

Nitrous oxide: A colorless, sweet-smelling gas used by dentists for mild anesthesia. It is sometimes called laughing gas because it makes some patients feel giddy or silly.

Oral surgeon: A dentist who specializes in surgical procedures of the mouth, including extractions.

Orthodontic treatment: The process of straightening teeth to correct their appearance and function.

Section 31.2

Wisdom Teeth

Reprinted with permission from the American Association of Oral and Maxillofacial Surgeons. © 1999. For additional information, visit www. aaoms.org.

Most people start getting their third molars (also called wisdom teeth) when they reach their late teens or early twenties. In many cases, the jaws are not large enough to accommodate these teeth and they remain under the gum (impacted).

What Is an Impacted Tooth?

When a tooth develops, it travels to its appropriate position in the dental arch. If the path to eruption through the gum is prevented due to the size of the jaw, the tooth will become partially or totally blocked (impacted).

How Serious Is an Impacted Tooth?

Serious problems can develop from partially blocked teeth such as infection, and possible crowding of and damage to adjacent teeth. More serious complications can develop when the sac that surrounds the impacted tooth fills with fluid and enlarges to form a cyst, causing an enlargement that hollows out the jaw and results in permanent damage to the adjacent teeth, jawbone, and nerves. Left untreated, a tumor may develop from the walls of these cysts and a more complicated surgical procedure would be required for removal.

Must the Tooth Come out If It Hasn't Caused Any Problems Yet?

No one can tell you when your impacted molar will cause trouble, but trouble will probably arise. When it does, the circumstances can be much more painful and the teeth can be more complicated to treat.

When Should I Have My Impacted Teeth Removed?

The key to timely attention to third molars is regular x-rays of the mouth. With the help of these pictures the oral and maxillofacial surgeon can frequently predict if the wisdom teeth are going to cause trouble, either in the near future or later in life. If so, chances are the oral and maxillofacial surgeon will recommend their removal rather than wait for trouble to occur.

Removal is easier in younger patients. Roots are not yet fully developed and the bone is less dense. In older patients, removal before complications develop is key to shorter recovery and healing time and minimizing discomfort after surgery.

What Happens after Surgery?

Generally after surgery the patient experiences some swelling and discomfort. However, with personalized postoperative instructions and medications, the oral and maxillofacial surgeon can reduce the possible discomfort following surgery.

Section 31.3

Tooth Replacements and Restorations

From *Gale Encyclopedia of Medicine, 2nd Edition,* by Bethany Thivierge, 5, Gale Group, © 2002, Gale Group. Reprinted by permission of The Gale Group.

Definition

A tooth restoration is any artificial substance or structure that replaces missing teeth or part of a tooth in order to protect the mouth's ability to eat, chew, and speak. Restorations include fillings, inlays, crowns, bridges, partial and complete dentures, and dental implants.

Purpose

Restorations have somewhat different purposes depending on their extensiveness. Fillings, inlays, and crowns are intended to repair damage to individual teeth. They replace tooth structure lost by decay or injury, protect the part of the tooth that remains, and restore the tooth's shape and function. Bridges, dentures, and implants are intended to protect the shape and function of the mouth as a whole.

Precautions

Some patients are allergic to the medications used for local anesthesia in dental restorations. In addition, many people in the general population are afraid of dental work. Most dentists in present-day practice can help patients with this specific fear.

Description

Fillings

Fillings are restorations that are done to repair damage caused by tooth decay (dental caries). Tooth decay occurs when microorganisms in the mouth convert sugar from food to acid, which attacks the tooth. The acid forms cavities that start in the hard outer surface of the tooth (the enamel) and may extend inward to the pulp, which contains the tooth's nerves and blood vessels. Left untreated, tooth decay may lead to inflammation and infection that may cause toothache and perhaps more serious complications.

To stop the decay process, the dentist removes the decayed portion of the tooth using a high-speed drill or an air abrasion system, shapes the cavity walls, and replaces the tooth structure with a filling of silver amalgam, composite resin, or gold. The filling is placed in the cavity as a liquid or soft solid. It sets within a few minutes and continues to harden over the next several hours. Silver amalgam is commonly used to fill cavities on the biting surfaces of the back teeth, because it is strong enough to withstand the tremendous pressures exerted by grinding and chewing. Composite resin is typically used to fill cavities in front teeth and any other teeth that are visible when the patient smiles, because its color can be matched to the tooth surface. Gold as a filling material is far less common, but is being increasingly used. Although it is more expensive and less easily applied, it does not trigger the sensitivity reactions that some patients have to silver amalgam.

Inlays

An inlay resembles a filling in that it fills the space remaining after the decayed portion of a tooth has been removed. The difference is that an inlay is shaped outside the patient's mouth and then cemented into place. After the decay is removed and the cavity walls are shaped, the dentist makes a wax pattern of the space. A model is cast from the wax pattern. An inlay, usually of gold, is made from this mold and sealed into the tooth with dental cement.

Crowns

The crown of a tooth is the portion that is covered by enamel. A restorative crown replaces this outer part to protect the tooth. This protection becomes necessary when a tooth cracks or has its entire structure weakened by decay. As with a filling or inlay, the dentist first removes the decayed portion of the tooth. The tooth is then prepared for a crown. It may be tapered on the outside edges to a peg, reinforced with a cast metal core, or rebuilt with both a cast metal core and a post. A wax impression of the prepared tooth and the teeth next to it is made. The new crown is made to fit this mold. The crown may be made of gold or stainless steel alone, metal with a veneer of tooth-colored porcelain or resin, or of porcelain or resin alone. The finished crown is then placed over the prepared tooth, adjusted, and cemented into place.

Bridges

Bridges are a type of restoration that is done when one or more permanent teeth are lost or pulled. The resulting gap must be filled in to prevent the remaining teeth from shifting. If the other teeth shift, they will affect the patient's bit (occlusion), which sometimes produces pain in the jaw joint. As the teeth move and become crooked, they also become more difficult to keep clean. The risk of tooth decay and gum disease increases, increasing the likelihood that additional teeth will be lost. A bridge is inserted to prevent this risk. Bridges are nonremovable appliances of one or more artificial teeth (pontics) anchored by crowns on the adjacent teeth (abutment teeth). The abutment teeth carry the pressure when the patient chews food.

Partial Dentures

A partial denture is similar to a bridge in that it fills a gap left by missing teeth with artificial teeth on a metal frame. A partial denture is removable, however. It attaches to a crown on the abutment tooth with a metal clasp or precision attachment. A partial denture is primarily used at the end of a row of natural teeth, where there is only one abutment tooth. The pressure exerted by chewing is shared by this abutment and the soft tissues of the gum ridge beneath the appliance.

Complete Dentures

Complete dentures may be worn when all of the top or bottom teeth have been lost. A complete denture consists of artificial teeth mounted in a plastic base molded to fit the remaining oral anatomy. It may or may not be held in place with a denture adhesive.

Implants

Dental implants are a means of securing crowns, bridges, and dentures in the mouth. A hard plastic or metal fixture is implanted through the soft tissue into the bone. Over time, the bone grows around this fixture, firmly anchoring it. The exposed end of this fixture is covered with a crown and may serve as a stable abutment for a bridge or denture.

Preparation

Before a restoration is placed in the mouth, the dentist removes all traces of decay and shapes the remaining tooth structure for the restoration. Fillings are the only restoration created within the tooth itself—the others are made up in a laboratory using a model of the tooth structure. Thus, a filling may be placed in a single dental visit, while the other restorations usually take several appointments. Temporary crowns and dentures are put in place after the tooth is shaped until the permanent restoration is delivered by the laboratory.

Aftercare

Fillings

Fillings need to time to harden for several hours after being placed, so the patient should chew food on the opposite side of the mouth for the first day.

Dentures

A partial or complete denture may take several weeks of getting used to. Inserting and removing the denture will take practice. Speaking clearly may be difficult at first—the patient may find it helpful to read out loud for practice. Eating may also feel awkward. The patient should begin by eating small pieces of soft foods. Very hard or sticky foods should be avoided.

Patients with dentures must work on good oral hygiene. Specialty brushes and floss threaders may be used to remove plaque and food from around crowns and bridges. Dentures should be removed and brushed daily with a specially designed brush and a denture cleaner or other mild soap.

The patient should see the dentist for an adjustment if there is any discomfort or irritation resulting from a restoration. Otherwise, the patient should see the dentist at least twice a year for an oral examination.

Risks

Restoration procedures typically require local anesthesia. Some people may have allergic reactions to the medication. A very small number of people are allergic to one or more of the metals used in a dental restoration. In most cases, the dentist can use another material.

Normal Results

A well-made restoration should feel comfortable and last a relatively long time with proper care. Artificial dental restorations only approximate the original tooth, however. A complete denture will never feel as comfortable or work as well as natural teeth. It is better, therefore, to prevent the need for restorative dental work than to replace teeth. Restorations are expensive, may require many appointments, and still need careful cleaning and attention.

Key Terms

Abutment teeth: A crowned tooth that stabilizes a bridge or partial denture.

Bridge: An appliance of one or more artificial teeth anchored by crowns on the adjacent teeth.

Complete denture: A full set of upper or lower teeth, mounted in a plastic base. Dentures are also called false teeth.

Crown: A protective shell that fits over the tooth.

Dental caries: A disease of the teeth in which microorganisms convert sugar in the mouth to acid that erodes the tooth.

Enamel: The hard outermost surface of a tooth.

Filling: Dental material that occupies the space remaining within a tooth after the decayed portion has been removed.

Implant: A fixture with one end implanted into the bone and the other end covered with a crown, often to serve as a stable abutment for a bridge or denture.

Inlay: A filling that is made outside of the tooth and then cemented into place.

Occlusion: The way upper and lower teeth fit together during biting and chewing.

Partial denture: A removable bridge that usually clasps onto only one abutment.

Pontic: An artificial tooth.

Pulp: The soft innermost layer of a tooth that contains its blood vessels and nerves.

Section 31.4

What to Do after Tooth Extraction

"Instructions to Patients Following Oral Surgery " is reprinted with permission from HIVdent, www.hivdent.org. © 2000 HIVdent. Available online at http://www.hivdent.org/_peag/faq-Instos; accessed May 2003.

- Leave the gauze in your mouth in place for at least 30 minutes. Keep a firm but steady pressure on the gauze and when you remove it, remove it **gently** without disturbing the blood clot.

- Place an ice bag or a cold towel on your face over the operated area for 4 to 6 hours. This will help prevent excess swelling. The earlier this is started the more effective it will be. You may remove the cold pack 15 minutes for every hour it is necessary for your comfort.

- Do not rinse your mouth the day of surgery. Rinsing may dislodge the blood clot and interrupt the normal process of healing. You are encouraged, however, to drink (swallow) fluids.

- Spit as little as possible. (Blood cannot clot if you are constantly spitting it out.) If abnormal bleeding occurs, fold a sponge, wet it, place it over the socket, and bite down for 30 minutes with even pressure. If abnormal bleeding persists, don't hesitate to call your oral surgeon.

- On the day following surgery rinse your mouth **gently** after each meal with warm salt water (1/2 teaspoon of salt in a glass of warm water). This should also be done at bedtime. It should be emphasized that this rinsing be done gently. Rinsing with a mouth wash four times per day is also recommended. In addition, discontinue ice, and start warm heat (warm moist towels) to the operative area.

- Follow your own inclinations as to diet, but for your own comfort, soft foods or liquids are indicated for the first 24 to 48 hours. Keep up your food intake and drink plenty of fluids.

- The teeth should be given their usual care except in the region of surgery.

- Please carefully follow the directions on any prescriptions you may have been given.

- Occasionally there is numbness following a difficult extraction. This numbness may last for several weeks or longer, but is almost always temporary.

- Small pieces of bone may work their way out through the gum following an extraction. This normal and usually requires no treatment.

- If suture removal is necessary, please be advised that this is a painless process. Please be sure you make an appointment for a postoperative checkup.

- If you have any difficulties, call your oral surgeon.

Chapter 32

Oral Surgery

Chapter Contents

Section 32.1

The Oral and Maxillofacial Surgeon

"The Oral and Maxillofacial Surgeon: A Partner in the Healthcare Team" is reprinted with permission from the American Association of Oral and Maxillofacial Surgeons. © 1999. For additional information, visit www. aaoms.org.

This section is about the specialty of oral and maxillofacial surgery and its role in patient care. Patients who present to the primary care provider with complaints of pain or dysfunction in the oral and maxillofacial region are often candidates for referral to an oral and maxillofacial surgeon.

The following information will provide helpful guidelines for establishing a working relationship with an oral and maxillofacial surgeon in your area.

Training and Scope of Practice

After four years of postgraduate dental education, an oral and maxillofacial surgeon completes four or more years of intensive, postdoctoral, hospital-based surgical residency training. Oral and maxillofacial surgery residents spend significant time rotating through related medical fields such as internal medicine, general surgery, anesthesiology, otolaryngology, plastic surgery, and emergency medicine.

Depending on the residency program, some surgeons may also opt to complete the necessary requirements to earn a medical or other advanced degree. Some may also subsequently complete fellowships in subspecialty areas.

The scope of oral and maxillofacial surgery encompasses the diagnosis, surgical and related management of diseases, injuries, and defects that involve both the functional and esthetic aspects of the oral and maxillofacial regions. This includes preventive, reconstructive, or emergency care for the teeth, mouth, jaws, and facial structures.

Office Surgery

Oral and maxillofacial surgeons can perform a wide variety of procedures in an office setting as well as in a hospital environment. Local anesthesia, nitrous oxide, intravenous sedation, and general anesthesia are options available in the oral and maxillofacial surgery office for the appropriate patient and treatment.

Office surgery can be the most efficient and cost-effective way to perform many procedures while maintaining maximum patient comfort and safety. In addition, many oral and maxillofacial surgeons perform laser surgery in the private office setting. A number of soft tissue procedures, such as biopsy of oral tissues, can be done quickly and with less postoperative discomfort by using laser techniques.

Dentoalveolar Surgery

A tooth that fails to emerge or fully break through the gum tissue is, by definition, impacted. This is a common problem associated with third molars, or wisdom teeth, as they are the last teeth to develop and erupt into the mouth. Other teeth, however, such as cuspids and bicuspids, can also become impacted. The usual symptoms associated with impacted teeth are pain, swelling, and signs of infection in the surrounding tissues. An impacted tooth
has the potential to cause permanent damage to adjacent teeth, gum tissue, and supporting bone structure. Impacted teeth are also associated with the development of cysts and tumors that can destroy large portions of the jaw. Many times impacted teeth are not addressed until symptoms are present, but early removal may be indicated if radiographs predict potential problems. Oral and maxillofacial surgeons have extensive training in the diagnosis and management of impacted teeth and in tooth extraction and dentoalveolar surgery.

Reconstructive Surgery

Inadequate bone structure in the upper and/or lower jaws can be a result of injury, ablative tumor surgery, or long-term denture wearing. Osseous grafts using either autologous bone or bone substitutes can be performed to improve both the quantity and quality of the hard tissue. Skin grafts and soft tissue corrections can be utilized to improve the architecture of the intraoral soft tissues. Through oral reconstructive surgery, a solid foundation can be provided for dental rehabilitation, which in turn aids nutrition and speech. If the patient is a good candidate, dental implants may be used to replace lost teeth and improve function. Implants can also be used to anchor intraoral and extraoral prostheses.

Dental Implants

Millions of Americans suffer from permanent tooth loss. Dental implants offer an excellent alternative to natural teeth. Dental implants are made of materials that are compatible with human bone and tissue. Small posts are attached to the implants and serve as stable anchors for artificial replacement teeth.

Working as a team member with the restorative dentist, the oral and maxillofacial surgeon can evaluate the patient and place implants in conjunction with necessary bone grafting of the jaw. Dental implant surgery is often done in the doctor's office, dependent upon the patient's individual needs.

Facial Infections

Infections in the maxillofacial region can develop into life-threatening emergencies if not treated promptly and effectively. Pain and swelling in the face, jaws, or neck may indicate an infection of dental or related origin. If the infection is severe, an oral and maxillofacial surgeon is able to work within the hospital setting to diagnose and treat the problem. Appropriate imaging studies and culture and antibiotic sensitivity tests are routinely done. Surgical treatment may include intraoral or extraoral incision and drainage as well as extraction of involved teeth. For less severe infections, evaluation and treatment may be done in the office setting.

Depending on the diagnosis and severity of the case, oral and maxillofacial surgeons may work with other specialists to provide comprehensive patient care.

Facial Trauma

Because of their expanded dental/medical background and hospital-based training, oral and maxillofacial surgeons are uniquely qualified to deal with injuries to the face, jaws, mouth, and teeth. Dental occlusion is the most important piece of the puzzle in dealing with complex facial fractures. Oral and maxillofacial surgeons have extensive training in repairing traumatic injuries, including fractures of the mandible, maxilla and orbits as well as closure of extraoral lacerations.

Childhood injuries resulting from skateboarding, sports or bicycle accidents often involve dental or maxillofacial trauma. Younger children often sustain damage to teeth or supporting structures from falls. Such traumatic injuries can usually be effectively treated in the oral and maxillofacial surgery office, avoiding costly emergency room visits. For the pediatric patient, various sedation techniques can be employed to deliver prompt and effective treatment in the private office setting.

Facial Pain

Oral and maxillofacial surgeons are trained to diagnose and treat complaints of facial pain. A common cause of facial pain and headaches is disease or dysfunction of the temporomandibular joint (TMJ). TMJ disorders have a wide range of symptoms that may include earaches, headaches, and limitation of jaw opening. Patients may also complain of clicking or grating sounds in the joint or pain on opening or closing the mouth.

Causes of TMJ dysfunction can be degenerative (osteoarthritis), traumatic (meniscal displacement or injury), inflammatory (rheumatoid arthritis), or stress-related. Some patients experience a combination of muscle and joint problems.

Diagnosis involves clinical examination, necessary imaging studies (radiograph, CT, MRI) and nerve blocks. Once a specific problem is identified, recommendations can then be made for treatment. Usually, conservative management (soft diet, anti-inflammatory drugs, physical and/or bite splint therapy) is the first step. With certain conditions, joint surgery may be an appropriate option.

Arthroscopic joint surgery is minimally invasive and has proven effective in the resolution of certain conditions involving TMJ pain and dysfunction. The procedure can be done on an outpatient-surgery basis at a hospital or ambulatory surgery center under general anesthesia. More complex joint surgery may be indicated for advanced conditions.

Oral Pathology

Differential diagnosis of pathology in the maxillofacial region is an important part of the practice of oral and maxillofacial surgery. If indicated, biopsies and/or other tests can be performed to arrive at a definitive diagnosis and appropriate treatment plan. Early detection and treatment of oral lesions greatly improve the patient's prognosis. Lesions may be managed medically or surgically excised.

Orofacial Deformities

Discrepancies in skeletal growth between the upper and lower jaws may lead to both functional and psychological difficulties. Functionally, this may involve problems with chewing, swallowing, speech, or temporomandibular joint (TMJ) function. Patients may also exhibit psychological difficulties stemming from esthetic and social concerns.

Some abnormalities may involve only misaligned teeth and can be corrected orthodontically with braces or other appliances. Serious growth disturbances require surgery to realign the upper and/or lower jaw into a more normal relationship. Common dentofacial deformities, including under or overdevelopment of the jaws (prognathism, micrognathia, retrognathia) or misaligned teeth (over-bite or under-bite), can cause difficulty in eating, swallowing, speaking, and breathing. Surgical correction of these problems (orthognathic surgery) is often performed in conjunction with treatment by an orthodontist and restorative dentist. Through careful diagnosis and surgical treatment planning, the outcome may be reasonably predicted. Orthognathic surgery is usually performed in a hospital or ambulatory surgical center under general anesthesia. The end result is a more balanced, functional skeletal relationship.

Congenital deformities like cleft lip and palate result when all or a portion of the oral-nasal cavity does not grow together during fetal development. As part of a team of healthcare specialists, oral and maxillofacial surgeons play an important role in the carefully orchestrated, multiple-stage correctional program for these patients. The goal: to facilitate the complete restoration of the jaw and facial structures, leading to normal function and appearance. Care and treatment must include consideration of function, appearance, nutrition, speech and hearing, as well as emotional and psychological development.

Snoring/Obstructive Sleep Apnea

Obstructive breathing patterns during sleep occur in approximately 45% of the population and can range from snoring to periods of true apnea. Obstructive sleep apnea can lead to excessive daytime sleepiness, poor work performance, and cardiovascular disorders such as hypertension, arrhythmias, and congestive heart failure. Oral and maxillofacial surgeons are trained in both the diagnosis and treatment of this condition. When conservative methods fail to correct the problem, surgery may be indicated.

Surgical procedures can involve the soft tissue of the oropharynx (palatopharyngoplasty, laser-assisted uvulopalatoplasty, radio frequency ablation) or the hard tissue of the lower jaw (mandibular and/ or chin advancement). Oral and maxillofacial surgeons have the expertise to work with other medical specialists to provide treatment for obstructive sleep apnea.

Cosmetic Maxillofacial Surgery

Because of their surgical and dental background, oral and maxillofacial surgeons are finely attuned to the importance of harmony between facial appearance and function. Before any cosmetic procedure is performed, the oral and maxillofacial surgeon will request a thorough medical history to evaluate the patient's overall general health. A careful physical exam will be conducted. The procedure to be performed will be discussed, as well as the anticipated results, expected changes in appearance, type of anesthesia to be used, and possible risks and complications.

Cosmetic maxillofacial surgery may be performed on an outpatient basis in the oral and maxillofacial surgeon's office, surgical facility, or surgery center, or on an inpatient basis in the hospital, depending upon the surgeon's and patient's preference. Surgery may be performed under general anesthesia, IV sedation, or local anesthesia.

An Important Link

Oral and maxillofacial surgeons are an important link in the referral network for primary care providers. Through appropriate referrals, patients can be provided with expedient and cost-effective health care for conditions relating to the specialty of oral and maxillofacial surgery.

Section 32.2

What Is Oral and Maxillofacial Surgery?

Reprinted with permission from the American Association of Oral and Maxillofacial Surgeons. © 1999. For additional information, visit www.aaoms.org.

An oral and maxillofacial surgeon is a specialist whose knowledge is built on the firmest of foundations—four years of dental education plus four or more years of postdoctorate in-hospital surgical residency training.

Oral and maxillofacial surgeons specialize in disorders of the mouth, teeth, jaws, and facial structures. They care for people with problem wisdom teeth, facial pain, and misaligned jaws. They treat accident victims suffering facial injuries, offering reconstructive and cosmetic solutions. They are concerned about helping children born with poorly shaped jaws and they care for patients with cancer. Their concern extends to their patients' total health.

Words of Wisdom on Impacted Teeth

A tooth that fails to emerge or fully break through the gum tissue is termed impacted. Often this happens to third molars, also known as wisdom teeth, as they are the last teeth to develop and appear in the mouth. A common problem associated with impacted wisdom teeth involves swelling, pain and infection of the surrounding gum tissue. An impacted wisdom tooth may cause permanent damage to adjacent teeth, gums, and supporting bone and may sometimes lead to the formation of cysts or tumors that can destroy large portions of the jaw.

Many problems with wisdom teeth can occur with few or no symptoms. Regular x-rays of the mouth can frequently predict if wisdom teeth will cause trouble.

Unequal Jaw Growth—A Cause for Concern

When an individual's jaw fails to grow properly, both functional and psychological difficulties may be experienced. Functionally, this abnormality may interfere with proper chewing, create difficulties swallowing, cause a speech defect, result in chronic mouth breathing and lead to jaw pain. Psychological difficulties that can accompany this kind of problem are also important considerations.

Some abnormalities may involve only misaligned teeth and can be corrected orthodontically with braces or other appliances. More serious problems may require surgery to move all or part of the upper jaw, lower jaw, or both into a more normal position.

Surgical correction of jaw irregularities (orthognathic surgery) is undertaken after thorough study and consultation with an orthodontist and restorative dentist. Once the precise nature of the abnormality is determined, the surgical strategy is planned and the outcome may be reasonably predicted. Surgery can be performed in a hospital or ambulatory surgical center under general anesthesia.

Corrective jaw surgery moves teeth and jaws into a new position that is more balanced, functional, and healthy.

Looking and Feeling Your Best

Cosmetic maxillofacial surgery can repair physical malformations resulting from disease, injury, burns, birth defects, or aging. It may also serve to restore normal function and improve individual appearance.

Because of their surgical and dental background, oral and maxillofacial surgeons are uniquely qualified in the treatment of the face, mouth, teeth, and jaws. Extensive education and training in surgical procedures involving both the soft tissue (skin and muscle) and hard tissue (bone and cartilage) of the maxillofacial area makes the oral and maxillofacial surgeon finely attuned to the importance of harmony between facial form and function.

Helping Denture Wearers Find the Perfect Fit

An estimated 24 million adult Americans are totally without teeth. Almost half of the adult population are missing at least one tooth. When someone is about to have dentures for the first time, an oral and maxillofacial surgeon can correct bony and soft tissue irregularities of the jaws to provide a good, solid foundation for dentures.

Long-time denture wearers frequently experience loss of supporting bone, and dentures may no longer fit comfortably. In these cases, the jawbone may require additional surgical treatment, and soft tissue corrections may also be necessary. In cases of severe shrinkage of the jawbone, an oral and maxillofacial surgeon may recommend a bone graft to add bone where little remains.

Regular checkups can ensure that dentures fit properly and will preserve the health of the mouth.

Dental Implants—A Unique Solution to Toothlessness

Tooth loss can result in shrinkage of gums and jawbones that can lead to pain from ill-fitting dentures, decreased chewing function, and subtle malnutrition. It can also be a source of emotional or psychological distress. Oral and maxillofacial surgeons are providing a unique solution to the problem of toothlessness with dental implants.

Dental implants are tooth root substitutes that are surgically placed in the jawbone and act as anchors to stabilize artificial teeth. They can replace one, some, or all missing teeth and help eliminate the instability associated with surface adhesives and removable bridges.

Individuals with adequate bone level and density who are not prone to infection and can maintain stringent oral hygiene are good candidates for dental implants.

No matter what your age, if you are missing one or more of your natural teeth, dental implants may be the solution for you. Youngsters who have lost teeth due to accidents, adults who are missing teeth due to infection, and seniors who are tired of uncomfortable dentures have had equally gratifying experiences with dental implants.

Tracking and Treating Facial Pain

Oral and maxillofacial surgeons are trained to recognize and treat a variety of facial pains. One common source of headache and facial pain is disease or dysfunction of the temporomandibular joint (TMJ). The TMJ is a small joint located in front of the ear where the skull and lower jaw meet. It is a ball and socket joint that allows the lower jaw to move and function.

TMJ disorders have a variety of symptoms. Individuals may complain of earaches, headaches, and limited ability to open the mouth. They may also complain of clicking or grating sounds in the joint and painful opening and closing of the mouth.

Arthritis is one cause of TMJ disorders. It can result from an injury or from grinding of the teeth at night. Another common cause of problems is displacement or dislocation of the disc that is located between the jawbone and the socket. Injury or rheumatoid arthritis can cause parts of the joint to fuse, preventing jaw movement altogether.

Stress can trigger pain in the jaw muscles that is very similar to that caused by TMJ problems. Frequent clenching or grinding of the teeth can cause painful spasms in the muscles and difficulty in jaw movement. Some patients may experience a combination of muscle and joint problems.

Once properly diagnosed, most TMJ disorders can be treated, in whole or at least in part, by self-care, oral medications, physical therapy, or use of a plastic bite splint. When a diagnosis indicates a specific problem with the joint, surgery may be an appropriate option. Arthroscopic joint surgery is minimally invasive and has proven effective in resolving advanced TMJ disorders. For more serious joint problems, complex surgery is available.

Seek Help at the First Sign of Trouble

Any suspicious lesion or growth on the face and neck, or in or around the mouth, should be checked out by an oral and maxillofacial surgeon without delay. Lumps and sores or reddish or whitish patches can be signs of oral cancer. Upon examination, an oral and maxillofacial surgeon can diagnose potential problems.

If needed, a biopsy is done; lab tests then determine if there is a malignancy. Remember, early detection and treatment of oral cancer greatly increase the chance of complete recovery. Don't ignore suspicious lumps or sores. If you discover something, make an appointment for a prompt examination.

Lessening the Trauma of Facial Injury

Because of their dental background, oral and maxillofacial surgeons are uniquely qualified to deal with any injury to the face, jaws, mouth, or teeth. Cuts and lacerations anywhere on the face require meticulous attention. If stitches are needed, placement must be precise to ensure a proper cosmetic result. When facial bones are broken, the experience and training of the oral and maxillofacial surgeon are invaluable.

For a fractured jaw, metal braces may be attached to the teeth and wires or strong rubber bands used to hold the jaws in place and allow the bones to heal. Patients with few or no teeth may need dentures or special dental splints to align and fix the fracture. Severe fractures can require surgery to wire together broken bones or secure them with metal plates.

All You Will Feel Is Relief

Pain is a sure sign something is wrong. Unfortunately, fear of pain often prevents people from seeking needed oral care. Oral and maxillofacial surgeons are trained in the most advanced anesthetic and pain control procedures. During surgery, one or more of the following can be used in controlling pain and anxiety: local anesthesia, nitrous oxide, intravenous sedation, and general anesthesia.

Prior to any surgery your oral and maxillofacial surgeon can review the type of anesthetic to be used, as well as the way you're likely to feel during the operation. The main goal is to ensure maximum patient comfort and safety.

Section 32.3

Corrective Jaw Surgery

Reprinted with permission from the American Association of Oral and Maxillofacial Surgeons. © 1999. For additional information, visit www.aaoms.org.

Jaw growth is a slow and gradual process. Occasionally, something may go wrong with this process and the upper and lower jaws may grow at different rates.

Unequal Jaw Growth—A Cause for Concern

One or both jaws may grow too much or too little. The resulting abnormality may interfere with proper teeth alignment, speaking, and chewing. The tongue and lips may be forced to move awkwardly during speech and swallowing in an attempt to compensate for the jaw malrelationship. There may be a speech defect or excessive mouth breathing.

An improper bite may threaten the long-term health of the gums and teeth. The jaw joint (TMJ) can also be adversely affected by a jaw malrelationship. In addition, jaws of different sizes—that don't match—can affect appearance.

Treatment

When unequal jaw growth is the source of the problem, corrective jaw surgery may be necessary. Orthodontic treatment (braces or other appliances) may also be needed to allow the teeth to align properly. Corrective jaw surgery involves moving all or part of the upper and/or lower jaw into a more favorable position. For example, the entire jaw can be moved backward if it's too large. The goal of treatment is to improve function and restore facial balance.

Some people have facial abnormalities involving just the upper face, cheek bones, and nose. These can also be surgically corrected. The bones are repositioned so the facial features are more symmetrical. This is usually accompanied by the return of normal breathing, speaking, and eating patterns.

After the jaws are moved into their new position, rubber bands or wires attached to the teeth may be used to fasten the jaws together during healing. Alternatively, rigid internal fixation with miniature screws and plates may be used to allow you to open and close your jaws sooner after corrective surgery.

Take a Closer Look

Take a closer look at your bite and appearance. Does your chin stick out? Does it recede? Do your teeth fit together properly? Do you have buck teeth? Are your teeth straight? If you suspect there's cause for concern, have your oral and maxillofacial surgeon examine your face and bite.

Section 32.4

Nutrition after Oral Surgery

"Nutrition" is reprinted with permission from the American Association of Oral and Maxillofacial Surgeons. © 1999. For additional information, visit www.aaoms.org.

After any type of surgery, the body automatically sets about the task of healing itself, starting a natural rebuilding process. But in order to heal as quickly as possible, the body requires sufficient nutrients—carbohydrates, proteins, fats, minerals, and vitamins—as well as adequate amounts of fluid. The oral and maxillofacial surgery patient has perhaps even greater difficulty getting proper nutrition because often the surgery has been in the mouth.

Good nutrition ensures the body will have all the nutrients the healing process requires and means eating the right foods and consuming a well-balanced diet. For an adult, normal daily nutrition would include a balanced intake of 2 cups of milk or dairy products, 4 or more servings of grain or cereals, 2 or more servings of meat or other sources of protein, and 3 or more servings of vegetables.

Sometimes Eating Right Is Easier Said Than Done

If you fail to give your body adequate nourishment, the result can be fatigue, infection, and delayed healing. In the case of multiple tooth extractions or when surgery is performed for dentures, chewing can be difficult. When jaws are wired shut, normal eating is nearly impossible and food must be consumed in liquid form.

A Good Blend of Taste and Nutrition

Since solid foods can't be chewed, they can be liquefied in a blender. And although the food may not always look appetizing, it can be tasty. Cooked servings of your favorite foods can be blended separately or in combinations to suit your taste. Normal seasonings can be added. But, best of all, you'll be getting your full supply of nutrients.

When and How Much to Eat

To ensure getting your recommended daily requirements of nutrients and calories and to satisfy your hunger, you may wish to eat more frequently than usual, consuming 5-6 meals per day. To determine how much food to put in the blender, place the desired portions on a plate, add seasonings, then transfer the portions individually or in combinations into the blender. To make the blended mixture the proper consistency, use either milk, juice, broth, or water as a thinner, choosing the liquid that will either add to the flavor or will have little effect on the flavor.

In liquid form, food can be taken through a large plastic straw, it can be sipped out of a cup, or, if you can open your mouth wide enough, you can eat it with a spoon.

To prevent oral hygiene problems for people with wired jaws, the blended food mixture can be strained to remove food fiber and particles. Food supplements and vitamins may be used to provide additional nutrients. There are several commercially prepared food supplements available that your surgeon may recommend.

Suggested Recipes

The following recipes are provided as examples of blended meals that ensure getting proper nutrients during oral and maxillofacial surgery convalescence. Supplement these selections with your own favorite recipes to meet your nutrient and calorie requirements (for active adult females, 2000 calories a day; for active adult males, 2700 calories per day). Snack suggestions are included to lend variety to your rehabilitation diet and to satisfy hunger between regularly scheduled meals.

Breakfast

Orange Cereal Drink
3 tablespoons oatmeal (no added salt)
1 cup water
1 tablespoon honey
1 large orange, peeled and cut into fine pieces
1 cup whole milk

Add oatmeal to rapidly boiling water and cook until consistency of thick cream soup. Remove from heat and add brown sugar and honey. Mix until well dissolved; allow mixture to cool. Add orange, mix well; add milk slowly; and beat mixture with fork or wire whisk.

Yield: 16 ounces or two 8-ounce servings. One 8-ounce serving contains 287 calories, 7 grams of protein, 50 grams of carbohydrate, and 15 grams of fat.

Cream of Wheat

1 cup cooked cream of wheat made with milk

1/2 to 3/4 cup milk

Butter and brown sugar to taste

1 tablespoon wheat germ

May be blended if necessary.

Yield: Two 6-ounce servings. One 6-ounce serving contains 136 calories, 21 grams of carbohydrate, 7 grams of protein, and 4 grams of fat; slightly more if butter and sugar are added.

Lunch or Dinner

Potato Meat Drink

3 ounces of a medium cooked ground beef patty (lean) or substitute 3 ounces of cooked meat or poultry

1 1/2 cup milk

1/4 cup cooked or canned vegetable

1 medium boiled potato or 1/2 cup mashed

1 teaspoon butter

1 1/2 teaspoon salt

Blend 3/4 cup milk and meat separately for 4 minutes. Stir in potato, vegetable, salt, and remaining milk and blend for one minute. Strain. Melt butter in top of double boiler. Add the strained blended mixture and heat for five minutes.

Yield: One serving contains 747 calories, 47 grams of carbohydrate, 45 grams of protein, and 42 grams of fat.

Below are other blended lunch and dinner combinations you may wish to try.

- chili con carne thinned with tomato juice
- grilled hamburger or hot dog with baked beans thinned with V-8 juice
- spaghetti and meatballs thinned with tomato juice

- chop suey with beef or pork thinned with broth
- lasagna or ravioli thinned with milk or tomato juice
- beef stew thinned with broth or tomato juice
- chunky canned soup thinned with broth or tomato juice

Snacks

Jell-O Shake
1 cup Jell-O
10 ounces milk

Blend.

Yield: 16 ounces or two 8-ounce servings. One 8-ounce serving contains 180 calories, 26 grams of carbohydrate, 7 grams of protein, and 5 grams of fat.

Eggnog
16 ounces milk
2 large eggs
1 teaspoon vanilla extract
1 scoop vanilla ice cream

Blend.

Yield: Two 10-ounce servings. One 10-ounce serving contains 334 calories, 22 grams of carbohydrate, 18 grams of protein, and 21 grams of fat.

Fruit Eggnog
2/3 cup orange juice (or juice of your choice)
2 teaspoons lemon juice
1 tablespoon sugar or honey
1 large egg

Blend for 1 minute.

Yield: 12 ounces. One 12-ounce serving contains 226 calories, 34 grams of carbohydrate, 8 grams of protein, and 6 grams of fat.

Cottrange Cocktail
1/2 cup cream style cottage cheese
2 ounces water

Cottrange Cocktail (continued)

1/2 cup orange juice

pinch of cinnamon

Blend for 2 minutes. Pour over ice and serve.

Yield: 8 ounces. One 8-ounce serving contains 175 calories, 17 grams of protein, 16 grams of carbohydrate, and 5 grams of fat.

Fruit Yogurt Beverage

8 ounces plain yogurt (2% milk)

1/2 cup concentrated grape juice (or juice of your choice)

Beat yogurt with frozen concentrate until blended.

Yield: 12 ounces. One 12-ounce serving contains 305 calories, 59 grams of carbohydrate, 9 grams of protein, and 4 grams of fat.

Recipe suggestions were provided by Gloria R. Singer, MS, RD (member of the American Dietetic Association).

For more information to meet your specific needs, contact a registered dietitian at the healthcare facility where your surgery was performed.

Chapter 33

Orthodontics

Chapter Contents

Section 33.1

Overview of Orthodontic Treatment (Braces)

"Tell Me About Orthodontic Treatment (Braces)" is reprinted with permission from the British Dental Health Foundation, www.britishdental health.org.uk. © 2003 British Dental Health Foundation.

What Is Orthodontic Treatment?

Orthodontic treatment is a way of straightening or moving teeth, to improve the appearance of the teeth and how they work. It can also help to look after the long-term health of the teeth, gums, and jaw joints, by spreading the biting pressure over all the teeth.

Why Should I Have Orthodontic Treatment?

Many people have crowded or crooked teeth. Orthodontic treatment will straighten the teeth or move them into a better position. This can not only improve their appearance but also the way the teeth bite together, while also making them easier to clean.

In some patients the upper front teeth can stick out and look unsightly. These prominent teeth are more likely to be damaged, but orthodontic treatment can move them back into line. In others, the way the upper and lower jaws meet can cause teeth to look unsightly and lead to an incorrect bite. Orthodontic treatment may be able to correct both.

When the teeth don't meet correctly, this can put strain on the muscles of the jaw, causing jaw and joint problems and in some cases headaches. Orthodontic treatment can help you to bite more evenly and reduce the strain.

At What Age Should I Have Orthodontic Treatment?

Orthodontic treatment is generally best carried out in children, but adults can have orthodontic treatment, too—and more and more are doing so. Age is less important than having the proper number of teeth. In children it may be necessary to wait for enough teeth to come through before starting treatment.

Who Carries out Orthodontics?

Any dentist may carry out orthodontic treatment. Or the dentist may send the person to a specialist who has extra qualifications. The specialist may be in a practice or in a hospital department and is called an orthodontist.

What Does It Involve?

The most important thing is to have a full examination. This will usually involve looking at your teeth, taking x-rays, and making plaster models of your teeth.

Your dentist or orthodontist will then discuss what treatment is possible. Once you are sure you want to go ahead, the treatment can begin as soon as you have enough permanent teeth.

How Is Treatment Carried out?

Orthodontic treatment can be done with many sorts of appliances, which most people know as braces.

What Is a Removable Appliance?

Simple treatment may be carried out with a removable appliance, a plate that can be taken out to be cleaned. It has delicate wires and springs attached, which move the teeth using gentle pressure.

What Is a Functional Appliance?

It is sometimes possible to change the way the jaws grow, using orthodontic appliances. These functional appliances use the power of your jaw muscles and can help with certain types of problems.

What Is a Fixed Appliance?

Often, teeth need to be guided more accurately than they can be using a removable plate, so fixed appliances are used. These have brackets and bands temporarily stuck to the teeth. A flexible wire joins all the brackets and allows the teeth to be moved. It is not possible for the patient to take the appliance out and so it is called a fixed appliance.

What Is Headgear?

As well as an appliance, it is sometimes necessary to wear headgear. You usually only need to wear it in the evening or at night. Your orthodontist will discuss whether it is necessary. It is very important to wear it in the way the orthodontist tells you otherwise treatment may not progress correctly.

What Are Elastics?

It may be necessary to attach delicate elastic bands to a fixed brace to help move the teeth. Your orthodontist will tell you if you need elastics.

What Are Invisible Braces?

They are tough, clear plastic aligners (molds) that are used to straighten teeth. Several sets of specially molded, slightly different aligners are made for each patient. Each set is worn for two weeks before being replaced with the next one. They are made from clear plastic, so they are nearly invisible. This means that no one need know you are straightening your teeth.

The aligners should be worn for 22 to 23 hours a day for the best results. They can be easily removed for eating, drinking, brushing, and flossing. You need to have all your adult teeth before you can have this treatment.

How Long Will It Take?

The length of treatment depends on how severe the problem is, and may take anything from a few months to two and a half years. Most people can be treated in one to two years.

What Happens When the Teeth Are in the Right Position?

When treatment is finished, the teeth need to be held in position for a time. This period is called retention, and the appliances that hold the teeth in place are called retainers.

The retainers hold newly straightened teeth in position while the surrounding gum and bone settles. The retainers can be removable or fixed depending on the original problem.

How Many Visits Will It Take?

Orthodontic appliances usually need adjusting every four to six weeks. Your orthodontist will tell you how often your appliance will need adjusting.

Will It Hurt?

All appliances may feel strange to begin with and can cause discomfort. If the problem doesn't go away, the orthodontist may be able to carry out adjustments to help. Teeth are usually uncomfortable immediately after adjustment but this will settle.

How Successful Will It Be?

Success depends on a partnership between the skills of the orthodontist and the enthusiasm and help of patient and parents. It is important to attend regularly and carry out any instructions given by the orthodontist.

The success of the treatment also depends on the commitment of the patient. For children's orthodontic treatment it is very important that the patient is as keen as the parent.

Can Orthodontics Damage My Teeth?

Your teeth can be damaged if they are not properly looked after during treatment. Appliances will not in themselves cause damage, but poor cleaning and too many sugary drinks and snacks can cause permanent damage. Brackets, wires, and braces can trap food and cause more plaque than usual to build up. So the teeth and appliance need to be cleaned very thoroughly.

Is Orthodontic Work Permanent?

Even after retention, it is normal for minor tooth movements to happen throughout life, so no permanent guarantee can be given. However, it is unusual for teeth to alter enough to need further treatment.

How Do I Go about Getting Orthodontic Treatment?

The first thing to do is to go along to your own dentist and get his or her advice. Your dentist will know whether you need treatment and make the necessary arrangements.

How Much Does It Cost?

If you decide to have treatment, the orthodontist will be able to estimate the cost of your treatment and give you details. It is always a good idea to discuss the cost fully before treatment and, if necessary, have the cost confirmed in writing to avoid any confusion.

How Do I Care for My Braces and Teeth?

It is important to continue to have your teeth checked by your dentist while having orthodontic treatment. You also need to take extra care of your teeth and mouth:

- Clean your teeth carefully every day, including between your teeth where you can't see. Appliances are delicate and you need to make sure you clean them carefully so that they do not break. Your dentist or hygienist will be able to show you the special techniques to use depending on the appliance you are wearing.

- Cut down on how often you have sugary foods and drinks. Avoid snacking on foods or drinks containing sugars and on fizzy drinks. Also, sticky and hard foods may damage the delicate orthodontic appliances.

- Brush your teeth twice a day with fluoride toothpaste and, if necessary, use a mouthwash. Your dentist or hygienist may recommend a fluoride toothpaste or application for you to use. Look for a product carrying an accreditation logo. This shows that the product has been checked by a panel of experts and does what it says on the packet.

Section 33.2

Questions and Answers about Orthodontic Care

"About Orthodontics: Facts About Orthodontics" is reprinted with permission of the American Association of Orthodontists, www.braces.org. © 1999 American Association of Orthodontists.

What Is Orthodontics?

Orthodontics is the branch of dentistry that specializes in the diagnosis, prevention, and treatment of dental and facial irregularities. The technical term for these problems is malocclusion, which means bad bite. The practice of orthodontics requires professional skill in the design, application, and control of corrective appliances—such as braces—to bring teeth, lips, and jaws into proper alignment and to achieve facial balance.

What Is an Orthodontist?

All orthodontists are dentists, but only about 6 percent of dentists are orthodontists. An orthodontist is a specialist in the diagnosis, prevention, and treatment of dental and facial irregularities. Orthodontists must first attend college, and then complete a four-year dental graduate program at a university dental school or other institution accredited by the Commission on Dental Accreditation of the American Dental Association (ADA). They must then successfully complete an additional two- to three-year residency program of advanced education in orthodontics. This residency program must also be accredited by the ADA. Through this training, the orthodontist learns the skills required to manage tooth movement (orthodontics) and guide facial development (dentofacial orthopedics).

Only dentists who have successfully completed this advanced specialty education may call themselves orthodontists.

What Is the American Association of Orthodontists?

The American Association of Orthodontists is the national organization of dental specialists who limit their practice to orthodontics and dentofacial orthopedics. Founded in 1900, the AAO is the oldest and largest dental specialty organization in the United States and Canada. To date, the AAO has more than 13,500 members, including more than 2,000 international members from outside North America. This membership consists of approximately 94 percent of all orthodontists who currently practice in the United States.

The AAO is dedicated to advancing the art and science of orthodontics and dentofacial orthopedics, improving the health of the public by promoting quality orthodontic care, and supporting the successful practice of orthodontics. All members must meet the specialty educational requirements as defined by the Commission on Dental Education of the American Dental Association.

The American Dental Association has recognized that "specialists are necessary to protect the public, nurture the art and science of dentistry, and improve the quality of care."

At What Age Can People Have Orthodontic Treatment?

Children and adults can both benefit from orthodontics, because healthy teeth can be moved at almost any age. Because monitoring growth and development is crucial to managing some orthodontic problems well, the American Association of Orthodontists recommends that all children have an orthodontic screening no later than age 7. Some orthodontic problems may be easier to correct if treated early. Waiting until all the permanent teeth have come in, or until facial growth is nearly complete, may make correction of some problems more difficult.

An orthodontic evaluation at any age is advisable if a parent, family dentist, or the patient's physician has noted a problem.

What Causes Orthodontic Problems (Malocclusions)?

Most malocclusions are inherited, but some are acquired. Inherited problems include crowding of teeth, too much space between teeth, extra or missing teeth, and a wide variety of other irregularities of the jaws, teeth, and face.

Acquired malocclusions can be caused by trauma (accidents), thumb, finger or dummy (pacifier) sucking, airway obstruction by tonsils and adenoids, dental disease or premature loss of primary (baby) or permanent teeth. Whether inherited or acquired, many of these problems affect not only alignment of the teeth but also facial development and appearance as well.

What Are the Most Commonly Treated Orthodontic Problems?

Crowding: Teeth may be aligned poorly because the dental arch is small and/or the teeth are large. The bone and gums over the roots of extremely crowded teeth may become thin and recede as a result of severe crowding. Impacted teeth (teeth that should have come in, but have not), poor biting relationships, and undesirable appearance may all result from crowding.

Overjet or protruding upper teeth: Upper front teeth that protrude beyond normal contact with the lower front teeth are prone to injury, often indicate a poor bite of the back teeth (molars), and may indicate an unevenness in jaw growth. Commonly, protruded upper teeth are associated with a lower jaw that is short in proportion to the upper jaw. Thumb and finger sucking habits can also cause a protrusion of the upper incisor teeth.

Deep overbite: A deep overbite or deep bite occurs when the lower incisor (front) teeth bite too close or into the gum tissue behind the upper teeth. When the lower front teeth bite into the palate or gum tissue behind the upper front teeth, significant bone damage and discomfort can occur. A deep bite can also contribute to excessive wear of the incisor teeth.

Open bite: An open bite results when the upper and lower incisor teeth do not touch when biting down. This open space between the upper and lower front teeth causes all the chewing pressure to be placed on the back teeth. This excessive biting pressure and rubbing together of the back teeth makes chewing less efficient and may contribute to significant tooth wear.

Spacing: If teeth are missing or small, or the dental arch is very wide, space between the teeth can occur. The most common complaint from those with excessive space is poor appearance.

Crossbite: The most common type of a crossbite is when the upper teeth bite inside the lower teeth (toward the tongue). Crossbites of both back teeth and front teeth are commonly corrected early due to biting and chewing difficulties.

Underbite or lower jaw protrusion: About 3 to 5 percent of the population has a lower jaw that is to some degree longer than the upper jaw. This can cause the lower front teeth to protrude ahead of the upper front teeth, creating a crossbite. Careful monitoring of jaw growth and tooth development is indicated for these patients.

Why Is Orthodontic Treatment Important?

Crooked and crowded teeth are hard to clean and maintain. This may contribute to conditions that cause not only tooth decay but also eventual gum disease and tooth loss. Other orthodontic problems can contribute to abnormal wear of tooth surfaces, inefficient chewing function, excessive stress on gum tissue and the bone that supports the teeth, or misalignment of the jaw joints, which can result in chronic headaches or pain in the face or neck.

When left untreated, many orthodontic problems become worse. Treatment by a specialist to correct the original problem is often less costly than the additional dental care required to treat more serious problems that can develop in later years.

The value of an attractive smile should not be underestimated. A pleasing appearance is a vital asset to one's self-confidence. A person's self-esteem often improves as treatment brings teeth, lips, and face into proportion. In this way, orthodontic treatment can benefit social and career success, as well as improve one's general attitude toward life.

How Do I Find Someone to Treat an Orthodontic Problem?

Ask your family dentist for a referral to an orthodontist, or call 1-800-STRAIGHT (787-2444) for the names of orthodontists near you.

I Recently Took My Child to an Orthodontist for an Orthodontic Screening. The Orthodontist Recommended Treatment. Should I Seek a Second Opinion?

Review the recommended treatment with your family dentist. If you would still like to compare your comfort level with another orthodontic office or simply hear another orthodontist's assessment of your child's problem, arrange for a second opinion. You may have already had more than one orthodontist recommended to you by family, friends, your dentist, or the AAO's referral service. Seeking out a member of the AAO assures that your second opinion is from an educationally qualified orthodontic specialist. You should feel confident in the orthodontist and his or her staff, and trust their ability to provide you the care and lifetime orthodontic value you seek.

What Does Orthodontic Treatment Cost?

The actual cost of treatment depends on several factors, including the severity of the patient's problem and the treatment approach selected. You will be able to thoroughly discuss fees and payment options before any treatment begins. Most orthodontists offer convenient payment plans to patients. Generally, treatment fees may be paid over the course of active treatment. Arrangements commonly offered in orthodontic offices may include an initial down payment with monthly installments, credit card payment, finance company agreements, and other innovative ways to make treatment affordable. Insurance plans or other employer-sponsored payment programs, such as direct reimbursement plans, may be helpful.

Dental schools with graduate orthodontic programs usually offer treatment to a limited number of patients at a reduced cost. The Dental School Listing includes telephone numbers and website addresses for dental schools with orthodontic graduate programs.

How Long Will Orthodontic Treatment Take?

In general, active treatment time with orthodontic appliances (braces) ranges from one to three years. Interceptive, or early treatment procedures, may take only a few months. The actual time depends on the growth of the patient's mouth and face, the cooperation of the patient, and the severity of the problem. Mild problems usually require less time, and some individuals respond faster to treatment than others. Use of rubber bands and/or headgear, if prescribed by the orthodontist, contributes to completing treatment as scheduled.

While orthodontic treatment requires a time commitment, patients are rewarded with healthy teeth, proper jaw alignment, and a beautiful smile that lasts a lifetime. Teeth and jaws in proper alignment look better, work better, contribute to general physical health, and can improve self-confidence.

What Will I Look Like after Completing Orthodontic Treatment?

The American Association of Orthodontists can provide you with a free computer-generated photograph that shows how your teeth might look after orthodontic treatment.

What Are Orthodontic Study Records?

Diagnostic records are made to document the patient's orthodontic problem and to help determine the best course of treatment. As orthodontic treatment will create many changes, these records are also helpful in determining progress of treatment. Complete diagnostic records typically include a medical/dental history, clinical examination, plaster study models of the teeth, photos of the patient's face and teeth, a panoramic or other x-rays of all the teeth, a facial profile x-ray, and other appropriate x-rays. This information is used to plan the best course of treatment, help explain the problem, and propose treatment to the patient and/or parents.

The profile x-ray, or cephalometric film, shows the facial form, growth pattern, and inclination of the front teeth (if teeth are tipped or tilted), which are essential in planning comprehensive treatment. Panoramic or other dental x-rays are used to locate impacted teeth, missing teeth, and shortened or damaged tooth roots, to determine the amount of bone supporting teeth, and to evaluate position and development of permanent teeth that have not yet come in, among other things. From the necessary records, a custom treatment plan is created for each patient.

How Is Treatment Accomplished?

Custom-made appliances, or braces, are prescribed and designed by the orthodontist according to the problem being treated. They may be removable or fixed (cemented and/or bonded to the teeth). They may be made of metal, ceramic, or plastic. By placing a constant, gentle force in a carefully controlled direction, braces can slowly move teeth through their supporting bone to a new desirable position.

Orthopedic appliances, such as headgear, Bionater, Herbst and maxillary expansion appliances, use carefully directed forces to guide the growth and development of jaws in children and/or teenagers. For example, an upper jaw expansion appliance can dramatically widen a narrow upper jaw in a matter of months. Over the course of orthodontic treatment, a headgear or Herbst appliance can dramatically reduce the protrusion of upper incisor teeth (the top four front teeth) or retrusion of the lower jaw (a lower jaw that is too far behind the upper jaw), while making upper and lower jaw lengths more compatible.

Are There Less Noticeable Braces?

Today's braces are generally less noticeable than those of the past when a metal band with a bracket (the part of the braces that hold the wire) was placed around each tooth. Now the front teeth typically have only the bracket bonded directly to the tooth, minimizing the tin grin. Brackets can be metal, clear or colored, depending on the patient's preference. In some cases, brackets may be bonded behind the teeth (lingual braces). Modern wires are also less noticeable than earlier ones. Some of today's wires are made of space-age materials that exert a steady, gentle pressure on the teeth, so that the tooth-moving process may be faster and more comfortable for patients. A type of clear orthodontic wire is currently in an experimental stage.

How Have New High-Tech Wires Changed Orthodontics?

In recent years, many advances in orthodontic materials have taken place. Braces are smaller and more efficient. The wires now being used are no longer just stainless steel. They are made of alloys of nickel, titanium, copper, and cobalt, and some of the wires are heat-activated. (The nickel-titanium alloy was originally engineered by NASA to automatically activate antennae or solar panels of spacecraft orbiting into the sun's rays.) These new kinds of wires cause the teeth to continue to move during certain phases of treatment, which may reduce the number of appointments needed to make adjustments to the wires.

How Do Braces Feel?

Most people have some discomfort after their braces are first put on or when adjusted during treatment. After the braces are on, teeth may become sore and may be tender to biting pressures for three to five days. Patients can usually manage this discomfort well with what-ever pain medication they might commonly take for a headache. The orthodontist will advise patients and/or their parents what, if any, pain relievers to take. The lips, cheeks, and tongue may also become irritated for one to two weeks as they toughen and become accustomed to the surface of the braces. Overall, orthodontic discomfort is short-lived and easily managed.

Do Teeth with Braces Need Special Care?

Patients with braces must be careful to avoid hard and sticky foods. They must not chew on pens, pencils, or fingernails because chewing on hard things can damage the braces. Damaged braces will almost always cause treatment to take longer, and will require extra trips to the orthodontist's office.

Keeping the teeth and braces clean requires more precision and time, and must be done every day if the teeth and gums are to be healthy during and after orthodontic treatment. Patients who do not keep their teeth clean may require more frequent visits to the dentist for a professional cleaning.

The orthodontist and staff will teach patients how to best care for their teeth, gums, and braces during treatment. The orthodontist will tell patients (and/or their parents) how often to brush, how often to floss, and, if necessary, suggest other cleaning aids that might help the patient maintain good dental health.

How Important Is Patient Cooperation during Orthodontic Treatment?

Successful orthodontic treatment is a two-way street that requires a consistent, cooperative effort by both the orthodontist and patient. To successfully complete the treatment plan, the patient must carefully clean his or her teeth, wear rubber bands, headgear, or other appliances as prescribed by the orthodontist, and keep appointments as scheduled. Damaged appliances can lengthen the treatment time and may undesirably affect the outcome of treatment. The teeth and jaws can only move toward their desired positions if the patient consistently wears the forces to the teeth, such as rubber bands, as prescribed. Patients who do their part consistently make themselves look good and their orthodontist look smart.

To keep teeth and gums healthy, regular visits to the family dentist must continue during orthodontic treatment. Adults who have a history of or concerns about periodontal (gum) disease might also see a periodontist (specialist in treating diseases of the gums and bone) on a regular basis throughout orthodontic treatment.

Chapter 34

Early Orthodontic Treatment

Why Should Children Have an Orthodontic Screening No Later Than Age 7?

By age 7, enough permanent teeth have come in and enough jaw growth has occurred that the dentist or orthodontist can identify current problems, anticipate future problems, and alleviate parents' concerns if all seems normal. The first permanent molars and incisors have usually come in by age 7, and crossbites, crowding, and developing injury-prone dental protrusions can be evaluated. Any ongoing finger sucking or other oral habits can be assessed at this time also.

Some signs or habits that may indicate the need for an early orthodontic examination are:

- early or late loss of baby teeth
- difficulty in chewing or biting
- mouth breathing
- thumb sucking
- finger sucking
- crowding, misplaced, or blocked out teeth
- jaws that shift or make sounds
- biting the cheek or roof of the mouth

"About Orthodontics: Orthodontic Treatment for Growing Children" is reprinted with permission of the American Association of Orthodontists, www. braces.org. © 1999 American Association of Orthodontists.

- teeth that meet abnormally or not at all
- jaws and teeth that are out of proportion to the rest of the face

An orthodontic screening no later than age 7 enables the orthodontist to detect and evaluate problems (if any), advise if treatment will be necessary, and determine the best time for that patient to be treated.

What Are the Benefits of Early Treatment?

For those patients who have clear indications for early orthodontic intervention, early treatment presents an opportunity to:

- guide the growth of the jaw
- regulate the width of the upper and lower dental arches (the arch-shaped jaw bone that supports the teeth)
- guide incoming permanent teeth into desirable positions
- lower risk of trauma (accidents) to protruded upper incisors (front teeth)
- correct harmful oral habits such as thumb or finger sucking
- reduce or eliminate abnormal swallowing or speech problems
- improve personal appearance and self-esteem, potentially simplify and/or shorten treatment time for later corrective orthodontics
- reduce likelihood of impacted permanent teeth (teeth that should have come in, but have not)
- preserve or gain space for permanent teeth that are coming in

What Is a Space Maintainer?

Baby molar teeth, also known as primary molar teeth, hold needed space for permanent teeth that will come in later. When a baby molar tooth is lost, an orthodontic device with a fixed wire is usually put between teeth to hold the space for the permanent tooth, which will come in later.

Why Do Baby Teeth Sometimes Need to Be Pulled?

Pulling baby teeth may be necessary to allow severely crowded permanent teeth to come in at a normal time in a reasonably normal location. If the teeth are severely crowded, it may be clear that some unerupted permanent teeth (usually the canine teeth) will either remain impacted (teeth that should have come in, but have not), or come in to a highly undesirable position. To allow severely crowded teeth to move on their own into much more desirable positions, sequential removal of baby teeth and permanent teeth (usually first premolars) can dramatically improve a severe crowding problem. This sequential extraction of teeth, called serial extraction, is typically followed by comprehensive orthodontic treatment after tooth eruption has improved as much as it can on its own.

After all the permanent teeth have come in, the pulling of permanent teeth may be necessary to correct crowding or to make space for necessary tooth movement to correct a bite problem. Proper extraction of teeth during orthodontic treatment should leave the patient with both excellent function and a pleasing look.

How Can a Child's Growth Affect Orthodontic Treatment?

Orthodontic treatment and a child's growth can complement each other. A common orthodontic problem to treat is protrusion of the upper front teeth ahead of the lower front teeth. Quite often this problem is due to the lower jaw being shorter than the upper jaw. While the upper and lower jaws are still growing, orthodontic appliances can be used to help the growth of the lower jaw catch up to the growth of the upper jaw. Abnormal swallowing may be eliminated. A severe jaw length discrepancy, which can be treated quite well in a growing child, might very well require corrective surgery if left untreated until a period of slow or no jaw growth. Children who may have problems with the width or length of their jaws should be evaluated for treatment no later than age 10 for girls and age 12 for boys. The AAO [American Association of Orthodontists] recommends that all children have an orthodontic screening no later than age 7 as growth-related problems may be identified at this time.

What Kinds of Orthodontic Appliances Are Typically Used to Correct Jaw-Growth Problems?

Correcting jaw-growth problems is done by the process of dentofacial orthopedics. Some of the more common orthopedic appliances used by orthodontists today that help the length of the upper and lower jaws become more compatible include:

Headgear: This appliance applies pressure to the upper teeth and upper jaw to guide the rate and direction of upper jaw growth and upper tooth eruption. The headgear may be removed by the patient and is usually worn 10 to 12 hours per day.

Herbst: The Herbst appliance is usually fixed to the upper and lower molar teeth and may not be removed by the patient. By holding the lower jaw forward and influencing jaw growth and tooth positions, the Herbst appliance can help correct severe protrusion of the upper teeth.

Bionator: This removable appliance holds the lower jaw forward and guides eruption of the teeth into a more desirable bite while helping the upper and lower jaws to grow in proportion with each other. Patient compliance in wearing this appliance is essential for successful improvement.

Palatal Expansion Appliance: A child's upper jaw may also be too narrow for the upper teeth to fit properly with the lower teeth (a crossbite). When this occurs, a palatal expansion appliance can be fixed to the upper back teeth. This appliance can markedly expand the width of the upper jaw.

The decision about when and which of these or other appliances to use for orthopedic correction is based on each individual patient's problem. Usually one of several appliances can be used effectively to treat a given problem. Patient cooperation and the experience of the treating orthodontist are critical elements in success of dentofacial orthopedic treatment.

I've Just Heard about the Herbst Appliance. How Could It Help My Child Who Has an Underdeveloped Lower Jaw?

For patients who have an underdeveloped lower jaw, it is important to begin orthodontic treatment several years before the lower jaw ceases to grow. One method of correcting an underdeveloped jaw uses an orthodontic appliance that repositions the lower jaw. These appliances influence the jaw muscles to work in a way that may improve forward development of the lower jaw. There are many appliances used by orthodontists today to treat underdeveloped lower jaws—such as the Frankel, headgears, Activator, Twin Block, Bionater, and Herbst appliances. Some are fixed (cemented to the teeth) and some are removable. You and your orthodontist can discuss which appliance is best for your child.

Can My Child Play Sports while Wearing Braces?

Yes. Wearing a protective mouthguard is advised while playing any contact sports. Your orthodontist can recommend a specific mouthguard.

Will My Braces Interfere with Playing Musical Instruments?

Playing wind or brass instruments, such as the trumpet, will clearly require some adaptation to braces. With practice and a period of adjustment, braces typically do not interfere with the playing of musical instruments.

Why Does Orthodontic Treatment Time Sometimes Last Longer Than Anticipated?

Estimates of treatment time can only be that—estimates. Patients grow at different rates and will respond in their own ways to orthodontic treatment. The orthodontist has specific treatment goals in mind, and will usually continue treatment until these goals are achieved. Patient cooperation, however, is the single best predictor of staying on time with treatment. Patients who cooperate by wearing rubber bands, headgear, or other needed appliances as directed, while taking care not to damage appliances, will most often lead to on-time and excellent treatment results.

Why Are Retainers Needed after Orthodontic Treatment?

After braces are removed, the teeth can shift out of position if they are not stabilized. Retainers provide that stabilization. They are designed to hold teeth in their corrected, ideal positions until the bones and gums adapt to the treatment changes. Wearing retainers exactly as instructed is the best insurance that the treatment improvements last for a lifetime.

Will My Child's Tooth Alignment Change Later?

Studies have shown that as people age, their teeth may shift. This variable pattern of gradual shifting, called maturational change, probably slows down after the early 20's, but still continues to a degree throughout life for most people. Even children whose teeth developed into ideal alignment and bite without treatment may develop orthodontic problems as adults. The most common maturational change is crowding of the lower incisor (front) teeth. Wearing retainers as instructed after orthodontic treatment will stabilize the correction. Beyond the period of full-time retainer wear, nighttime retainer wear can prevent maturational shifting of the teeth.

What about the Wisdom Teeth (Third Molars)? Should They Be Removed?

In about three out of four cases where teeth have not been removed during orthodontic treatment, there are good reasons to have the wisdom teeth removed, usually when a person reaches his or her mid- to late-teen years. Careful studies have shown, however, that wisdom teeth do not cause or contribute to the progressive crowding of lower incisor teeth that can develop in the late teen years and beyond. Your orthodontist, in consultation with your family dentist, can determine what is right for you.

Chapter 35

Adult Orthodontic Treatment

Can Orthodontic Treatment Do for Me What It Does for Children?

Healthy teeth can be moved at almost any age. Many orthodontic problems can be corrected as easily and as well for adults as children. Orthodontic forces move the teeth in the same way for both a 75-year-old adult and a 12-year-old child. Complicating factors, such as lack of jaw growth, may create special treatment planning needs for the adult.

One in five orthodontic patients is an adult. The AAO [American Association of Orthodontists] estimates that nearly 1,000,000 adults in the United States and Canada are receiving treatment from an orthodontist. To learn about correction of a specific problem, please consult your family dentist or an orthodontist.

How Does Adult Treatment Differ from That of Children and Adolescents?

Adults are not growing and may have experienced some breakdown or loss of their teeth and bone that supports the teeth. Orthodontic treatment may then be only a part of the patient's overall treatment plan. Close coordination may be required between the orthodontist,

---

oral surgeon, periodontist, endodontist, and family dentist to assure that a complicated adult orthodontic problem is managed well and complements all other areas of the patient's treatment needs. Below are the most common characteristics that can cause adult treatment to differ from treatment for children.

No jaw growth: Jaw problems can usually be managed well in a growing child with an orthopedic, growth-modifying appliance. However, the same problem for an adult may require jaw surgery. For example, if an adult's lower jaw is too short to match properly with the upper jaw, a severe bite problem may result. The limited amount that the teeth can be moved with braces alone may not correct this bite problem. Bringing the lower teeth forward into a proper bite relationship could require jaw surgery, which would lengthen the lower jaw and bring the lower teeth forward into the proper bite. Other jaw-width or jaw-length discrepancies between the upper and lower jaws might also require surgery for bite correction if tooth movement alone cannot correct the bite.

Gum or bone loss (periodontal breakdown): Adults are more likely to have experienced damage or loss of the gum and bone supporting their teeth (periodontal disease). Special treatment by the patient's dentist or a periodontist may be necessary before, during, and/or after orthodontic treatment. Bone loss can also limit the amount and direction of tooth movement that is advisable.

Worn, damaged, or missing teeth: Worn, damaged, or missing teeth can make orthodontic treatment more difficult, but more important for the patient to have. Teeth may gradually wear and move into positions where they can be restored only after precise orthodontic movement. Damaged or broken teeth may not look good or function well even after orthodontic treatment unless they are carefully restored by the patient's dentist. Missing teeth that are not replaced often cause progressive tipping and drifting of other teeth, which worsens the bite, increases the potential for periodontal problems, and makes any treatment more difficult.

I Have Painful Jaw Muscles and Jaw Joints. Can an Orthodontist Help?

Jaw muscle and jaw joint discomfort is commonly associated with bruxing, that is, habitual grinding or clenching of the teeth, particularly at night. Bruxism is a muscle habit pattern that can cause severe wearing of the teeth and overloading and trauma to the jaw joint structures. Chronically or acutely sore and painful jaw muscles may accompany this bruxing habit. An orthodontist can help diagnose this problem. Your family dentist or orthodontist may also place a bite splint or nightguard appliance that can protect the teeth and help jaw muscles relax, substantially reducing the original pain symptoms. Sometimes structural damage can require joint surgery and/or restoration of damaged teeth.

My Family Dentist Said I Need to Have Some Missing Teeth Replaced, but I Need Orthodontic Treatment First. Why?

Your dentist is probably recommending orthodontics so that he or she might treat you in the best manner possible to bring you to optimal dental health. Many complicated tooth restorations, such as crowns, bridges, and implants, can be best accomplished when the remaining teeth are properly aligned and the bite is correct.

When permanent teeth are lost, it is common for the remaining teeth to drift, tip, or shift. This movement can create a poor bite and uneven spacing that cannot be restored properly unless the missing teeth are replaced. Tipped teeth usually need to be straightened so they can stand up to normal biting pressures in the future.

My Teeth Have Been Crooked for More Than 50 Years. Why Should I Have Orthodontic Treatment Now?

Orthodontic treatment, when indicated, is a positive step—especially for adults who have endured a long-standing problem. Orthodontic treatment can restore good function. Teeth that work better usually look better, too. And a healthy, beautiful smile can improve self-esteem, no matter the age.

Chapter 36

Crowns and Bridges

Chapter Contents

Section 36.1

Crowns

"What Are Crowns?" © 2003 Academy of General Dentistry. Reprinted with permission from the Academy of General Dentistry. For additional oral health topics, toll free access to a directory of members in your zip code area and other consumer services, see page 557 of this *Sourcebook* or contact the Academy of General Dentistry, 211 E. Chicago Avenue, Suite 900, Chicago, IL 60611, 312-440-4300, or visit their website at www.agd.org.

A crown is a restoration that covers, or caps, a tooth to restore it to its normal shape and size, strengthening and improving the appearance of a tooth. Crowns are necessary when a tooth is generally broken down and fillings won't solve the problem. If a tooth is cracked, a crown holds the tooth together to seal the cracks so the damage doesn't get worse. Crowns are also used to support a large filling when there isn't enough of the tooth remaining, attach a bridge, protect weak teeth from fracturing, restore fractured teeth, or cover badly shaped or discolored teeth.

How Is a Crown Placed?

To prepare the tooth for a crown, it is reduced so the crown can fit over it. An impression of teeth and gums is made and sent to the lab for the crown fabrication. A temporary crown is fitted over the tooth until the permanent crown is made. On the next visit, the dentist removes the temporary crown and cements the permanent crown onto the tooth.

Will It Look Natural?

Yes. The dentist's main goal is to create crowns that look like natural teeth. That is why dentists take an impression. To achieve a certain look, a number of factors are considered, such as the color, bite, shape, and length of your natural teeth. Any one of these factors alone can affect your appearance.

If you have a certain cosmetic look in mind for your crown, discuss it with your dentist at your initial visit. When the procedure is complete, your teeth will not only be stronger, but they may be more attractive.

Why Choose Crowns and Not Veneers?

Crowns require more tooth structure removal, hence, they cover more of the tooth than veneers. Crowns are stationary and are customarily indicated for teeth that have sustained significant loss of structure, or to replace missing teeth. Crowns may be placed on natural teeth or dental implants.

What Is the Difference between a Cap and a Crown?

There is no difference between a cap and a crown.

How Long Do Crowns Last?

Crowns should last approximately 5 to 8 years. However, with good oral hygiene and supervision most crowns will last for a much longer period of time. Some damaging habits like grinding your teeth, chewing ice, or fingernail biting may cause this period of time to decrease significantly.

How Should I Take Care of My Crowns?

To prevent damaging or fracturing the crowns, avoid chewing hard foods, ice, or other hard objects. You also want to avoid teeth grinding. Besides visiting your dentist and brushing twice a day, cleaning between your teeth is vital with crowns. Floss or interdental cleaners (specially shaped brushes and sticks) are important tools to remove plaque from the crown area where the gum meets the tooth. Plaque in that area can cause dental decay and gum disease.

Section 36.2

Bridges

"Dental Bridges" is reprinted with permission from
www.aboutcosmeticdentistry.com. © 2003 About Cosmetic Dentistry.

What Is a Dental Bridge?

A dental bridge is a false tooth, known as a pontic, which is fused between two porcelain crowns to fill in the area left by a missing tooth. The two crowns holding it in place are attached onto your teeth on each side of the false tooth. This is known as a fixed bridge. This procedure is used to replace one or more missing teeth. Fixed bridges cannot be taken out of your mouth as you might do with removable partial dentures.

In areas of your mouth that are under less stress, such as your front teeth, a cantilever bridge may be used. Cantilever bridges are used when there are teeth on only one side of the open space. Bridges can reduce your risk of gum disease, help correct some bite issues, and even improve your speech. Bridges require your commitment to serious oral hygiene, but will last as many ten years or more.

Who Is a Candidate for Dental Bridges?

If you have missing teeth and have good oral hygiene practices, you should discuss this procedure with your cosmetic dentist. If spaces are left unfilled, they may cause the surrounding teeth to drift out of position. Additionally, spaces from missing teeth can cause your other teeth and your gums to become far more susceptible to tooth decay and gum disease.

Overview of the Dental Bridge Procedure

If you have a space from a missing tooth, a bridge will be custom made to fill in the space with a false tooth. The false tooth is attached by the bridge to the two other teeth around the space—bridging them together.

How Is a Dental Bridge Accomplished?

Your cosmetic dentist will prepare the teeth on either side of the space for the false tooth. You will be given a mild anesthetic to numb the area, and the cosmetic dentist will remove an area of each abutment (teeth on either side of the space) to accommodate for the thickness of the crown. When these teeth already have fillings, part of the filling may be left in place to help as a foundation for the crown.

The dentist will then make an impression, which will serve as the model for which the bridge, false tooth, and crowns will be made by a dental laboratory. A temporary bridge will be placed for you to wear until your bridge is ready at your next visit. This temporary bridge will serve to protect your teeth and gums.

On your second appointment, the temporary bridge will be removed. Your new permanent bridge will be fitted and checked and adjusted for any bite discrepancies. Your new bridge will then be cemented to your teeth.

Types of Dental Bridges

There are three types of dental bridges.

Traditional Fixed Bridge

A dental bridge is a false tooth, known as a pontic, which is fused between two porcelain crowns to fill in the area left by a missing tooth. There are two crowns holding it in place that are attached onto your teeth on each side of the false tooth. This is known as a fixed bridge. This procedure is used to replace one or more missing teeth. Fixed bridges cannot be taken out of your mouth as you might do with removable partial dentures.

Resin Bonded Bridges

The resin bonded bridge is primarily used for your front teeth. Because it is less expensive, this bridge is best used when the abutment teeth are healthy and don't have large fillings. The false tooth is fused to metal bands that are bonded to the abutment teeth with a resin that is hidden from view. This type of bridge reduces the amount of preparation on the adjacent teeth.

Cantilever Bridges

In areas of your mouth that are under less stress, such as your front teeth, a cantilever bridge may be used. Cantilever bridges are used when there are teeth on only one side of the open space. This procedure involves anchoring the false tooth to one side over one or more natural and adjacent teeth.

How Much Do Dental Bridges Cost?

The average cost of a single fixed bridge depends on many factors, from which region you're in to how many and which type of bridges are needed. Typically dental bridge cost ranges from $500 to $900 per tooth. Dental insurance typically pays for about half of the cost of the bridge.

Pros and Cons of a Dental Bridge

Advantages of dental bridges: Bridges are natural in appearance and usually require only two visits to your dentist. If you maintain good oral hygiene, your fixed bridge should last as many as ten years or more.

Disadvantages of having a dental bridge: It is common for your teeth to be mildly sensitive to extreme temperatures for a few weeks after the treatment. The buildup of bacteria formed from food acids on your teeth and gums can become infected if proper oral hygiene is not followed.

Chapter 37

Dental Implants

Life's simple pleasures can cause problems and pain for the millions of adults who suffer from permanent tooth loss.

Men and women of all ages are self-conscious about their dentures, bridges, or missing teeth. Some have difficulty speaking because their dentures slip or click.

For others, the irritation and pain caused by dentures are constant reminders of the limitations they feel. Many are concerned about their appearance and may feel that their tooth loss has aged them before their time.

Some regularly decline invitations to social events because they are unwilling to face the uncertainties of eating, speaking, and laughing in public. Many can no longer enjoy their favorite foods or the social interaction with family and friends that accompanies special meals.

A Unique Solution to a Troublesome Problem

Now, more and more people are putting an end to these problems by choosing dental implants, a revolutionary way to replace missing teeth. Dental implants offer an excellent alternative to the limitations of conventional dentures, bridges, and missing teeth.

Dental implants are changing the way people live. With them, people are rediscovering the comfort and confidence to eat, speak, laugh, and enjoy life.

Reprinted with permission from the American Association of Oral and Maxillofacial Surgeons. © 1999. For additional information, visit www.aaoms.org.

Why Are People Choosing Dental Implants?

A national survey of oral and maxillofacial surgeons found that patient interest and demand has grown significantly.

The survey found:

- Dental implant use has nearly tripled since 1986 and is expected to continue to rise rapidly.

- People of all ages are turning to dental implants to replace a single tooth, several teeth, or a full set of dentures.

- Leading reasons cited for choosing dental implants are to restore normal eating and speaking abilities; to enhance facial appearance and confidence; and to increase denture retention.

- The reasons for the increased demand are growing public awareness of the significant functional and esthetic advantages of dental implants over conventional dentures and bridges and the availability of data on the long-term success of dental implants.

Experts predict that the demand for the procedure will continue to grow as people become more familiar with the benefits of dental implants.

An Alternative to Natural Teeth

Dental implants are a great option for patients missing natural teeth because they act as a secure anchor for artificial replacement teeth and eliminate the instability associated with surface adhesives and removable bridges.

Your natural teeth absorb biting pressure of up to 540 pounds per square inch. Long-time denture wearers can often absorb no more than 50 pounds per square inch. Dental implants, when properly placed, can withstand 450 pounds per square inch of biting pressure.

Dental implants are made of materials that are compatible with human bone and tissue. The subperiosteal implants are surgically placed directly into the jawbone. Small posts are then attached to the implants which protrude through the gums. These posts provide stable anchors for artificial replacement teeth.

Based on patient needs, a single tooth, a partial bridge, or a full set of replacement teeth are fitted to the implants and locked in place over the protruding posts. In appearance and in function, implants are the closest thing to natural teeth and a good alternative to conventional dentures.

Implants eliminate the day-to-day frustrations and pain of ill-fitting dentures. They allow people to enjoy a healthy and varied diet without the restrictions many denture wearers face. With a sense of renewed self-confidence, many people rediscover the excitement of an active lifestyle shared with family and friends and the chance to speak clearly and comfortably with coworkers.

For all these reasons, people with dental implants often say they feel better, they look better, and they live better.

What to Expect

An oral and maxillofacial surgeon can determine if you are a candidate for dental implants. You will be evaluated based upon a number of things including dental health, lifestyle, jawbone quality and oral hygiene habits. In close consultation with your own dentist, the oral and maxillofacial surgeon can plan your dental implant treatment program.

Dental implant surgery is often done in an oral and maxillofacial surgeon's office. In some cases, the procedure is done in a hospital or ambulatory surgery center. In any event, an oral and maxillofacial surgeon can determine the most appropriate setting based on your individual needs.

For most patients, the placement of dental implants involves two surgical procedures. First, the implants are surgically placed into your jawbone. These small devices make up the framework needed to securely hold replacement teeth. For the first three to six months following surgery, the implants are beneath the surface of the gums, gradually bonding with the jawbone.

During this time, you should be able to wear temporary dentures and eat a soft diet. Some patients do report minor pain and swelling immediately after the procedure but most experience no change in their daily routines.

While the implants are bonding with the jawbone, new replacement teeth are fashioned by your dentist. The replacement teeth must clip onto the implants, fit securely in the mouth, and withstand the day-to-day movement and pressure created by chewing and speaking. So, it is important that they are created by a dentist with proper training in restorative techniques.

Once the implants have bonded to the jawbone, the second phase of the procedure begins. At this time, the oral and maxillofacial surgeon uncovers the implants and attaches small posts which will act as anchors for the artificial teeth.

The posts protrude through the gum line but are not visible when artificial teeth are attached. The entire process, from evaluation to completion, generally takes six to eight months. During this time, most patients do not experience any disruption in their normal business and social activities.

Because dental implants are made of materials that are compatible with human bone, there is little chance for an allergic reaction in the body. However, implants can fail when proper oral hygiene techniques are not used. Dental implants require special individual care. Proper brushing, flossing, rinsing, and regular checkups are critical to the long-term success of your implants.

A Team Effort

Though dental implants are a relatively simple procedure, they generally warrant the expertise of two dental professionals—an oral and maxillofacial surgeon and a restorative dentist.

Working as a team, the oral and maxillofacial surgeon and restorative dentist can determine if you are a candidate for implants and design an appropriate treatment plan. A restorative dentist, with training in dental implants, creates the replacement teeth. The doctor prepares the necessary molds and works with a dental laboratory to make sure that the denture or bridge will meet the particular needs of each patient. Additionally, dental implant patients should see a dentist for routine follow-up care and maintenance.

An oral and maxillofacial surgeon is a dental specialist who surgically treats the mouth and jaw area. Following dental school, an oral and maxillofacial surgeon completes several additional years of training in a hospital residency program and is trained to administer and monitor all types of anesthesia needed for oral and maxillofacial surgery procedures.

Start a New Way of Living Today

If you are among the millions of Americans who suffer from permanent tooth loss, you can eliminate the problems and pain caused by dentures, bridges, or missing teeth. You can begin to rediscover the joy of eating healthy, speaking clearly, and laughing comfortably.

Take the first step. Get the facts about dental implants. See your dentist or a member of the American Association of Oral and Maxillofacial Surgeons. With their training and expertise, they can determine if dental implants are right for you.

Chapter 38

Dentures

Chapter Contents

Section 38.1

Understanding Dentures

"Frequently Asked Questions: Dentures" is reprinted with permission of the American Dental Association. © 2003 American Dental Association. For additional information, visit www.ada.org.

What's the Difference between Conventional Dentures and Immediate Dentures?

Complete dentures are called conventional or immediate according to when they are made and when they are inserted into the mouth.

Immediate dentures are inserted immediately after the removal of the remaining teeth. To make this possible, the dentist takes measurements and makes the models of the patient's jaws during a preliminary visit.

An advantage of immediate dentures is that the wearer does not have to be without teeth during the healing period. However, bones and gums can shrink over time, especially during the period of healing in the first six months after the removal of teeth. When gums shrink, immediate dentures may require rebasing or relining to fit properly. A conventional denture can then be made once the tissues have healed. Healing may take at least six to eight weeks.

What Is an Overdenture?

A removable denture that fits over a small number of remaining natural teeth or implants. The natural teeth must be prepared to provide stability and support for the denture. Your dentist can determine if an overdenture would be suitable for you.

What Will Dentures Feel Like?

New dentures may feel awkward for a few weeks until you become accustomed to them. The dentures may feel loose while the muscles of your cheek and tongue learn to keep them in place.

It is not unusual to experience minor irritation or soreness. You may find that saliva flow temporarily increases. As your mouth becomes accustomed to the dentures, these problems should diminish.

One or more follow-up appointments with the dentist are generally needed after a denture is inserted. If any problem persists, particularly irritation or soreness, be sure to consult your dentist.

Will Dentures Make Me Look Different?

Dentures can be made to closely resemble your natural teeth so that little change in appearance will be noticeable. Dentures may even improve the look of your smile and help fill out the appearance of your face and profile.

Will I Be Able to Eat with My Dentures?

Eating will take a little practice. Start with soft foods cut into small pieces. Chew slowly using both sides of your mouth at the same time to prevent the dentures from tipping. As you become accustomed to chewing, add other foods until you return to your normal diet.

Continue to chew food using both sides of the mouth at the same time. Be cautious with hot or hard foods and sharp-edged bones or shells.

Will Dentures Change How I Speak?

Pronouncing certain words may require practice. Reading out loud and repeating troublesome words will help. If your dentures click while you're talking, speak more slowly.

You may find that your dentures occasionally slip when you laugh, cough, or smile. Reposition the dentures by gently biting down and swallowing. If a speaking problem persists, consult your dentist.

How Long Should I Wear My Dentures?

Your dentist will provide instructions about how long dentures should be kept in place. During the first few days, you may be advised to wear them most of the time, including while you sleep.

After the initial adjustment period, you may be instructed to remove the dentures before going to bed. This allows gum tissues to rest and promotes oral health. Generally, it is not desirable that the tissues be constantly covered by denture material.

Should I Use a Denture Adhesive?

Denture adhesive can provide additional retention for well-fitting dentures. Denture adhesives are not the solution for old, ill-fitting dentures. A poorly fitting denture, which causes constant irritation over a long period, may contribute to the development of sores. These dentures may need a reline or need to be replaced. If your dentures begin to feel loose, or cause pronounced discomfort, consult with your dentist immediately.

How Do I Take Care of My Dentures?

Dentures are very delicate and may break if dropped even a few inches. Stand over a folded towel or a basin of water when handling dentures. When you are not wearing them, store your dentures away from children and pets.

Like natural teeth, dentures must be brushed daily to remove food deposits and plaque. Brushing helps prevent dentures from becoming permanently stained and helps your mouth stay healthy. It's best to use a brush designed for cleaning dentures. A toothbrush with soft bristles can also be used. Avoid using hard-bristled brushes that can damage dentures.

Some denture wearers use hand soap or mild dishwashing liquid, which are both acceptable for cleaning dentures. Avoid using other powdered household cleansers, which may be too abrasive. Also, avoid using bleach, as this may whiten the pink portion of the denture.

Your dentist can recommend a denture cleanser. Look for denture cleansers with the ADA Seal of Acceptance. Products with the ADA Seal have been evaluated for safety and effectiveness.

The first step in cleaning dentures is to rinse away loose food particles thoroughly. Moisten the brush and apply denture cleanser. Brush every surface, scrubbing gently to avoid damage. Dentures may lose their shape if they are allowed to dry out. When they are not worn, dentures should be placed in a denture cleanser soaking solution or in water. Your dentist can recommend the best method. Never place dentures in hot water, which could cause them to warp.

Ultrasonic cleaners are also used to care for dentures. However, using an ultrasonic cleaner does not replace a thorough daily brushing.

Can I Make Minor Adjustments or Repairs to My Dentures?

You can seriously damage your dentures and harm your health by trying to adjust or repair your dentures. A denture that is not made to fit properly can cause irritation and sores.

See your dentist if your dentures break, crack, chip, or if one of the teeth becomes loose. A dentist can often make the necessary adjustments or repairs on the same day. A person who lacks the proper training will not be able to reconstruct the denture. This can cause greater damage to the denture and may cause problems in your mouth. Glue sold over the counter often contains harmful chemicals and should not be used on dentures.

Will My Dentures Need to Be Replaced?

Over time, dentures will need to be relined, rebased, or remade due to normal wear. To reline or rebase a denture, the dentist uses the existing denture teeth and refits the denture base or makes a new denture base. Dentures may need to be replaced if they become loose and the teeth show signs of significant wear. Dentures become loose because a mouth naturally changes with age. Bone and gum ridges can recede or shrink, causing jaws to align differently. Shrinking ridges can cause dentures to fit less securely. Loose dentures can cause health problems, including sores and infections. A loose denture also makes chewing more difficult and may change your facial features. It's important to replace worn or poorly fitting dentures before they cause problems.

Must I Do Anything Special to Care for My Mouth?

Even with full dentures, you still need to take good care of your mouth. Every morning, brush your gums, tongue, and palate with a soft-bristled brush before you put in your dentures. This removes plaque and stimulates circulation in the mouth. Selecting a balanced diet for proper nutrition is also important for maintaining a healthy mouth.

How Often Should I Schedule Dental Appointments?

Your dentist will advise you about how often to visit. Regular dental check-ups are important. The dentist will examine your mouth to see if your dentures continue to fit properly. The dentist also examines your mouth for signs of oral diseases including cancer.

With regular professional care, a positive attitude and persistence, you can become one of the millions of people who wear their dentures with a smile.

Section 38.2

Removable Partial Dentures

"Frequently Asked Questions: Removable Partial Dentures" is reprinted with permission of the American Dental Association. © 2003 American Dental Association. For additional information, visit www.ada.org.

How Do You Wear a Removable Partial Denture?

Removable partial dentures usually consist of replacement teeth attached to pink or gum-colored plastic bases, which are connected by metal framework. Removable partial dentures attach to your natural teeth with metal clasps or devices called precision attachments. Precision attachments are generally more esthetic than metal clasps and they are nearly invisible. Crowns on your natural teeth may improve the fit of a removable partial denture and they are usually required with attachments. Dentures with precision attachments generally cost more than those with metal clasps. Consult with your dentist to find out which type is right for you.

How Long Will It Take to Get Used to Wearing a Denture?

For the first few weeks, your new partial denture may feel awkward or bulky. However, your mouth will eventually become accustomed to wearing it. Inserting and removing the denture will require some practice. Follow all instructions given by your dentist. Your denture should fit into place with relative ease. Never force the partial denture into position by biting down. This could bend or break the clasps.

How Long Should I Wear the Denture?

Your dentist will give you specific instruction about how long the denture should be worn and when it should be removed. Initially, you may be asked to wear your partial denture all the time. Although this may be temporarily uncomfortable, it is the quickest way to identify those denture parts that may need adjustment. If the denture puts too much pressure on a particular area, that spot will become sore. Your dentist will adjust the denture to fit more comfortably. After making adjustments, your dentist will probably recommend that you take the denture out of your mouth before going to bed and replace it in the morning.

Will It Be Difficult to Eat with a Partial Denture?

Replacing missing teeth should make eating a more pleasant experience. Start out by eating soft foods that are cut into small pieces. Chew on both sides of the mouth to keep even pressure on the denture. Avoid foods that are extremely sticky or hard. You may want to avoid chewing gum while you adjust to the denture.

Will the Denture Change How I Speak?

It can be difficult to speak clearly when you are missing teeth. Consequently, wearing a partial denture may help. If you find it difficult to pronounce certain words with your new denture, practice reading out loud. Repeat the words that give you trouble. With time, you will become accustomed to speaking properly with your denture.

How Do I Take Care of My Denture?

Handling a denture requires care. It's a good idea to stand over a folded towel or a sink of water just in case you accidentally drop the denture. Brush the denture each day to remove food deposits and plaque. Brushing your denture helps prevent the appliance from becoming permanently stained. It's best to use a brush that is designed for cleaning dentures. A denture brush has bristles that are arranged to fit the shape of the denture. A regular, soft-bristled toothbrush is also acceptable. Avoid using a brush with hard bristles, which can damage the denture.

Your dentist can recommend a denture cleaner. Look for denture cleansers with the American Dental Association (ADA) Seal of Acceptance.

Products with the ADA Seal have been evaluated for safety and effectiveness.

Some people use hand soap or mild dishwashing liquid to clean their dentures, which are both acceptable. Other types of household cleaners and many toothpastes are too abrasive and should not be used for cleaning dentures.

Clean your dentures by thoroughly rinsing off loose food particles. Moisten the brush and apply the denture cleaner. Brush all denture surfaces gently to avoid damaging the plastic or bending the attachments.

A denture could lose its proper shape if it is not kept moist. At night, the denture should be placed in soaking solution or water. However, if the appliance has metal attachments, they could be tarnished if placed in soaking solution. Your dentist can recommend the proper method for keeping your dentures in good shape.

Will My Denture Need Adjusting?

Over time, adjusting the denture may be necessary. As you age, your mouth naturally changes, which can affect the fit of the denture. Your bone and gum ridges can recede or shrink, resulting in a loose-fitting denture. Dentures that do not fit properly should be adjusted by your dentist. Loose dentures can cause various problems, including sores or infections. See your dentist promptly if your denture becomes loose.

Can I Make Minor Adjustments or Repairs to My Denture?

You can do serious harm to your denture and to your health by trying to adjust or repair your denture. A denture that is not made to fit precisely by a dentist can cause irritation and sores. Using a do-it-yourself kit can damage the appliance beyond repair. Glues sold over-the-counter often contain harmful chemicals and should not be used on a denture.

If your denture no longer fits properly, if it breaks, cracks, or chips, or if one of the teeth becomes loose, see your dentist immediately. In many cases, dentists can make necessary adjustments or repairs, often on the same day. Complicated repairs may require that the denture be sent to a special dental laboratory.

Must I Do Anything Special to Take Care of My Mouth?

Brushing twice a day and cleaning between your teeth daily help prevent tooth decay and gum disease that can lead to tooth loss. Pay special attention to cleaning teeth that fit under the denture's metal clasps. Plaque that becomes trapped under the clasps will increase the risk of tooth decay. Your dentist or dental hygienist can demonstrate how to properly brush and clean between teeth. Selecting a balanced diet for proper nutrition is also important.

How Often Should I See My Dentist?

Your dentist will advise you on the frequency of dental visits. Regular dental checkups and having your teeth professionally cleaned are vital for maintaining a healthy smile.

How Can I Fill the Gap?

A bridge—a device used to replace missing teeth—attaches artificial teeth to adjacent natural teeth, called abutment teeth. Bridges can be applied either permanently (fixed bridges), or they can be removable.

Fixed bridges are applied by either placing crowns on the abutment teeth—to provide support for artificial teeth—or by bonding the artificial teeth directly to the abutment teeth. Removable bridges are attached to the teeth by either metal clasps or by precision attachments.

Section 38.3

Maintaining Denture Fit and Comfort

Reprinted with permission from the American Association of Oral and Maxillofacial Surgeons. © 1999. For additional information, visit www.aaoms.org.

After years of comfortably wearing dentures, you may come to find that they don't fit the way they once did. Advances in surgical procedures and materials now allow oral and maxillofacial surgeons to help the patient without teeth to eat, speak, and smile without worrying about slipping or uncomfortable dentures.

Over time, the shape and size of the jawbone changes, beginning when a tooth is lost. These changes can result in dentures that slip and click and even cause pain. The irritation caused by ill-fitting dentures can produce further changes in the bone or the gum tissues. After years of shrinkage, many patients are left without enough jawbone to support dentures at all.

Treatment Options Exist

Preservation and restoration of the jawbone begins at the time of extraction of teeth. Bone and soft tissue grafting techniques performed in conjunction with extractions may decrease or prevent bone loss under dentures. Oral and maxillofacial surgeons have developed many procedures for treating the patient without teeth who suffers with the social and physical problems caused by ill-fitting dentures. Your oral and maxillofacial surgeon will explore these options with you before deciding on a treatment plan.

If shrinkage of the jawbone has taken place and some ridge height and width remains, the oral and maxillofacial surgeon may use bone or bone substitute to build up the jawbone. Depending on the degree of shrinkage, this treatment sometimes can be completed in the office.

Another treatment option which your oral and maxillofacial surgeon may consider is called a vestibuloplasty. If enough jawbone remains below the muscle attachments of the lip, cheeks, and tongue, firm tissue can be grafted over the bone to provide a larger ridge. This usually requires taking tissue from the roof of the mouth or thigh.

After careful evaluation of your problem, the oral and maxillofacial surgeon may decide that implants are necessary to support a denture and restore proper function.

Maintenance Is Important

Many people stop going to their dentist after dentures are fitted. Regular checkups are still the best insurance that your mouth is healthy. Changes in the gums and jawbone can occur under a denture, especially as a result of chronic irritation.

Overgrowth of tissues in some areas, or sores on the gum, is also common. In addition, your dentist or oral and maxillofacial surgeon will sometimes see early warning signs of generalized disease. It is also important to be aware of changes in oral tissue due to cigarette smoking or alcohol consumption so that alterations in these habits can prevent future problems.

Exploring your options with your dentist and oral and maxillofacial surgeon will allow you to function without worrying about your dentures and will preserve the health of your mouth.

Chapter 39

Jaw and Oromandibular Disorders

Chapter Contents

Section 39.1

Temporomandibular Disorders (Jaw Disorders)

"Frequently Asked Questions—TMD/TMJ (Jaw Disorders)" is a brochure published by the U.S. Department of Health and Human Services, National Women's Health Information Center, 1998. Available online at www.4woman.gov/faq/TMDTMJJawDisorders.htm; accessed May 2003.

What Is TMD?

TMD, or temporomandibular disorders, are a group of conditions affecting the temporomandibular joint (TMJ) and the muscles involved in chewing.

These disorders occur more frequently in women than men, and it has been estimated that approximately 10 million women in the U.S. suffer from chronic face or jaw joint pain. There are many possible causes of these disorders, and diagnosis can be confusing and difficult. Treatment is usually conservative and reversible, and may require many different medical specialists. Occasionally injections and surgery are necessary for chronic pain and disability.

What Is TMJ?

The temporomandibular joint's name is derived from the two bones that it connects. It joins the bone at the side of the head (temporal bone) to the lower jaw (mandible). This joint can be felt on either side of the head when placing a finger in front of each ear and opening the mouth.

Upon opening the mouth, the rounded end at the top of the lower jaw, known as the condyle, will glide along a groove in the temporal bone. Upon closing the mouth, the condyle will slide back to its original position.

In order to preserve a smooth gliding motion, a very thin soft disc lies between the condyle and the temporal bone. This disc acts as a shock absorber for the TMJ during daily functions such as chewing, talking, and yawning. It is during these actions that the TMJ and its surrounding muscles may be affected, resulting in any one of a number of uncomfortable conditions including TMD.

TMD Categories

Researchers have found that temporomandibular disorders generally fall into three main categories:

- **Myofascial pain.** This is the most common form of TMD, which involves discomfort or pain in the muscles that control jaw function, as well as the neck and shoulder muscles.

- **Internal derangement of the TMJ.** This involves a dislocated jaw, displaced disc, or injury to the condyle.

- **Degenerative joint disease.** This includes diseases such as osteoarthritis or rheumatoid arthritis in the TMJ.

What Are the Causes of TMD?

Severe injury to the jaw or TMJ can cause TMD. For example, a heavy blow can fracture the bones associated with the joint or damage the disc. This may result in a disruption of smooth jaw motion causing pain or locking of the jaw during movement. Other causes of TMD are less clear. A poor bite (malocclusion), orthodontic treatment, jaw clenching, teeth grinding, as well as physical and mental stress have all been linked to TMD.

Unfortunately, their roles as definite causes have not yet been determined.

What Are the Signs and Symptoms of TMD?

Pain, particularly in the chewing muscles and/or the TMJ, is the most common symptom of TMD. Other symptoms include the following:

- Limited movement or locking of the jaw

- Radiating pain to the face, neck, or shoulders

- Painful clicking, popping, or grating sounds in the jaw joint when opening or closing the mouth

- Sudden major changes in the way that the upper and lower teeth fit together

- Headaches, earaches, dizziness, and hearing problems may also be related to TMD.

It is important to understand that occasional discomfort in the jaw or chewing muscles is quite common. It is usually temporary in duration, and is not generally a cause for concern.

A common sensation in the general population is clicking or popping of the TMJ. Upon opening and/or closing the mouth, one may hear or feel a clicking or popping of the jaw joint. Researchers believe that most people who have clicking or popping of the TMJ probably have a displaced disc within the joint. If the displaced disc causes no pain or locking of the jaw, then typically no treatment is required.

How Do You Diagnose TMD?

Since the causes and symptoms of TMD are often unclear, diagnosis can be confusing and difficult. In about 90% of cases, the combination of the patient's description of symptoms, dental and medical history, and a physical examination of the face and jaw, can provide useful information for the diagnosis of these disorders.

The physical examination involves feeling the TMJ and chewing muscles for pain or tenderness; listening for clicking, popping, or grating sounds during jaw movement; and observing any limited motion or locking of the jaw while opening or closing the mouth.

Routine dental and TMJ x-rays are not always useful in the diagnosis of TMD, but may be helpful in few patients. Other x-ray techniques such as arthrography (x-rays of the joint using a dye), and magnetic resonance imaging (MRI, which pictures the soft tissues) are usually needed only when the practitioner strongly suspects a condition such as osteoarthritis or internal derangement of the TMJ, or when significant pain persists over time and symptoms have not improved with previous treatment.

How Do You Treat TMD?

Since most of the discomfort of TMD is temporary, treatment is usually conservative and reversible. Conservative non-surgical treatments do no invade the tissues of the face, jaw, or joint. Reversible treatments do not cause permanent, or irreversible, changes to the position of the jaws or teeth. Researchers strongly recommend using the most conservative, reversible treatments possible before considering any invasive treatments.

Simple self-care practices such as special relaxation and stress-reduction techniques can be used in order to help patients relieve the pain that is often a TMD symptom. Eating soft foods, applying moist heat packs, and avoiding extreme jaw movements are useful measures that can help ease TMD symptoms. Other conservative, reversible treatments include physical therapy that focuses on gentle muscle stretching, and the short-term use of muscle relaxants and anti-inflammatory drugs. Occasionally, a psychiatric/psychological or neurological condition is believed to be the cause of TMD, and then referrals to the appropriate clinicians are recommended.

In some cases, an oral appliance, known as a splint, may be necessary. The splint is a plastic mouth guard that fits over the upper or lower teeth. It acts to help reduce clenching or grinding of the teeth, thereby easing muscle tension. It should not be used for a long period of time, nor should it increase pain, or cause permanent changes in a person's bite.

Other less conservative treatments of TMD include injecting medications directly into the joint or affected muscles, removing scar or destroyed tissue from the TMJ, or conducting surgery on the jaw bone to improve the relationship between upper and lower teeth (orthognathic surgery).

Surgical treatments are often irreversible and as with most surgical procedures, there are usually significant risks involved. Surgery may result in an increased level of pain, discomfort, or cause permanent damage to the jaw and TMJ. Typically, conservative therapy is recommended prior to any surgical procedure. Only if multiple conservative therapies have failed should surgery be considered.

Prior to any surgery, it is strongly advised that one clearly understands the reason for this type of treatment, its benefits, and possible risks. Furthermore, one should seek at least a second opinion prior to consenting to any possibly irreversible surgical procedure.

Section 39.2

Oromandibular Dystonia

Reprinted with permission from the Dystonia Medical Research Foundation, www.dystonia-foundation.org. © 2000 Dystonia Medical Research Foundation.

What Is It?

Oromandibular dystonia is a focal dystonia characterized by forceful contractions of the jaw and tongue causing difficulty in opening and closing the mouth and often affecting chewing and speech.

Symptoms

Oromandibular is often associated with dystonia of the cervical muscles (cervical dystonia/spasmodic torticollis), eyelids (blepharospasm), or larynx (spasmodic dysphonia). The combination of upper and lower dystonia is sometimes called cranial-cervical dystonia. When oromandibular is combined with blepharospasm, it may be referred to as Meige's Syndrome named after Henry Meige, the French neurologist who first described the symptoms in detail in 1910.

The symptoms usually begin between the ages of 40 and 70 years old and appear to be more common in women than in men.

Oromandibular dystonia may be a continuous disorder that persists even during sleep, or it may be task-specific, occurring only during activities such as speaking or chewing.

Difficulty in swallowing is a common aspect of oromandibular dystonia if the jaw if affected, and spasms in the tongue can also make it difficult to swallow.

If oromandibular dystonia causes any type of impairment, it is because muscle contractions interfere with normal function. Features such as cognition, strength, and the senses, including vision and hearing, are normal. Although dystonia is not fatal, it is a chronic disorder and prognosis is difficult to predict.

Cause

Oromandibular dystonia is believed to be due to abnormal functioning of the basal ganglia, which are deep brain structures involved with the control of movement. The basal ganglia assists in initiating and regulating movement. What goes wrong in the basal ganglia is still unknown. An imbalance of dopamine, a neurotransmitter in the basal ganglia, may underlie several different forms of dystonia, but much more research needs to be done for a better understanding of the brain mechanisms involved with dystonia.

Cases of inherited cranial dystonia have been reported, usually in conjunction with early-onset generalized dystonia that is associated with the DYT1 gene.

Oromandibular dystonia may be secondary, or symptomatic, occurring in association with other disorders such as tardive dystonia, Wilson's disease, Parkinson's disease, and X-linked dystonia-parkinsonian syndrome.

Diagnosis

Diagnosis of blepharospasm is based on information from the affected individual and the physical and neurological examination. At this time, there is no test to confirm diagnosis of oromandibular, and, in most cases, laboratory tests are normal.

Oromandibular dystonia should not be mistaken for temporomandibular joint disease (TMJ) which is an arthritic condition, and not dystonia.

Treatment

Treatment for dystonia is designed to help lessen the symptoms of spasms, pain, and disturbed postures and functions. Most therapies are symptomatic, attempting to cover up or release the dystonic spasms. No single strategy will be appropriate for every case.

The goal of any treatment is to achieve the greatest benefits while incurring the fewest risks. It is to allow you to lead a fuller, more productive life by reducing the effects of dystonia. Establishing a satisfactory regimen requires patience on the part of both the affected individual and the physician.

The approach for treatment of dystonia is usually three-tiered: oral medications, botulinum toxin injections, and surgery. These therapies may be used alone or in combination.

Complementary care, such as physical therapy and speech therapy, may also have a role in the treatment management depending on the form of dystonia.

For many people, supportive therapy provides an important adjunct to medical treatment.

Although there is currently no known cure for dystonia, we are gaining a better understanding of dystonia through research and are developing new approaches to treatments.

Medications

A multitude of drugs has been studied to determine benefit for people with oromandibular dystonia, but none appear to be uniformly effective.

About one-third of people's symptoms improved when treated with oral medications such as Klonopin (clonazepam), Artane (trihexyphenidyl), diazepam (Valium), tetrabenazine, and Lioresal (baclofen), but the degree of improvement is usually unsatisfactory and at the expense of side effects.

Botulinum Toxin Injections

Dystonia in the jaw can affect various muscles. Botulinum toxin injections are most effective when the correct muscles are injected. If the jaw muscles are injected, the facial muscles should not be affected, but injections into the face muscles may affect expressions. About 70 percent of people with oromandibular experience some reduction of spasm and improvement of chewing and speech after injection of botulinum toxin into the masseter, temporalis, and lateral pterygoid muscles. Botulinum toxin injections are most effective in jaw-closure dystonia, whereas treating jaw-opening dystonia is more challenging, benefiting less people.

Side effects such as swallowing difficulties, slurred speech, and excess weakness in injected muscles may occur, but these side effects are usually transient and well tolerated.

Surgery

The structure of the jaw is so complex that at this time denervation (cutting a nerve) surgery for oromandibular dystonia cannot be done.

Complementary Therapy

The use of sensory tricks may also be effective in dealing with oromandibular. Some of the most common tricks include touching the lips or chin, chewing gum, talking, biting on a toothpick, or putting a finger near an eye or underneath the chin to keep the jaw closed. Different sensory tricks work for different people, and if a person finds a sensory trick that works, it usually continues to work.

Speech and swallowing therapy may lessen spasms, improve range of motion, strengthen unaffected muscles, and facilitate speech and swallowing.

Support

By educating yourself, you have taken the first step in dealing with dystonia. Dystonia and its emotional offshoots affect every aspect of a person's life—how we think, the way we act, and how we cope.

Stress is an inevitable part of life, and although it clearly does not cause dystonia, it can aggravate dystonia symptoms. Stress-reduction programs such as relaxation techniques, meditation, and journal writing may be beneficial.

Sometimes depression can be a byproduct of dystonia. It, too, can aggravate symptoms and make them worse, but often, treating depression can result in an improvement of dystonia. It is important to remember that depression is a disease; it is treatable and not a reflection of one's self.

Thousands of people are experiencing similar symptoms, and you are not alone in coping with dystonia. Reassurance from family, friends, and others who have dystonia is beneficial. Support groups offer encouragement, camaraderie, and information about new treatments and medical advances. The Dystonia Medical Research Foundation maintains a network of support groups throughout North America along with many online resources.

Chapter 40

Bruxism

When you look in on your sleeping child, you want to hear the sweet sounds of sweet dreams: easy breathing and perhaps an occasional sigh. But some parents hear the harsher sounds of gnashing and grinding teeth, called bruxism.

Bruxism is common among young children. Read on to find out what causes bruxism and how you can help your child.

What Is Bruxism?

Bruxism is the medical term for the grinding of teeth or the clenching of jaws, especially during deep sleep or while under stress. It comes from the Greek word "brychein," which means to gnash the teeth. Three out of every 10 kids will grind or clench, experts say, with the highest incidence in children under 5.

What Causes Bruxism?

"We don't know exactly why bruxism happens," says Dr. Eugene Howden, a pediatric dentist in Chapel Hill, North Carolina. "There have been many studies done, but we can't find a cause." There are

This information was provided by KidsHealth, one of the largest resources online for medically reviewed health information written for parents, kids, and teens. For more articles like this one, visit www.KidsHealth.org or www. TeensHealth.org. © 2001 The Nemours Center for Children's Health Media, a division of The Nemours Foundation.

anatomical and psychological catalysts, however, that can be a factor in whether a child has bruxism.

In some cases, bruxism is related to a child's growth and development. Some children grind because the top and bottom teeth are not aligned properly. Others do it as a response to pain, such as an earache or teething. Your child might grind her teeth as a way to ease the pain, just as she might rub a sore muscle. "These are fairly common causes for grinding," says Dr. Dan Howell, a dentist in Cary, North Carolina. "Most kids outgrow them."

Stress—usually nervous tension or anger—is another cause. For instance, your child may be worrying about a test at school or experiencing a change in routine (a new sibling or a new teacher) —and she may find that troubling. Even arguing with parents and siblings can cause enough stress to get her teeth grinding or jaw clenching.

Some children who are hyperactive also experience bruxism.

Effects of Bruxism

Generally, bruxism doesn't hurt a child's teeth. Many cases go undetected with no adverse effects, though some may result in mild morning headaches or earaches. Most often, however, the condition can be more bothersome to you and others in your home because of the grinding sound.

In some extreme circumstances, nighttime grinding and clenching can wear down tooth enamel, chip teeth, increase temperature sensitivity, and cause severe facial pain and jaw problems, such as temporomandibular joint disease (TMJ). Most children who grind, however, do not have TMJ problems unless their grinding and clenching is chronic.

Diagnosis

Lots of kids grind their teeth and are not even aware of it, so it is often siblings or parents who identify the problem. Dr. Howden advises parents to watch for indicators. "Usually, mom or dad will notice that their kids make a lot of grinding noises when they're asleep. Or their kids might complain that their jaw or face is sore in the morning."

If your child sucks her thumb, bites her fingernails, gnaws on pencils and toys, or chews the inside of her cheeks, she may also be grinding at night.

If you suspect your child is grinding her teeth, visit your child's dentist. The dentist will examine your child's teeth for chipped enamel and unusual wear and tear as well as spray air and water on the teeth to check for unusual sensitivity.

If your dentist detects damage, he or she will ask your child a few questions, such as:

- How do you feel before bed?
- Are you worried about anything at home or school?
- Are you angry with someone?
- What do you do before bed?

The exam will help your child's dentist determine whether her grinding is caused by anatomical (misaligned teeth) or psychological (stress) forces. With that information, your child's dentist can devise an effective treatment plan.

Treatment

"The best thing to do is to wait it out and see if your child outgrows it," Dr. Howell says. A combination of parental observation and dental visits should keep the problem in check.

In some cases, however, dentists prescribe a special night guard. These guards are similar to the protective mouthpieces worn by football players. They are molded to your child's teeth to ensure a good fit.

Night guards are prescribed if grinding and clenching make your child's face and jaw sore, or if her teeth are being damaged. Though they may take some getting used to, your child—and you—will begin to see positive results soon.

What Can I Do to Help?

Whether the cause is physical or psychological, your child may be able to control her bruxism by relaxing before bedtime. Taking a warm bath or shower, listening to a few minutes of slow music, or reading a book can help calm your child. Find a relaxing activity she likes and make that a part of her nightly bedtime routine.

For bruxism that's caused by stress, you'll need to find out what's upsetting your child and find a way to fix that. Talking to her about how she feels can clue you in to situations that might be troubling her. Once identified, you can work with her to relieve those stresses. For example, if she's worried about being away from home for her first camping trip, reassure her that you will be nearby if anything happens or that she will have a lot of fun with her friends.

If the issue is more complicated, such as moving to a new town, talk to her about what is concerning her and try to ease her fears. If you have any concerns about your child's emotional state, consult your child's doctor.

In rare cases, however, these basic stress relievers are not enough to stop bruxism. If your child is having trouble sleeping or is acting differently than usual, your child's dentist or doctor may suggest a psychological assessment. This can help determine the cause of your child's stress and set a course of treatment.

Duration

Usually childhood bruxism is outgrown by adolescence. Most kids stop grinding when they lose their baby teeth because permanent teeth are much more sensitive to pain.

A few children continue to grind into adolescence. And if the bruxism is caused by stress, it will continue until the stress is relieved.

Prevention

Because some bruxism is a child's natural reaction to growth and development, most cases cannot be prevented. Stress-induced bruxism can be avoided, however, by talking with your child regularly about her feelings and helping her deal with stress in her life.

Note: All information on KidsHealth is for educational purposes only. For specific medical advice, diagnoses, and treatment, consult your doctor.

Chapter 41

Cosmetic Dentistry

Chapter Contents

Section 41.1

What You Should Know about Cosmetic Dentistry

From "Cosmetic Dentistry: It Can Really Make a Difference," © 2001 California Dental Association. Reprinted with Permission. For more information, visit the website of the California Dental Association at www.cda.org. As a public service, the California Dental Association also maintains a consumer information website at www.smilecalifornia.org.

Have you ever asked yourself, "Could my smile be brighter?" or "Is it possible for me to get my discolored (or misshaped or chipped or crooked) teeth to look good?" Thanks to the wonders of modern cosmetic dentistry, the answer is very likely to be, "Not only is it possible, but in many cases, it's quick, painless, and surprisingly affordable."

You may be able to spruce your mouth up with one, maybe two, of the vast array of cosmetic dental procedures available these days.

Bleaching lightens teeth that have been stained or discolored by food and age or darkened as a result of injury. There are two ways to professionally bleach teeth. Your dentist can apply a bleaching solution to one or more of your teeth per visit, over the course of several appointments. Or you can be fitted with a custom-made bleaching tray that you wear for a couple of hours every night at home under a dentist's guidance. This process can take anywhere from one to six weeks.

Bonding involves applying a tooth-colored plastic putty called composite resin to the surface of your chipped, broken, or discolored teeth. The composite resin can also fill in gaps between your teeth and protect roots that are exposed due to gum recession. The entire procedure is virtually painless and is usually completed in one visit. However, complex cases may require several appointments.

Porcelain veneers are thin, custom-made, tooth-colored shells that cover the front of your teeth. Once applied, they correct or camouflage misaligned, poorly shaped, damaged, or discolored teeth. The process of applying veneers usually involves two visits to your dentist.

If your teeth are a bit overcrowded or uneven, they can be slightly contoured in a procedure called enamel shaping or cosmetic recontouring. For instance, if one of your teeth looks much longer than the rest, some enamel can be removed and your tooth can be reshaped. The process is usually quick and painless.

Recent advances in orthodontic treatment, such as less visible and more effective brackets and wires, now make straightening crooked teeth more palatable for many adults. How long you'll have to wear them depends on the severity of your problem, the health of your teeth, gums, and supporting bone, and your age.

A lost tooth or teeth can be replaced with dental implants. Dental implants are artificial teeth that are attached directly into your jaw. They're much more secure and natural looking than dentures or bridgework, but they can be expensive and the entire process can be quite lengthy. Long-time denture wearers also benefit from implants by having their loose-fitting dentures secured to a specially designed implant attachment.

If you're feeling somewhat self-conscious about your teeth, talk to your dentist about these cosmetic dentistry options.

Section 41.2

Porcelain Veneers

"Tell Me About Veneers" is reprinted with permission from the British Dental Health Foundation, www.britishdentalhealth.org.uk. © 2003 British Dental Health Foundation.

What Is a Veneer?

A veneer is a thin layer of porcelain made to fit over the front surface of a tooth, like a false fingernail fits over a nail. Sometimes a natural color composite material is used instead of porcelain.

When Would I Need a Veneer?

Veneers can improve the color, shape, and position of your teeth. A precise shade of porcelain can be chosen to give the right color to improve a single discolored or stained tooth or to lighten front teeth (usually the upper ones) generally. A veneer can make a chipped tooth look intact again. The porcelain covers the whole of the front of the tooth with a thicker section replacing the broken part. Veneers can also be used to close small gaps, when orthodontics (braces) are not suitable. If one tooth is slightly out of position, a veneer can sometimes be fitted to bring it into line with the others.

What Are the Advantages of Veneers?

Veneers make teeth look natural and healthy. Because they are very thin and are held in place by a special strong bond (rather like super glue) very little preparation of the tooth is needed.

How Are Teeth Prepared for a Veneer?

Some of the shiny outer enamel surface of the tooth may be removed, to make sure that the veneer can be bonded permanently in place later. The amount of enamel removed is tiny and will be the same as the thickness of the veneer to be fitted, so that the tooth stays the same size. A local anesthetic (injection) may be used to make sure that there is no discomfort, but often this is not necessary. Once the tooth has been prepared, the dentist will take an impression (mold). This will be given to the dental technician, along with any other information needed to make the veneer. The color of the surrounding teeth is matched on a shade guide to make sure that the veneer will look entirely natural.

How Long Will It Take?

A veneer takes at least two visits: the first to prepare the tooth and to match the shade, and the second to fit it. Before bonding it in place, your dentist will show you the veneer on your tooth to make sure you are happy with it. Bonding a veneer in place is done with a special adhesive, which holds it firmly on the tooth.

Will I Need a Temporary Veneer between Visits?

Because the preparation of the tooth is so slight you will probably not need a temporary veneer. The tooth will look very much the same after preparation, but will feel slightly less smooth.

What Happens after the Veneer Is Fitted?

Only minor adjustments can be made to the veneer after it is fitted. It is usually best to wait a little while to get used to it before any changes are made. Your dentist will probably want to check and polish it a week or so after it is fitted, and make sure that you are happy with it.

How Much Will It Cost?

The cost of a veneer varies. It is important to discuss charges and treatment options with your dentist before starting treatment.

How Long Will a Veneer Last?

Veneers should last for many years; but they can chip or break, just as your own teeth can. Your dentist will tell you how long each individual veneer should last. Small chips can be repaired, or a new veneer fitted if necessary.

What about Alternatives?

A natural-colored filling material can be used for minor repairs to front teeth. This is excellent where the tooth supports the filling, but may not work so well for broken tooth corners. There will always be a join between the tooth and the filling material. Crowns are used for teeth which need to be strengthened—either because they have broken, have been weakened by a very large filling, or have had root canal treatment.

Section 41.3

Tooth Whitening Systems

Reprinted with permission from the American Dental Hygienists'
Association Website, www.adha.org. © 2003.

Why Do My Teeth Have Stains and Discolorations?

Most stains are caused by age, tobacco, coffee, or tea. Other types
of stains can be caused by antibiotics, such as tetracycline; or too much
fluoride.

What Treatments Are Used for Stained Teeth?

Ask your oral health care professional about tooth-whitening options. They include a number of over-the-counter whitening systems,
whitening toothpastes, and the latest high-tech option—laser tooth
whitening. For maximum whitening, experts agree that peroxide is
usually the way to go.

Supervised bleaching procedures that are done in the office and
at home have become among the most popular treatment options. In
some cases, the procedure is performed entirely in the office, using a
light or heat source to speed up the bleaching process. In other cases,
an oral health care professional gets the procedure started during an
office visit and then gives you what you need to complete it at home.
Still another popular procedure is one that you complete entirely at
home.

At-home procedures, sometimes called nightguard vital bleaching, consist of placing a bleaching solution, usually a peroxide mixture, in a tray (nightguard) that has been custom fitted for your mouth
by an oral health care professional. The bleaching solutions may
vary in potency and may be worn for an hour or throughout the night.
Your oral health care professional can advise you on the appropriate
type of application and the length of time needed to whiten your
teeth, based on the severity of tooth discoloration and your specific
needs.

How Effective Are Bleaching Systems?

Bleaching is effective in lightening most stains caused by age, tobacco, coffee, and tea. Based on clinical studies, 96 percent of patients with these kinds of stains experience some lightening effect. Other types of stains, such as those produced by tetracycline use or fluorosis (too much fluoride), respond to bleaching less reliably. And one cosmetic dentist points out that bleaching systems are not fully predictable. If you have a tooth-colored filling when your teeth are bleached, the filling will stay yellow—dental restorations do not change color when tooth whitener is applied.

Are There Any Side Effects to Tooth Bleaching?

In some studies, patients have experienced uncomfortable short-term side effects when having teeth bleached. Hydrogen peroxide can increase temperature sensitivity in the teeth, particularly at higher concentrations, and nightguards often cause gum irritation.

And overzealous use of over-the-counter home bleaching products can wear away tooth enamel, especially with solutions that contain acid. Therefore, bleaching is a procedure best done under the care of an oral health care professional.

Still, the general health risks of bleaching systems are minimal as far as your body is concerned. Applications are controlled so that you don't swallow hydrogen peroxide.

What's Available?

While research continues into all types of bleaching systems, tooth bleaching is sure to continue to grow in popularity. Here's a selection of what's currently available.

- At-home bleaching kits—the most popular whitening option. Mouth trays are usually made in one office visit, and your oral health care professional will provide a whitening brand suitable to your needs. Some trays are worn for an hour, others through the night. Kits range in price from $300 to $500.

- Bonding—a composite resin that is molded onto the teeth to change their color and to reshape them. The resin material can stain and chip over time. Bonding can usually be done in one office visit for $300 to $700 per tooth.

- Porcelain veneers—these shell-like facings can be bonded onto stained teeth. They are used to reshape and/or lengthen teeth as well as to whiten. Veneers require at least two office visits and cost $700 to $1,200 per tooth.

- Whitening toothpastes—While some whitening toothpastes effectively keep the teeth cleaner and, therefore, looking whiter, some are more abrasive than others. The stronger toothpastes rely on abrasion to remove external stains as opposed to actually changing the color of teeth. The key is to study a product's ingredients, look at your teeth to see if it changes their color, and consult your oral health care professional for customized advice.

Note: Before using any whitening procedure, ADHA recommends that you first be evaluated by an oral health care professional to determine which application and program are best for you.

Section 41.4

Enamel Microabrasion

Reprinted with permission from the American Academy of Pediatric Dentistry, www.aapd.org. © 2002.

What Is Microabrasion?

In microabrasion, dentists carefully rub a compound on the teeth to remove superficial stains and discoloration.

Why Are My Child's Teeth Discolored?

A number of conditions can cause discoloration of permanent teeth. For example, trauma to a baby tooth, an infection around a baby tooth, and high fevers or prolonged chronic illnesses during childhood can cause discolorations. Fluoride can also cause some white or brown discolorations of teeth when a child receives a high dose over a period of time.

Some teeth have a deeper, irreversible stain or discoloration, the result of trauma, root canal therapy, or medications such as tetracycline. These deep stains are not improved by microabrasion.

Will Microabrasion Work for My Child?

The success of microabrasion depends on a number of factors, especially the type and extent of discoloration. So, it is difficult to predict when microabrasion will remove a discoloration completely from a tooth. Pediatric dentists have learned that brown or dark stains are removed readily in most cases. White discolorations are often improved; sometimes they are totally eliminated. Other times, white discolorations are very persistent and not removed completely with microabrasion.

Some teeth have a speckled appearance, showing a lot of white spots all over the tooth. These teeth may be improved with microabrasion. By removing the bright white spots, the teeth will have a slightly darker, but more even, natural color.

What If Microabrasion Doesn't Work?

Microabrasion is a safe, minimal treatment of discolored teeth. Attempting microabrasion does not eliminate any of the alternatives for treatment. Other treatments for discolored teeth are plastic or porcelain veneers or porcelain crowns. These options are less affordable and more extensive than microabrasion because they require some tooth preparation. So, it's wise to consider microabrasion as your first choice of treatment for discolored teeth.

Part Five

Health Conditions
That Affect Oral Care

Chapter 42

Oral Conditions in Children with Special Needs

Children with special health care needs may experience a variety of oral conditions and problems.

Problems with Oral Development

Tooth Eruption

Tooth eruption may be delayed, accelerated, or inconsistent in children with growth disturbances. Gums may appear red or bluish-purple

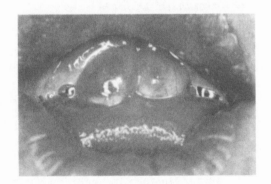

Figure 42.1. A child with tooth eruption problems.

Excerpted from a brochure published by the National Institute of Dental and Craniofacial Research (NIDCR)/National Oral Health Information Clearinghouse, November 2002. Available online at www.nohic.nidcr.nih.gov/pubs/oral_conditions/index.htm; accessed May 2003.

before erupting teeth break through into the mouth. Eruption depends on genetics, growth of the jaw, muscular action, and other factors. Children with Down syndrome may show delays of up to 2 years. Health care providers should offer information about the variability in tooth eruption patterns and refer you to an oral health care provider for additional questions.

Malocclusion

Malocclusion, a poor fit between the upper and lower teeth, and crowding of teeth occur frequently in people with developmental disabilities. Nearly 25 percent of the more than 80 craniofacial anomalies that can affect oral development are associated with mental retardation. Muscle dysfunction contributes to malocclusion, particularly in people with cerebral palsy. Teeth that are crowded or out of alignment are more difficult to keep clean, contributing to periodontal disease and dental caries. Health care providers should refer you to an orthodontist or pediatric dentist for evaluation and specialized instruction in daily oral hygiene.

Tooth Anomalies

Tooth anomalies are variations in the number, size, and shape of teeth. People with Down syndrome, oral clefts, ectodermal dysplasia, or other conditions may experience congenitally missing, extra, or malformed teeth. Consult an oral health care provider for dental treatment planning during a child's growing years.

Developmental Defects

Developmental defects appear as pits, lines, or discoloration in the teeth. Very high fever or certain medications can disturb tooth formation and defects may result. Many teeth with defects are prone to dental caries, are difficult to keep clean, and may compromise appearance. Health care providers should refer you to an oral health care provider for evaluation of treatment options and advice on keeping teeth clean.

Problems from Oral Trauma

Trauma to the face and mouth occur more frequently in people who have mental retardation, seizures, abnormal protective reflexes, or muscle incoordination. People receiving restorative dental care should be observed closely to prevent chewing on anesthetized areas. If a tooth is avulsed or broken, take the patient and the tooth to a dentist

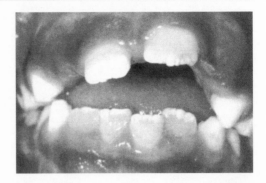

Figure 42.2. A child with malocclusion.

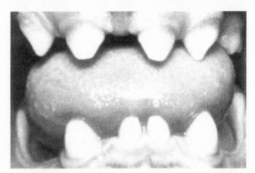

Figure 42.3. A child with tooth anomalies.

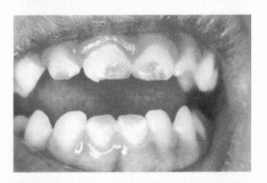

Figure 42.4. A child with developmental tooth defects.

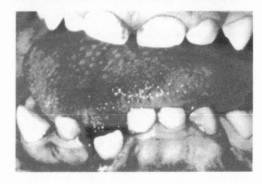

Figure 42.5. A child with oral trauma.

immediately. Talk to a health care provider about ways to prevent trauma and what to do when it occurs.

Bruxism

Bruxism, the habitual grinding of teeth, is a common occurrence in people with cerebral palsy or severe mental retardation. In extreme cases, bruxism leads to tooth abrasion and flat biting surfaces. Refer to a dentist for evaluation; behavioral techniques or a bite guard may be recommended.

Problems from Oral Infections

Tooth Decay

Dental caries, or tooth decay, may be linked to frequent vomiting or gastroesophageal reflux, less than normal amounts of saliva, medications containing sugar, or special diets that require prolonged bottle feeding or snacking. When oral hygiene is poor, the teeth are at increased risk for caries. Talk to a health care provider about daily oral hygiene, including frequent rinsing with plain water and use of a fluoride-containing toothpaste or mouth rinse. Explain the need for supervising children to avoid swallowing fluoride. Talk to an oral health care provider and/or gastroenterologist for prevention and treatment. Prescribe sugarless medications when available.

Viral Infections

Viral infections are usually due to the herpes simplex virus. Children rarely get herpetic gingivostomatitis or herpes labialis before 6 months of age. Herpetic gingivostomatitis is most common in young children, but may occur in adolescents and young adults. Viral infections can be painful and are usually accompanied by a fever. Counsel the parent/caregiver about the infectious nature of the lesions, the need for frequent fluids to prevent dehydration, and methods of symptomatic treatment.

Gum Disease

Early, severe periodontal (gum) disease can occur in children with impaired immune systems or connective tissue disorders and inadequate oral hygiene. Simple gingivitis results from an accumulation of bacterial plaque and presents as red, swollen gums that bleed easily.

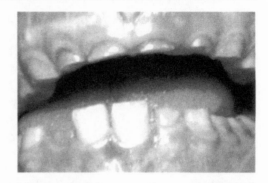

Figure 42.6. A child with bruxism.

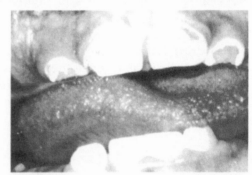

Figure 42.7. A child with tooth decay.

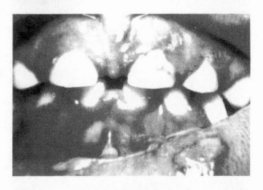

Figure 42.8. A child with oral problems due to viral infections.

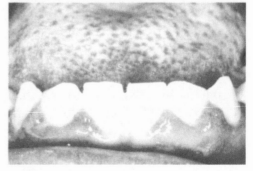

Figure 42.9. A child with gum disease.

Periodontitis is more severe and leads to tooth loss if not treated. Professional cleaning by an oral health care provider, systemic antibiotics, and instructions on home care may be needed to stop the infection. Talk to your child's doctor about how you can help with daily toothbrushing and flossing. Frequent appointments with an oral health care provider may be necessary.

Problems from Gingival Overgrowth

Gingival overgrowth may be a side effect from medications such as calcium channel blockers, phenytoin sodium, and cyclosporine. Poor oral hygiene aggravates the condition and can lead to superimposed infections. Severe overgrowth can impair tooth eruption, chewing, and appearance. Refer to an oral health care provider for prevention and treatment. A preventive regimen of antimicrobial rinses and frequent appointments may be needed. Consider alternative medications if possible.

Figure 42.10. A child with gingival overgrowth.

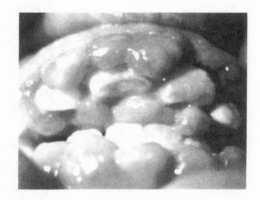

Suggested Reading

Helpin ML, Rosenberg HM. Dental care: Beyond brushing and flossing. *Children with Disabilities.* 4th ed. Baltimore: Brookes Publishing Co., 1997, 643–656.

Pinkham JR, et al. *Pediatric Dentistry. Infancy Through Adolescence.* 3rd ed. Philadelphia: WB Saunders Company, 1999.

Rutkauskas JS, ed. Practical considerations in special patient care. *Dental Clinics of North America.* 38(3):361–584, 1994.

Chapter 43

Oral Care for Children with Arthritis

Children with arthritis may have limited jaw movement, which can make brushing and flossing their teeth difficult. Your child's dentist may suggest various toothbrush handles, electric toothbrushes, floss holders, toothpicks, and rinses that will help your child maintain healthy teeth and gums.

Medications may also affect your child's oral health and development. Always inform you dentist about the status of your child's disease and the medications he or she is taking. The dentist will consider these when planning any treatment, general anesthesia, sedation, or oral surgery. Older children who have had joint replacements may require an antibiotic before dental treatment.

The joint in front of the ears, where the lower jaw connects to the base of the skull, is called the temporomandibular joint (TMJ). Arthritis may affect this joint in the same way it does others, by causing pain, stiffness, and altered growth. Jaw exercises and therapy may be recommended for the pain and stiffness. If the lower jaw does not develop properly, it may create an overbite. Your child's dentist may recommend an early consultation with an orthodontist if this occurs. Surgery is also sometimes necessary for this condition.

A child with active arthritis may not always have the stamina for even routine dental work. If possible, schedule appointments when your child has the most stamina or schedule shorter appointments.

Excerpted from *Arthritis in Children*, © 2001. Reprinted with permission of the Arthritis Foundation, 1330 Peachtree St., Atlanta GA 30309. For free copies of Arthritis Foundation brochures, call 800-282-7800, or visit www.arthritis.org.

Chapter 44

Oral Care for Children with Cleft Lip or Cleft Palate

Cleft lip and cleft palate comprise the fourth most common birth defect in the United States. One of every 700 newborns is affected by cleft lip and/or cleft palate.

A cleft lip is a separation of the two sides of the lip. The separation often includes the bones of the upper jaw and/or upper gum. A cleft palate is an opening in the roof of the mouth in which the two sides of the palate did not fuse, or join together, as the unborn baby was developing.

Cleft lip and cleft palate can occur on one side (unilateral cleft lip and/or palate), or on both sides (bilateral cleft lip and/or palate). Because the lip and the palate develop separately, it is possible for the child to have a cleft lip, a cleft palate, or both cleft lip and cleft palate.

Cleft lip and cleft palate are congenital defects, or birth defects, which occur very early in pregnancy. The majority of clefts appear to be due to a combination of genetics and environmental factors. The risks of recurrence of a cleft condition are dependent upon many factors, including the number of affected persons in the family, the closeness of affected relatives, the race and sex of all affected persons, and the severity of the clefts.

This chapter includes text reprinted with permission from "About Cleft Lip & Palate," published 1990, reviewed annually; "Dental Care of a Child with Cleft Lip and Palate," published 1988, reviewed annually; and "Missing Tooth Fact Sheet," published 1997, reviewed annually. © Cleft Palate Foundation. For additional information, call 1-800-24-CLEFT or visit www.cleftline.org. Graphics provided courtesy of the Cleft Palate Foundation, 1-800-24-CLEFT, www.cleftline.org.

A child born with a cleft frequently requires several different types of services, e.g., surgery, dental/orthodontic care, and speech therapy, all of which need to be provided in a coordinated manner over a period of years. This coordinated care is provided by interdisciplinary

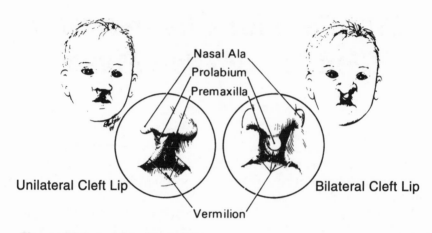

Figure 44.1. A child with cleft lip.

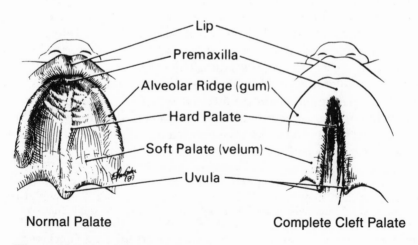

Figure 44.2. A child with cleft palate.

cleft palate/craniofacial teams comprised of professionals from a variety of health care disciplines who work together on the child's total rehabilitation.

Dental Care of a Child with Cleft Lip and Palate

How Does Cleft Lip/Palate Affect the Teeth?

A cleft of the lip, gum (alveolus), and/or palate in the front of the mouth can produce a variety of dental problems. These may involve the number, size, shape, and position of both the baby teeth and the permanent teeth. The teeth most commonly affected by the clefting process are those in the area of the cleft, primarily the lateral incisors. Clefts occur between the cuspid (eye tooth) and the lateral incisor. In some cases the lateral incisor may be entirely absent. In other cases there may be a twinning (twin = two) of the lateral incisor so that one is present on each side of the cleft. In still other cases the incisor, or other teeth, may be present but may be poorly formed with an abnormally shaped crown and/or root. Finally, the teeth in the area of the cleft may be displaced, resulting in their erupting into abnormal positions. Occasionally the central incisors on the cleft side may have some of the same problems as the lateral incisor.

What Does This Mean for Future Dental Care?

A child with a cleft lip/palate requires the same regular preventive and restorative care as the child without a cleft. However, since children with clefts may have special problems related to missing, malformed, or malpositioned teeth, they require early evaluation by a dentist who is familiar with the needs of the child with a cleft.

Early Dental Care

With proper care, children born with a cleft lip and/or palate can have healthy teeth. This requires proper cleaning, good nutrition, and fluoride treatment. Appropriate cleaning with a small, soft-bristled toothbrush should begin as soon as teeth erupt. Oral hygiene instructions and preventative counseling can be provided by a pediatric dentist or a general dentist. Many dentists recommend that the first dental visit be scheduled at about one year of age or even earlier if there are special dental problems. The early evaluation is usually provided through the Cleft Palate Team. Routine dental care with a local dentist begins at about three years of age. The treatment recommended depends upon many factors. Some children require only preventative care while others will need fillings or removal of a tooth.

Orthodontic Care

The first orthodontic evaluation may be scheduled even before the child has any teeth. The purpose of this visit is to assess facial growth, particularly the growth of the jaws. Later as teeth begin to erupt, the orthodontist will make plans for the child's short and long-term dental needs. For example, if a child's upper teeth do not fit together (occlude) properly with the lower teeth, the orthodontist may suggest an early period of treatment to correct the relationship of the upper jaw to the lower jaw. It is not unusual for this initial period of treatment to be followed by a long rest period when the orthodontist monitors facial growth and dental development. With the eruption of the permanent teeth, the final phase of orthodontics completes alignment of the teeth.

Coordinated Dental/Surgical Care

Coordination of treatment between the surgeon and dental specialist is important since several procedures may be completed during the same period of anesthesia. Restorations or dental extractions can be scheduled at the same time as other surgery.

Coordination between the surgeon and the orthodontist becomes most important in the management of the bony defect in the upper jaw that may result from the cleft. Reconstruction of the cleft defect may be accomplished with a bone graft performed by the surgeon. The orthodontist may place an appliance on the teeth of the upper jaw to prepare for the bone graft. A retainer is usually placed after the bone graft until full braces are applied.

When the child approaches adolescence the orthodontist and the surgeon again coordinate their efforts if the teeth do not meet properly because the jaws are in abnormal positions. If the tooth relations cannot be made normal by orthodontics alone, a combined approach of both orthodontics and surgical repositioning of the jaws is necessary. Such surgery is usually performed after the pubertal growth spurt is completed.

Prosthodontic Care

The maxillofacial prosthodontist is a dental specialist who makes artificial teeth and dental appliances to improve the appearance of individuals with cleft and to meet their functional requirements for eating and speaking. The prosthodontist may make a dental bridge to replace missing teeth. Oral appliances called speech bulbs or palatal lifts may help close the nose from the mouth so that speech will sound more normal. The prosthodontist must also coordinate treatment with the surgeon and/or the orthodontist to assure the best possible result. When a speech bulb or palatal lift is developed, the prosthodontist usually coordinates treatment with the speech pathologist. For the child or adult who wears one of these appliances, the care of the teeth holding the appliance is of particular importance.

How Can I Get the Best Care for My Child?

Children with cleft lip and/or palate require the coordinated services of a number of specialists. For this reason many parents seek care for their child at a cleft palate or craniofacial treatment center. At such a center evaluation, treatment planning, and care are provided by an experienced, multidisciplinary team composed of representatives from a variety of dental, medical, and other health care specialties. Even if you do not have such a center locally, the care your child will receive in such a center may be well worth the inconvenience of traveling to another city.

Parent/patient support groups are located throughout the country. You might want to join one to obtain support and practical help from others who share common problems. To obtain a list of cleft palate-craniofacial centers and parent/patient support groups in your region contact the Cleft Palate Foundation.

Missing Teeth in Children with Cleft Lip or Cleft Palate

Patients with cleft lip or cleft lip and palate are often born with a missing tooth, most often the lateral incisor (immediately next to the front central incisor). This may occur unilaterally or bilaterally, but special planning is needed to solve the functional and cosmetic problems the absence creates.

Who Will Be Involved in Dealing with the Missing Tooth?

Several dental specialists will be most important in planning treatment. Orthodontists align improperly placed teeth, whereas prosthodontists can replace missing teeth in a variety of ways. Oral and maxillofacial surgeons perform surgery to the teeth, mouth, and surrounding areas of the head and face. Coordinated planning by all specialists involved is necessary for the best result.

What Role Does the Orthodontist Play in Replacing a Missing Tooth?

The large majority of patients with clefts will require full orthodontic treatment, especially if the cleft has passed through the tooth-bearing ridge. Goals of treatment will be to line up the teeth in the upper arch, create an arch form that is harmonious with the lower dental arch, and line up the midline of the upper arch with that of the lower arch. When a tooth is missing, the upper midline is usually shifted, so this must be corrected. A space is often opened up and maintained for later replacement of the missing lateral incisor.

During orthodontic treatment, an artificial tooth may be attached to the orthodontic wire as a temporary replacement for the lateral incisor. When the braces are removed, a removable retainer with an artificial tooth serves to maintain the space and improve speech and appearance until a definitive restoration is made.

Is the Missing Tooth Always Replaced?

In many instances, the space for the lateral incisor will be orthodontically and/or surgically closed by moving the canine forward into the space normally occupied by the lateral incisor. This will then require modification of the canine to make it appear as a lateral incisor. This may be accomplished by adding plastic or porcelain filling material or a porcelain crown to reshape its appearance.

What Options Are Available for Permanent Replacement of the Lateral Incisor?

Treatment options for the permanent replacement of the lateral incisor depend upon whether or not the cleft has been repaired with a bone graft. In a non-grafted dental arch, there are two options for replacement.

First, a removable partial denture may be used to replace the missing tooth. Although this option may be made to look acceptable, it has several disadvantages. The removable prosthesis must cover most of the palate for support. This may cause irritation on the roof of the mouth or at the gum line where it rests. Many patients also object to the extra bulk and removable nature of the partial denture and report that it feels unnatural. This type of prosthesis is best as a temporary replacement as described above.

The second option in a patient without a bone graft is a fixed bridge. The missing tooth is restored with an artificial one connected to crowns (caps) on teeth on each side of the cleft. Because there is loss of supporting bone at each tooth on either side of the cleft, two teeth on each side must usually be crowned to give adequate support to the bridge. This type of prosthesis is not removable. Its contours and appearance look and feel more natural than a removable partial denture. However, it does require grinding down the support teeth in order to crown them and connect them to the artificial tooth. Cleaning between the crowned teeth also becomes more difficult since they are connected.

Can a Fixed Bridge Be Made Immediately after Braces?

In a teenager or young adult, the nerves and blood vessels in the tooth pulps are rather large. Drilling down these teeth for crowns may expose the pulps and require root canal therapy. Therefore, this type of treatment must usually wait until adulthood when the pulps are smaller.

What Options Are Available for a Patient Who Has Had a Bone Graft?

Bone grafting the cleft site in the upper jaw creates a more normal arch and eliminates special restorative considerations relative to the cleft. A conventional fixed bridge as described above may be used. In many cases, only one tooth on either side of the cleft needs to be crowned, since the graft has stabilized the arch and added bone. If the teeth that hold the bridge are not otherwise in need of restoration, a resin-bonded fixed bridge may be chosen. This type of bridge requires much less tooth reduction of adjacent teeth, and there is no danger of nerve involvement.

A porcelain replacement tooth is held in place by metal extensions cemented to the backs of the adjacent teeth. This is a more conservative restoration with regard to tooth preparation but still requires connecting teeth together.

The most natural, lifelike restoration for a patient with a bone graft is a single porcelain crown attached to an osseointegrated dental implant. This involves a surgical procedure where a titanium screw the size and shape of a tooth's root is inserted into the bone at the site of the missing tooth. It is covered by the gum for six months while the bone bonds to the implant surface. Then the implant is uncovered and an artificial tooth (crown) is attached. While this procedure does require minor surgery, it does not require cutting down or crowning any other teeth. Cleaning is also easier because the replacement tooth is not connected to any other teeth. This restoration does give the most natural result but does require that sufficient bone is present in order to hold the screw.

In summary:

- Finding the best treatment for a missing tooth requires cooperation and planning among several specialists

- A variety of options for successful tooth replacement are available

- Patients with missing teeth and/or their parents should thoroughly discuss treatment options with the multidisciplinary team before making a decision.

Chapter 45

Oral Care for People Undergoing Cancer Treatment

Chapter Contents

Section 45.1

Head and Neck Radiation Treatment and Your Mouth

"Oral Complications of Cancer Treatment: Head and Neck Radiation Treatment and Your Mouth" is a brochure published by the National Institute of Dental and Craniofacial Research (NIDCR)/National Oral Health Information Clearinghouse, NIH Publication Number 02-4362, July 2002. Available online at www.nohic.nidcr.nih.gov/campaign/rad_bro. htm; accessed May 2003.

Are You Being Treated with Radiation for Cancer in Your Head or Neck?

If so, this chapter can help you. While head and neck radiation helps treat cancer, it can also cause other things to happen in your mouth called side effects. Some of these problems could cause you to delay or stop treatment.

This chapter will tell you ways to help prevent mouth problems so you'll get the most from your cancer treatment.

To help prevent serious problems, see a dentist at least 2 weeks before starting radiation.

How Does Head and Neck Radiation Affect the Mouth?

Doctors use head and neck radiation to treat cancer because it kills cancer cells. But radiation to the head and neck can harm normal cells, including cells in the mouth. Side effects include problems with your teeth and gums; the soft, moist lining of your mouth; glands that make saliva (spit); and jaw bones.

It's important to know that side effects in the mouth can be serious.

- The side effects can hurt and make it hard to eat, talk, and swallow.

- You are more likely to get an infection, which can be dangerous when you are receiving cancer treatment.

- If the side effects are bad, you may not be able to keep up with your cancer treatment. Your doctor may need to cut back on your cancer treatment or may even stop it.

What Mouth Problems Does Head and Neck Radiation Cause?

You may have certain side effects in your mouth from head and neck radiation. Another person may have different problems. Some problems go away after treatment. Others last a long time, while some may never go away.

- Dry mouth
- A lot of cavities
- Loss of taste
- Sore mouth and gums
- Infections
- Jaw stiffness
- Jaw bone changes

Why Should I See a Dentist?

You may be surprised that your dentist is important in your cancer treatment. If you go to the dentist before head and neck radiation begins, you can help prevent serious mouth problems. Side effects often happen because a person's mouth is not healthy before radiation starts. Not all mouth problems can be avoided but the fewer side effects you have, the more likely you will stay on your cancer treatment schedule.

It's important for your dentist and cancer doctor to talk to each other before your radiation treatment begins. Be sure to give your dentist your cancer doctor's phone number.

When Should I See a Dentist?

You need to see the dentist at least 2 weeks before your first radiation treatment. If you have already started radiation and didn't go to a dentist, see one as soon as possible.

What Will the Dentist and Dental Hygienist Do?

- Check your teeth.

- Take x-rays.
- Take care of mouth problems.
- Show you how to take care of your mouth to prevent side effects.
- Show you how to prevent and treat jaw stiffness by exercising the jaw muscles 3 times a day. Open and close the mouth as far as possible (without causing pain) 20 times.

What Can I Do to Keep My Mouth Healthy?

You can do a lot to keep your mouth healthy during head and neck radiation. The first step is to see a dentist before you start cancer treatment. Once your treatment starts, it's important to look in your mouth every day for sores or other changes. These tips can help prevent and treat a sore mouth.

Keep Your Mouth Moist

- Drink a lot of water.
- Suck ice chips.
- Use sugarless gum or sugar-free hard candy.
- Use a saliva substitute to help moisten your mouth.

Clean Your Mouth, Tongue, and Gums

- Brush your teeth, gums, and tongue with an extra-soft toothbrush after every meal and at bedtime. If it hurts, soften the bristles in warm water.
- Use a fluoride toothpaste.
- Use the special fluoride gel that your dentist prescribes.
- Don't use mouthwashes with alcohol in them.
- Floss your teeth gently every day. If your gums bleed and hurt, avoid the areas that are bleeding or sore, but keep flossing your other teeth.
- Rinse your mouth several times a day with a solution of 1/4 teaspoon baking soda and 1/8 teaspoon salt in one cup of warm water. Follow with a plain water rinse.
- Dentures that don't fit well can cause problems. Talk to your cancer doctor or dentist about your dentures.

If Your Mouth Is Sore, Watch What You Eat and Drink

- Choose foods that are good for you and easy to chew and swallow.
- Take small bites of food, chew slowly, and sip liquids with your meals.
- Eat moist, soft foods such as cooked cereals, mashed potatoes, and scrambled eggs.
- If you have trouble swallowing, soften your food with gravy, sauces, broth, yogurt, or other liquids.
- Sipping liquids with your meal will make eating easier.

Call Your Doctor or Nurse When Your Mouth Hurts

- Work with them to find medicines to help control the pain.
- If the pain continues, talk to your cancer doctor about stronger medicines.

Remember to Stay away from

- Sharp, crunchy foods, like taco chips, that could scrape or cut your mouth
- Foods that are hot, spicy, or high in acid, like citrus fruits and juices, which can irritate your mouth
- Sugary foods, like candy or soda, that could cause cavities
- Toothpicks, because they can cut your mouth
- All tobacco products
- Alcoholic drinks

Do Children Get Mouth Problems, Too?

Head and neck radiation cause other side effects in children, depending on the child's age.

Problems with teeth are the most common. Permanent teeth may be slow to come in and may look different from normal teeth. Teeth may fall out. The dentist will check your child's jaws for any growth problems.

Before radiation begins, take your child to a dentist. The dentist will check your child's mouth carefully and pull loose teeth or those that may become loose during treatment. Ask the dentist or hygienist what you can do to help your child with mouth care.

Remember

- Visit your dentist before your head and neck radiation treatment starts.

- Take good care of your mouth during treatment.

- Talk to your dentist about using fluoride gel to help prevent all the cavities that head and neck radiation causes.

- Talk regularly with your cancer doctor and dentist about any mouth problems you have during and after head and neck radiation treatment.

Section 45.2

Chemotherapy and Your Mouth

"Oral Complications of Cancer Treatment: Chemotherapy and Your Mouth" is a brochure published by the National Institute of Dental and Craniofacial Research (NIDCR)/National Oral Health Information Clearinghouse, NIH Publication Number 02-4361, July 2002. Available online at www.nohic.nidcr.nih.gov/campaign/chmo_bro.htm; accessed May 2003.

Are You Being Treated with Chemotherapy for Cancer?

If so, this chapter can help you. While chemotherapy helps treat cancer, it can also cause other things to happen in your body called side effects. Some of these problems affect the mouth and could cause you to delay or stop treatment.

This chapter will tell you ways to help prevent mouth problems so you'll get the most from your cancer treatment.

To help prevent serious problems, see a dentist at least 2 weeks before starting chemotherapy.

How Does Chemotherapy Affect the Mouth?

Chemotherapy is the use of drugs to treat cancer. These drugs kill cancer cells, but they may also harm normal cells, including cells in the mouth. Side effects include problems with your teeth and gums; the soft, moist lining of your mouth; and the glands that make saliva (spit).

It's important to know that side effects in the mouth can be serious.

- The side effects can hurt and make it hard to eat, talk, and swallow.

- You are more likely to get an infection, which can be dangerous when you are receiving cancer treatment.

- If the side effects are bad, you may not be able to keep up with your cancer treatment. Your doctor may need to cut back on your cancer treatment or may even stop it.

What Mouth Problems Does Chemotherapy Cause?

You may have certain side effects in your mouth from chemotherapy. Another person may have different problems. The problems depend on the chemotherapy drugs and how your body reacts to them. You may have these problems only during treatment or for a short time after treatment ends.

- Painful mouth and gums
- Dry mouth
- Burning, peeling, or swelling tongue
- Infection
- Change in taste

Why Should I See a Dentist?

You may be surprised that your dentist is important in your cancer treatment. If you go to the dentist before chemotherapy begins, you can help prevent serious mouth problems. Side effects often happen because a person's mouth is not healthy before chemotherapy starts. Not all mouth problems can be avoided but the fewer side effects you have, the more likely you will stay on your cancer treatment schedule.

It's important for your dentist and cancer doctor to talk to each other about your cancer treatment. Be sure to give your dentist your cancer doctor's phone number.

When Should I See a Dentist?

You need to see the dentist at least 2 weeks before chemotherapy begins. If you have already started chemotherapy and didn't go to a dentist, see one as soon as possible.

What Will the Dentist and Dental Hygienist Do?

- Check your teeth.
- Take x-rays.
- Take care of mouth problems.
- Show you how to take care of your mouth to prevent side effects.

What Can I Do to Keep My Mouth Healthy?

You can do a lot to keep your mouth healthy during chemotherapy. The first step is to see a dentist before you start cancer treatment. Once your treatment starts, it's important to look in your mouth every day for sores or other changes. These tips can help prevent and treat a sore mouth.

Keep Your Mouth Moist

- Drink a lot of water.
- Suck ice chips.
- Use sugarless gum or sugar-free hard candy.
- Use a saliva substitute to help moisten your mouth.

Clean Your Mouth, Tongue, and Gums

- Brush your teeth, gums, and tongue with an extra-soft toothbrush after every meal and at bedtime. If brushing hurts, soften the bristles in warm water.
- Use a fluoride toothpaste.
- Don't use mouthwashes with alcohol in them.
- Floss your teeth gently every day. If your gums bleed and hurt, avoid the areas that are bleeding or sore, but keep flossing your other teeth.

- Rinse your mouth several times a day with a solution of 1/4 teaspoon baking soda and 1/8 teaspoon salt in one cup of warm water. Follow with a plain water rinse.

- Dentures that don't fit well can cause problems. Talk to your cancer doctor or dentist about your dentures.

If Your Mouth Is Sore, Watch What You Eat and Drink

- Choose foods that are good for you and easy to chew and swallow.

- Take small bites of food, chew slowly, and sip liquids with your meals.

- Eat soft, moist foods such as cooked cereals, mashed potatoes, and scrambled eggs.

- If you have trouble swallowing, soften your food with gravy, sauces, broth, yogurt, or other liquids.

- Sipping liquids with your meals will make eating easier.

Call Your Doctor or Nurse When Your Mouth Hurts

- Work with them to find medicines to help control the pain.

- If the pain continues, talk to your cancer doctor about stronger medicines.

Remember to Stay away from

- Sharp, crunchy foods, like taco chips, that could scrape or cut your mouth

- Foods that are hot, spicy, or high in acid, like citrus fruits and juices, which can irritate your mouth

- Sugary foods, like candy or soda, that could cause cavities

- Toothpicks, because they can cut your mouth

- All tobacco products

- Alcoholic drinks

Do Children Get Mouth Problems, Too?

Chemotherapy causes other side effects in children, depending on the child's age.

Problems with teeth are the most common. Permanent teeth may be slow to come in and may look different from normal teeth. Teeth may fall out. The dentist will check your child's jaws for any growth problems.

Before chemotherapy begins, take your child to a dentist. The dentist will check your child's mouth carefully and pull loose teeth or those that may become loose during treatment. Ask the dentist or hygienist what you can do to help your child with mouth care.

Remember

- Visit your dentist before your cancer treatment starts.

- Take good care of your mouth during treatment.

- Talk regularly with your cancer doctor and dentist about any mouth problems you have.

Section 45.3

Three Good Reasons to See a Dentist If You Have Cancer

"Oral Complications of Cancer Treatment: Three Good Reasons to See a Dentist (Tip Sheet)" is a brochure published by the National Institute of Dental and Craniofacial Research (NIDCR)/National Oral Health Information Clearinghouse, July 2002. Available online at www.nohic.nidcr. nih.gov/campaign/tip_sht.htm; accessed May 2003.

Prior to cancer treatment, you should see a dentist to:

- Feel better: Your cancer treatment may be easier if you work with your dentist and hygienist. Make sure you have a pretreatment dental checkup.

- Save teeth and bones: A dentist will help protect your mouth, teeth, and jaw bones from damage caused by radiation and chemotherapy. Children also need special protection for their growing teeth and facial bones.

- Fight cancer: Doctors may have to delay or stop your cancer treatment because of problems in your mouth. To fight cancer best, your cancer care team should include a dentist.

Protect Your Mouth during Cancer Treatment

Brush Gently, Brush Often

- Brush your teeth—and your tongue—gently with an extra-soft toothbrush.
- If your mouth is very sore, soften the bristles in warm water.
- Brush after every meal and at bedtime.

Floss Gently—Do It Daily

- Floss once a day to remove plaque.
- If your gums bleed and hurt, avoid the areas that are bleeding or sore, but keep flossing your other teeth.

Keep Your Mouth Moist

- Rinse often with water.
- Don't use mouthwashes with alcohol in them.
- Use a saliva substitute to help moisten your mouth.

Eat and Drink with Care

- Choose soft, easy-to-chew foods.
- Protect your mouth from spicy, sour, or crunchy foods.
- Choose lukewarm foods and drinks instead of hot or icy cold foods and drinks.
- Avoid alcoholic drinks.

Keep Trying to Quit Using Tobacco

- Ask your cancer care team to help you stop smoking or chewing tobacco.
- People who quit smoking or chewing tobacco have fewer mouth problems.

When Should You Call Your Cancer Care Team about Mouth Problems?

Take a moment each day to check how your mouth looks and feels. Call your cancer care team when:

- you first notice a mouth problem
- an old problem gets worse
- you notice any changes you're not sure about

Tips for Mouth Problems

Sore mouth, sore throat: To help keep your mouth clean, rinse often with ¼ teaspoon of baking soda and 1/8 teaspoon of salt in 1 cup of warm water. Follow with a plain water rinse. Ask your cancer care team about medicines that can help with the pain.

Dry mouth: Rinse your mouth often with water, use sugar-free gum or candy, and talk to your dentist about saliva substitutes.

Infections: Call your cancer care team right away if you see a sore, swelling, bleeding, or a sticky, white film in your mouth.

Eating problems: Your cancer care team can help by giving you medicines to numb the pain from mouth sores and showing you how to choose foods that are easy to swallow.

Bleeding: If your gums bleed or hurt, avoid flossing the areas that are bleeding or sore, but keep flossing other teeth. Soften the bristles of your toothbrush in warm water.

Stiffness in chewing muscles: Three times a day, open and close your mouth as far as you can without pain. Repeat 20 times.

Vomiting: Rinse your mouth after vomiting with 1/4 teaspoon of baking soda in 1 cup of warm water.

Cavities: Brush your teeth after meals and before bedtime. Your dentist might have you put fluoride on your teeth to help prevent cavities.

Chapter 46

Diabetes and Oral Health

What Are Diabetes Problems?

Too much sugar in the blood for a long time causes diabetes problems. This high blood sugar can damage many parts of the body, such as the heart, blood vessels, and kidneys. Diabetes problems can be scary, but there is a lot you can do to prevent them or slow them down.

This chapter is about tooth and gum problems caused by diabetes. You will learn the things you can do each day and during each year to stay healthy and prevent diabetes problems.

What Should I Do Each Day to Stay Healthy with Diabetes?

- Follow the healthy eating plan that you and your doctor or dietitian have worked out. Eat your meals and snacks at around the same times each day.

- Be active a total of 30 minutes most days. Ask your doctor what activities are best for you.

- Take your diabetes medicine at the same times each day.

"Prevent Diabetes Problems: Keep Your Teeth and Gums Healthy" is a brochure published by the National Institute of Diabetes and Digestive and Kidney Diseases (NIDDK), NIH Publication Number 00-4280, May 2000. Available online at www.niddk.nih.gov/health/diabetes/pubs/complications/teeth/teeth. htm; accessed May 2003.

- Check your blood sugar every day. Each time you check your blood sugar, write the number in your record book. Call your doctor if your numbers are too high or too low for 2 to 3 days.

- Check your feet every day for cuts, blisters, sores, swelling, redness, or sore toenails.

- Brush and floss your teeth and gums every day.

- Don't smoke.

How Can Diabetes Hurt My Teeth and Gums?

Tooth and gum problems can happen to anyone. A sticky film full of germs (also called plaque) builds up on your teeth. High blood sugar helps germs (bacteria) grow. Then you can get red, sore, and swollen gums that bleed when you brush your teeth.

People with diabetes can have tooth and gum problems more often if their blood sugar stays high. High blood sugar can make tooth and gum problems worse. You can even lose your teeth.

Smoking makes it more likely for you to get a bad case of gum disease, especially if you have diabetes and are age 45 or older.

Red, sore, and bleeding gums are the first sign of gum disease. This can lead to periodontitis. Periodontitis is an infection in the gums and the bone that holds the teeth in place. If the infection gets worse, your gums may pull away from your teeth, making your teeth look long.

Call your dentist if you think you have problems with your teeth or gums.

How Do I Know If I Have Damage to My Teeth and Gums?

If you have one or more of these problems, you may have tooth and gum damage from diabetes:

- Red, sore, swollen gums.

- Bleeding gums.

- Gums pulling away from your teeth so your teeth look long.

- Loose or sensitive teeth.

- Bad breath.

- A bite that feels different.

- Dentures (false teeth) that do not fit well.

How Can I Keep My Teeth and Gums Healthy?

- Keep your blood sugar as close to normal as possible.

- Use dental floss at least once a day. Flossing helps prevent the buildup of plaque on your teeth. Plaque can harden and grow under your gums and cause problems. Using a sawing motion, gently bring the floss between the teeth, scraping from bottom to top several times.

- Brush your teeth after each meal and snack. Use a soft tooth-brush. Turn the bristles against the gum line and brush gently. Use small, circular motions. Brush the front, back, and top of each tooth.

- Brush and floss your teeth and gums every day.

- If you wear false teeth, keep them clean.

- Ask the person who cleans your teeth to show you the best way to brush and floss your teeth and gums. Ask this person about the best toothbrush and toothpaste to use.

- Call your dentist right away if you have problems with your teeth and gums.

- Call your dentist if you have red, sore, or bleeding gums; gums that are pulling away from your teeth; a sore tooth that could be infected; or soreness from your dentures.

- Get your teeth and gums cleaned and checked by your dentist twice a year.

- If your dentist tells you about a problem, take care of it right away.

- Be sure your dentist knows that you have diabetes.

- If you smoke, talk to your doctor about ways to quit smoking.

How Can My Dentist Take Care of My Teeth and Gums?

- By cleaning and checking your teeth and gums twice a year.

- By helping you learn the best way to brush and floss your teeth and gums.

- By telling you if you have problems with your teeth or gums and what to do about them.

- By making sure your false teeth fit well.

Plan ahead. You may be taking a diabetes medicine that can make your blood sugar too low. This very low blood sugar is called hypoglycemia. If so, talk to your doctor and dentist before the visit about the best way to take care of your blood sugar during the dental work. You may need to bring some diabetes medicine and food with you to the dentist's office.

If your mouth is sore after the dental work, you might not be able to eat or chew for several hours or days. For guidance on how to adjust your normal routine while your mouth is healing, ask your doctor.

- What foods and drinks you should have.

- How you should change your diabetes medicines.

- How often you should check your blood sugar.

For More Information

Diabetes Teachers (nurses, dietitians, pharmacists, and other health professionals): To find a diabetes teacher near you, call the American Association of Diabetes Educators toll-free at 800-TEAMUP4 (800-832-6874), or look on the Internet at http://www. aadenet.org and click on Find an Educator.

Recognized Diabetes Education Programs (teaching programs approved by the American Diabetes Association): To find a program near you, call toll-free at 800-DIABETES (800-342-2383), or see http://www.diabetes.org/education/edustate2.asp on the Internet.

Dietitians: To find a dietitian near you, call the American Dietetic Association's National Center for Nutrition and Dietetics toll-free at 800-366-1655, or look on the Internet at http://www.eatright.org and click on Find a Dietitian.

Government: The National Institute of Dental and Craniofacial Research (NIDCR) is part of the National Institutes of Health. To learn more about tooth and gum problems, write or call NIDCR's information clearinghouse, the National Oral Health Information Clearinghouse (NOHIC), at 1 NOHIC Way, Bethesda, MD 20892-3500, (301) 402-7364; or see http://www.nohic.nidcr.nih.gov on the Internet.

Chapter 47

Oral Care for People with Latex Allergies

Since the late 1980's, there has been a significant increase in the number of allergic reactions to natural rubber latex. The Food and Drug Administration attributes this rise to a ten-fold increase in the use of latex gloves. While only 1% to 6% of the general population is allergic to latex, the prevalence in healthcare workers and others whose occupations involve exposure to rubber products is around 10%. Children and adolescents with spina bifida also have an increased incidence because of their frequent exposure to latex products from birth.

Natural rubber latex (NRL) is manufactured from the sap of the *Havea brasiliensis* rubber tree. Some individuals are allergic to the proteins found in this natural rubber. During the production of commercial latex, several chemicals are added to the natural rubber. These chemicals also cause some individuals to have allergic reactions to latex products.

Three types of reactions can occur with the use of natural rubber latex. Irritant contact dermatitis is the most common reaction to latex products. It is caused by the chemicals added to NRL during manufacturing. The chemicals directly injure the skin resulting in redness, swelling, dryness, itching, and burning. This reaction can also occur from the powder added to latex gloves. Irritant contact dermatitis is not a true allergy and the symptoms disappear within several hours after removal of the stimulus. Allergic contact dermatitis is a delayed type of immunological response resulting from the chemicals used in the manufacture of the latex product. The chemicals penetrate the skin resulting in an allergic reaction. Symptoms such as redness and swelling occur between 24 to 48 hours after exposure and can last for several days. This delayed type of allergic response accounts for approximately 80% of the true allergic reactions to latex. Latex allergy is an immediate hypersensitivity response to proteins found in natural rubber latex. The response begins within minutes of exposure to the allergen (protein) and can take the form of an urticaria (hives) if exposure is through the skin, or respiratory symptoms (wheezing, runny nose, sneezing) if the allergen is inhaled. In some cases, an anaphylactic reaction (facial swelling, difficulty in breathing, and a severe drop in blood pressure) may occur if the protein is introduced directly into the blood. This immediate type of hypersensitivity or true allergic reaction to NRL is most likely to be found in those individuals who have multiple allergies and are frequently exposed to NRL products. Because of a similarity of proteins, individuals allergic to latex may also be sensitive to foods such as chestnuts, bananas, kiwi fruit, and avocados. Patients should be informed of this potential cross allergenicity.

As a result of the chemical similarity between natural rubber and gutta-percha, the material used in filling the root canal, questions have arisen concerning its use in patients with a history of natural rubber latex. To date, there's only one report of a supposed allergic reaction to gutta-percha. There is, however, no definitive proof that the patient had a true allergic reaction to the gutta-percha. In patients with a true immediate hypersensitivity to natural rubber latex, a consultation with the patient's allergist should be made prior to initiating the obturation phase of treatment. The contents of dental gutta-percha and the technique to be used should be discussed with the physician. A complete medical history and dental history should include identifying patients with a history of latex allergy or those at high risk for being allergic. Precautions must be taken to safely treat these patients. Hypoallergenic gloves and rubber dams in which the manufacturer has removed allergy-causing chemicals can be substituted. If, however, the patient has an immediate type of allergy to the proteins found in natural latex, vinyl, or nitride rubber gloves and dams must be used. In addition, thought should be given to treating the patient as the first appointment in the day in order to minimize exposure to airborne particles of latex. Special latex-free rooms may be necessary for the most severe cases.

Latex Allergies and Dental Procedures

Patients with a history of latex allergy or a high risk for being allergic can be identified through their medical and dental history. Patients should verbally notify their dentists of their medical condition prior to their appointment, especially if there is potential for an allergic reaction to latex.

Relationship between Latex Allergy and Endodontic (Root Canal) Procedures

Endodontists use gloves and rubber dams to ensure safe and successful endodontic treatment. These products often contain latex. Precautions can and must be taken to safely treat patients with latex allergies. Special gloves and rubber dams from which the manufacturer has removed allergy-causing chemicals can be substituted. If, however, the patient has an immediate type of allergy to natural latex proteins, the endodontist must use vinyl or nitrile rubber gloves and dams instead. In patients with a true immediate hypersensitivity to natural rubber latex, the endodontist should consult with the patient's allergist prior to treatment. The physician, patient, and endodontist should all be involved in any decisions made concerning the dental materials and techniques used in performing the endodontic treatment. With proper precautions, a patient with a history of latex allergy can safely receive endodontic treatment and save a tooth which might otherwise be lost.

References

American Academy of Allergy and Immunology. Task force of allergic reactions to latex. *J Allergy Clin Immunol* 1993; 92:16–18.

American Association of Nurse Anesthetists. Latex Allergy Protocol. *J of Am Assc of Nurse Anesthetists* 1993;61:223–4.

Beezhold DH, Kostyal DA, Wiseman J. The transfer of protein allergens from latex gloves: a study of influencing factors. *AORN Journal* 1994;59:605–13.

Bernstein, M. An overview of latex allergy and its implications for emergency nurses. *J Emerg Nurs* 1996;22:29–36.

Birmingham, PK, Dsida, RM, Grayhack, JJ, Han, Jianping, Wheeler, M., Pongracic, JA, Cote, CJ & Hall, SC. Do latex precautions in children with myelodysplasia reduce intraoperative allergic reactions? *Journal of Pediatric Orthopaedics* 1996;16:799–802.

Boxer MB, Grammer LC, Orfan N. Gutta-percha allergy in a health care worker with latex allergy. *J Allergy Clin Immunol* 1994;93:943–4.

Capriles-Hulett A, Sanchez-Borges M, Von-Scanzoni C & Medina JR. Very low frequency of latex and fruit allergy in patients with spina bifida from Venezuela: influence of socioeconomic factors. *Ann Allergy, Asthma & Immunol* 1995;75:62–4.

Charous BL. The puzzle of latex allergy: some answers, still more questions. *Ann Allergy* 1994;73:277–80.

Emans JB. Allergy to latex in patients who have myelodysplasia. *JBJS* 1992;74A:1103–9.

Frankland AW. Food reactions in pollen and latex allergic patients. *Clinical and Experimental Allergy*. 1995;25:580–581.

Gazelius B, Olgart L, Wrangsjo K. Unexpected symptoms to root filling with gutta-percha. *Int Endod J* 1986;19:202–4.

Holzman RS. Latex allergy: an emerging operating room problem. *Anesth Analg* 1993;76:633–41.

Kelly KJ, Management of the latex-allergic patient. *Immunol & Allergy Clinics of N America* 1995;15:139–57.

Kelly KJ, Kurup VP, Reijula KE, Fink JN. The diagnosis of natural rubber latex allergy. *J Allergy Clin Immunol* 1994;93:813–6.

Kwittken PL, Becker J, Oyefara B, Danziger R, Pawlowski NA, Sweinberg S. Latex hypersensitivity reactions despite prophylaxis. *Allergy Proc* 1992;13:123–7.

Kwittken PL, Sweinberg SK, Campbell DE & Pawlowski NA. Latex hypersensitivity in children: clinical presentation and detection of latex-specific immunoglobulin E. *Pediatrics* 1995;95:693–9.

Landwehr LP & Boguniewicz M. Current perspectives on latex allergy. *J Pediatrics* 1996;128:305–12.

Latex (Natural Rubber) allergy in spina bifida patients. *Spina Bifida Spotlight*; Spina Bifida Association of America, 1996.

Leger R. Meeropol E. Children at risk: latex allergy and spina bifida. *J Pediatric Nurs* 1992;7:371–6.

Meeropol E. Latex allergy update: clinical guidelines and unresolved issues. *J Wound, Ostomy and Continence Nurs* 1996;23:193–196.

Meeropol E, Leger R, Frost J. Latex allergy in patients with myelodysplasia and in health care providers: A double jeopardy. *Urol Nurs* 1993;13:39–44.

Meeropol E, Romanczuk A. Rubber on the rebound: two MCH nurses talk about latex allergy. *MCN* 1996;21:38–39.

Preventing allergic reactions to natural rubber latex in the workplace. *Nosh Alert*, U.S. Department of Health and Human Resources, Pub 97-135, August 1997.

Romanczuk A. Latex use with infants and children: it can cause problems *MCN* 1993;18:208–12.

Schwartz HA, Zurowski D. Anaphylaxis to latex in intravenous fluids. *J Allergy Clin Immunol* 1993;92:358–9.

Schwartz HJ. Latex: A potential hidden "food" allergen in fast food restaurants. *J Allergy Clin Immunol* 1995;95:139–40.

Shapiro E, Kelly KJ, Setlock MA, Suwalski KL, Meyers P. Complications of latex allergy. *Dialogues Pediatr Urol* 1992;15(3):1–8.

Slater JE. Rubber anaphylaxis. *N Engl J Med* 1989;320:1126–30.

Slater JE. Latex allergy—what do we know? [editorial] *J Allergy Clin Immunol* 1992;90:279–81.

Sorva R, Makinen-Kiljunen S, Suvillehto K, Juntunen-Backman K & Haahtela T. Latex allergy in children with no known risk factor for latex sensitization. *Pediatric Allergy and Immunology* 1995;6:36–38.

Vassallo SA, Thurston TA, Kim SH & Todres ID. Allergic reaction to latex from stopper of a medication vial. *Anesth Analg* 1995;80:1057–8.

Williams PB, Buhr MP, Weber RW, Volz MA, Koepke JW, Selner JC. Latex allergen in respirable particulate air pollution. *J Allergy Clin Immunol* 1995;95:88–93.

Chapter 48

Oral Care for
People with Hemophilia

Making time for dental care with all of the other demands of a hectic life can be a challenge. But oral health is particularly important for people with hemophilia.

Good dental care is important for everyone, but it is particularly important for people with hemophilia. "Oral health impacts overall health, making it even more critical for people with hemophilia to have good dental habits," stresses Dr. Mary Hayes, dentist at Rush Presbyterian Hemophilia Treatment Center in Chicago, Illinois.

Admittedly, it's not always easy to make time for dental care. "There are so many issues to deal with when you have a chronic illness like hemophilia, and dental care is not usually the top priority," says Karen Ridley, dental hygienist for the University of Michigan and Michigan State University (MSU) Comprehensive Hemophilia Treatment Centers. "Other matters take precedence and financial issues can affect whether a family will seek out dental care as well."

Dr. Hayes agrees. "It's understandable that families who are dealing with hemophilia have so much on their plate that dental care often falls to the bottom of the list," she says. "But it needs to be given a much higher priority, because it's so important to health overall. Ideally, dental care should start early, when the child is young and a good preventive program can be put into effect."

Excerpted from "Beyond Brushing and Flossing: Dental Care for People with Hemophilia" © 2003. Reprinted with permission from the Hemophilia Galaxy Web site (www.HemophiliaGalaxy.com), Baxter Healthcare Corporation.

That's because years of neglect can make even a routine visit problematic. Dental professionals recall many a sad tale that could have been prevented by following dental hygiene basics. "We saw a patient recently who needed thousands of units of factor concentrate just to have his teeth cleaned," says Ridley. "If he had taken care of his teeth and gone to his dentist for regular checkups, this would never have happened."

Dr. Hayes remembers treating a three-year-old who had bleeding gums and cavities from baby bottle tooth decay (caused by leaving the bottle in an infant's mouth when he goes to sleep). "The parents were giving him lots of antifibrinolytic agent (a product that helps clots stay in the mouth) and he was still bleeding. I instructed the parents to brush his teeth twice daily, which toughened up the gums, and he's fine now—no need for any additional treatment for the gums and the cavities were also restored. His good brushing routine will prevent additional decay from occurring." (Note: Use of antifibrinolytic agents is not recommended for inhibitor patients using Factor VIII bypassing therapy, due to the increased possibility of thrombotic risk)

A team effort between the dental care provider, the hemophilia treatment center, and the patient is well worth the effort, says Ridley. "Hemophilia doesn't cause dental disease, and the person with hemophilia can maintain a healthy mouth and a beautiful smile for life."

Find a Dental Home

"Having a dental home is essential, so if you have a crisis or an accident, you're already evaluated and set up," says Dr. Hayes. "An accident is not a good way to meet someone for the first time.

People with hemophilia need a dentist to help them manage a variety of dental issues, from infection and extraction of baby teeth and wisdom teeth to treating infected and cracked teeth, and of course, periodontal or gum disease."

The first step is to contact your HTC [hemophilia treatment center], where a dentist might already be part of the comprehensive team. If not, your HTC can help locate a dentist in your area who is familiar with bleeding disorders. You also can try a local dental school or hospital.

"There's a growing number of dentists who treat people with special needs like hemophilia," says Dr. Hayes. "If your dentist is not familiar with hemophilia, but is interested and willing to treat you, open the lines of communication. He or she may be overly concerned about your condition, so you should assure the dentist that dealing with it is a normal part of your routine."

Then make sure your dentist contacts your HTC to obtain essential information about your hemophilia. "It's important for the dentist to be aware of the effects of poor dental health on hemophilia," says Dr. Hayes. He or she should know whom to contact on your HTC team and get access to your medical records, if necessary.

"The dentist will take a comprehensive medical history during your first visit, and you should be open and thorough about your condition," says Dr. Hayes. "Inform the dentist if you're on prophylactic therapy and how you treat a minor bleeding episode."

Communication should be two-way, says Dr. Hayes. Dentists are responsible for telling patients about the risks of any procedure, especially the administration of local anesthetic. "Because the injection sometimes needs to be given back in an area with major blood vessels, patients should understand the risk beforehand."

But don't let fear of what might happen prevent you from asking for and receiving needed care. "Parents should be aware that their child's dental care should not be compromised in any way because of hemophilia," says Janet Mulherin, dental hygienist for Indiana Hemophilia and Thrombosis Center. "Dentists may sometimes delay working on a child because of the bleeding disorder, and that should not happen."

Visit Your Dental Home Regularly

Once you have a dental care provider who is familiar with your condition and knows how to treat you, be sure to visit regularly. The importance of routine care cannot be emphasized enough, according to Mulherin. "Regular visits mean you'll deal with small issues rather than large ones," she says. "It pays for itself because you're not dealing with the emotional and financial costs of emergency root canals or extractions."

How often you visit is up to you and your dentist. "Just like how often you need to clean your teeth, it's different for each patient," says Ridley. "Older patients with periodontal disease need to be seen more often than a 10-year-old with good hygiene habits.

That's why you should see the dentist as often as your dentist thinks is necessary."

Getting to the Root of the Problem

What you do in between visits makes all of the difference between a healthy mouth and dental problems. Brushing and flossing are important for everyone, but neglecting these basics has a more profound impact on people with hemophilia.

The roots of the teeth are surrounded by bone, which is covered by soft tissue known as the gingival, or gums. If gum disease, or gingivitis, occurs, spontaneous bleeding is one of the first signs.

"That's a much more difficult problem for people with hemophilia, because they'll bleed longer," explains Dr. Hayes. "It's why maintaining healthy gums and minimizing exposure to periodontal disease is very important."

To prevent gum disease, you need to brush your teeth and floss regularly. Sometimes, people with hemophilia fear that brushing and flossing will result in mouth bleeds. But dental experts are quick to provide reassurance.

"Healthy gums do not generally bleed during brushing and flossing, even in the person with hemophilia," emphasizes Ridley. "The only time some bleeding might occur is if you're overly aggressive with the toothbrush when brushing.

"But don't stop brushing, because that bleeding is likely caused by plaque, and you definitely want to scrub that off," she continues.

"Just be aware that if bleeding continues for more than 20 minutes or stops and then starts again, it's time to call your hemophilia treatment center."

Most important to remember, according to Ridley: "Bleeding gums are a sign of dental disease. Treating with factor concentrate or other therapies may temporarily stop the bleeding, but not the disease, so please see your dentist or dental hygienist."

Attack the Plaque

Plaque, the most common cause of dental disease, is a sticky, colorless film of bacteria that forms on the tooth surface. Plaque formation is no different for people with hemophilia. "If you're experiencing a mouth bleed, however, you may notice more plaque at that time," says Ridley.

The best way to attack the plaque is to floss your teeth regularly. Flossing removes plaque that the toothbrush can't reach, enabling you to clean between the teeth and under the gum line, where bits of food and bacteria get trapped.

The gums might bleed slightly when you begin regular flossing. It usually will stop within a week, if flossing is kept up every day, and does not usually require treatment with factor concentrate. "As plaque is removed and gums get healthier, bleeding will decrease," says Ridley. "Of course, you should contact your HTC if you have any concerns about continued bleeding."

If you have joint damage in your elbows, you might have difficulty flossing due to limited elbow motion. "Ask your dentist about special flossing devices, like a floss holder," advises Ridley. Various types of interdental cleaners also can help. Since plaque causes both cavities and periodontal disease, flossing is essential. The good news is that "once-a-day, thorough plaque removal can help you prevent dental disease, keep a healthy smile, and protect your teeth for a lifetime," says Ridley.

Chapter 49

Oral Care in People with Respiratory Diseases and Conditions

Chronic lung-disease sufferers should be especially fastidious about brushing and flossing their teeth. That is the message delivered in a study just published in the *Journal of Periodontology* conducted by oral biologists from the University at Buffalo.

The researchers found an association between chronic respiratory disease and periodontal disease in an analysis of data from a large national database, the Third National Health and Nutrition Examination Survey, known as NHANES III. The results add to a growing body of evidence that poor oral health is linked to a number of chronic diseases.

Frank Scannapieco, D.M.D., Ph.D., associate professor of oral biology in UB's School of Dental Medicine and lead author of the study, said the mechanism linking oral health and lung disease isn't clear, but that bacteria in the mouth likely are to blame.

"Accumulation of disease-causing organisms associated with gum disease may increase the risk for serious lower-respiratory-tract infection in susceptible subjects," said Scannapieco.

"It is possible that bacteria that normally stick to the teeth are sloughed into the saliva and may be breathed into the upper airways, changing that environment and paving the way for other germs to infect the lower airways. Oral conditions likely work together with other factors, such as smoking, environmental pollutants, allergies, and genetics to make existing lung problems worse."

Scannapieco's earlier work with pneumonia in hospitalized patients suggested a potential association between respiratory diseases and poor oral health, and led him to investigate whether such a relationship exists in the general population. For the analysis, he used data from 13,792 participants in NHANES III who were at least 20 years old and had at least six natural teeth.

Questionnaires completed by participants included items about their history of respiratory disease. The physical examination measured each person's forced expiratory volume (FEV1), or how much air a person can blow out in one second, a measure of lung health and function.

A dental examination assessed the loss of gum attachment supporting the teeth, amount of gum bleeding, number of cavities and number of teeth.

Analyzing these two sets of data for a relationship, the researchers found that lung function appeared to diminish as the amount of gum-attachment loss increased. Results also showed a decline in respiratory function as oral health worsened.

"We aren't saying that if you don't brush, you'll develop lung disease," said Scannapieco. "We're saying that if you already have lung disease, taking care of your teeth and gums is especially important. It's possible that improved oral health is one factor that may help prevent progression of this disease, which is responsible for 2.2 million deaths a year worldwide."

Alex W. Ho, M.S., oral-biology statistician, was the co-author of the study.

The work was supported in part by grants from the U.S. Health Service and the National Institute of Dental and Craniofacial Research.

Part Six

Disorders of the Mouth

Chapter 50

Oral Cancer

Chapter Contents

Section 50.1

What You Need to Know about Oral Cancer

"What You Need To Know About™ Oral Cancer," is published by the National Cancer Institute, NIH Publication Number 97-1574, posted September 1998; updated September 2002. Available online at www.cancer.gov/cancerinfo/wyntk/oral; accessed May 2003.

Introduction

The National Cancer Institute (NCI) has written this chapter to help people with oral cancer and their families and friends better understand this disease. We hope others will also read it to learn more about oral cancer.

This chapter describes symptoms, diagnosis, and treatment. It also has information about rehabilitation and about sources of support to help patients cope with oral cancer.

The Oral Cavity

This chapter deals with cancer of the oral cavity (mouth) and the oropharynx (the part of the throat at the back of the mouth). The oral cavity includes many parts: the lips; the lining inside the lips and cheeks, called the buccal mucosa; the teeth; the bottom (floor) of the mouth under the tongue; the front two-thirds of the tongue; the bony top of the mouth (hard palate); the gums; and the small area behind the wisdom teeth. The oropharynx includes the back one-third of the tongue, the soft palate, the tonsils, and the part of the throat behind the mouth. Salivary glands throughout the oral cavity make saliva, which keeps the mouth moist and helps digest food.

What Is Cancer?

Cancer is a group of diseases. It occurs when cells become abnormal and divide without control or order. More than 100 different types of cancer are known.

Like all organs of the body, the mouth and throat are made up of many kinds of cells. Cells normally divide in an orderly way to produce more cells only when the body needs them. This process helps keep the body healthy.

Cells that divide when new cells are not needed form too much tissue. The mass of extra tissue, called a tumor, can be benign or malignant.

Benign tumors are not cancer. They can usually be removed, and in most cases, they don't grow back. Most important, the cells in benign tumors do not invade other tissues and do not spread to other parts of the body. Benign tumors usually are not a threat to life.

Malignant tumors are cancer. They can invade and damage nearby tissues and organs. Also, cancer cells can break away from a malignant tumor and enter the bloodstream or the lymphatic system. This is how cancer spreads and forms secondary tumors in other parts of the body. The spread of cancer is called metastasis.

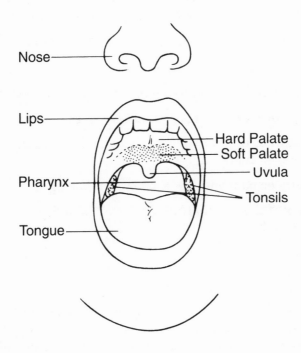

***Figure 50.1.** The oral cavity.*

When oral cancer spreads, it usually travels through the lymphatic system. Cancer cells that enter the lymphatic system are carried along by lymph, an almost colorless, watery fluid containing cells that help the body fight infection and disease. Along the lymphatic channels are groups of small, bean-shaped organs called lymph nodes (sometimes called lymph glands). Oral cancer that spreads usually travels to the lymph nodes in the neck. It can also spread to other parts of the body. Cancer that spreads is the same disease and has the same name as the original (primary) cancer.

Early Detection

Regular checkups that include an examination of the entire mouth can detect precancerous conditions or the early stages of oral cancer. Your doctor and dentist should check the tissues in your mouth as part of your routine exams.

Symptoms

Oral cancer usually occurs in people over the age of 45 but can develop at any age. These are some symptoms to watch for:

- A sore on the lip or in the mouth that does not heal
- A lump on the lip or in the mouth or throat
- A white or red patch on the gums, tongue, or lining of the mouth
- Unusual bleeding, pain, or numbness in the mouth
- A sore throat that does not go away, or a feeling that something is caught in the throat
- Difficulty or pain with chewing or swallowing
- Swelling of the jaw that causes dentures to fit poorly or become uncomfortable
- A change in the voice
- Pain in the ear

These symptoms may be caused by cancer or by other, less serious problems. It is important to see a dentist or doctor about any symptoms like these, so that the problem can be diagnosed and treated as early as possible.

Diagnosis and Staging

If an abnormal area has been found in the oral cavity, a biopsy is the only way to know whether it is cancer. Usually, the patient is referred to an oral surgeon or an ear, nose, and throat surgeon, who removes part or all of the lump or abnormal-looking area. A pathologist examines the tissue under a microscope to check for cancer cells.

Almost all oral cancers are squamous cell carcinomas. Squamous cells line the oral cavity. If the pathologist finds oral cancer, the patient's doctor needs to know the stage, or extent, of the disease in order to plan the best treatment. Staging tests and exams help the doctor find out whether the cancer has spread and what parts of the body are affected.

A patient who needs a biopsy may want to ask the doctor these questions:

- How much tissue will be removed for the biopsy?

- How long will the biopsy take? Will I be awake? Will it hurt?

- How should I care for the biopsy site afterward?

- How soon will I know the results?

- If I do have cancer, who will talk with me about treatment? When?

Staging generally includes dental x-rays and x-rays of the head and chest. The doctor may also want the patient to have a CT (or CAT) scan. A CT scan is a series of x-rays put together by a computer to form detailed pictures of areas inside the body. Ultrasonography is another way to produce pictures of areas in the body. High-frequency sound waves (ultrasound), which cannot be heard by humans, are bounced off organs and tissue. The pattern of echoes produced by these waves creates a picture called a sonogram. Sometimes the doctor asks for MRI (magnetic resonance imaging), a procedure in which pictures are created using a magnet linked to a computer. The doctor also feels the lymph nodes in the neck to check for swelling or other changes. In most cases, the patient will have a complete physical examination before treatment begins.

Treatment

After diagnosis and staging, the doctor develops a treatment plan to fit each patient's needs. Treatment for oral cancer depends on a number of factors. Among these are the location, size, type, and extent of the tumor and the stage of the disease. The doctor also considers the patient's age and general health. Treatment involves surgery, radiation therapy, or, in many cases, a combination of the two. Some patients receive chemotherapy, treatment with anticancer drugs.

For most patients, it is important to have a complete dental exam before cancer treatment begins. Because cancer treatment may make the mouth sensitive and more easily infected, doctors often advise patients to have any needed dental work done before treatment begins.

Most people with cancer want to learn all they can about their disease and their treatment choices so they can take an active part in decisions about their medical and dental care. The doctor is the best person to answer their questions. Also, the patient may want to talk with the doctor about taking part in a research study of new treatment methods. Such studies, called clinical trials, are designed to improve cancer treatment.

Many patients find it useful to make a list of questions before seeing the doctor. Taking notes can make it easier to remember what the doctor says. Some patients also find that it helps to have a family member or friend with them—to take part in the discussion, to take notes, or just to listen.

Before treatment begins, the patient may want to ask the doctor these questions:

- What are my treatment choices? Which do you recommend for me? Why?

- What are the risks and possible side effects of each treatment?

- What are the expected benefits of each kind of treatment?

- What can be done about side effects?

- Would a clinical trial be appropriate for me?

There is a lot to learn about cancer and its treatment. Patients do not need to ask all their questions or understand all the answers at once. They will have many chances to ask the doctor to explain things that are not clear and to ask for more information.

Planning Treatment

Treatment decisions can be complex. Before starting treatment, the patient may want to have another doctor review the diagnosis and treatment plan. A short delay will not reduce the chance that treatment will be successful. There are a number of ways to find a doctor for a second opinion:

- The patient's doctor or dentist may suggest a specialist who treats oral cancer.

- The Cancer Information Service, at 1-800-4-CANCER, can tell callers about cancer centers and other NCI-supported programs in their area.

- Patients can get the names of specialists from their local medical or dental society, a nearby hospital, or a medical or dental school.

- The Directory of Medical Specialists lists doctors' names along with their specialty and their background. This resource is available in most public libraries.

Methods of Treatment

Patients with oral cancer may be treated by a team of specialists. The medical team may include an oral surgeon; an ear, nose, and throat surgeon; a medical oncologist; a radiation oncologist; a prosthodontist; a general dentist; a plastic surgeon; a dietitian; a social worker; a nurse; and a speech therapist.

Surgery to remove the tumor in the mouth is the usual treatment for patients with oral cancer. If there is evidence that the cancer has spread, the surgeon may also remove lymph nodes in the neck. If the disease has spread to muscles and other tissues in the neck, the operation may be more extensive.

Before surgery, the patient may want to ask the doctor these questions:

- What kind of operation will it be?

- How will I feel after the operation? If I have pain, how will you help me?

- Will I have trouble eating?

- Where will the scars be? What will they look like?

- Do you expect that there will be long-term effects from the surgery?

- Will there be permanent changes in my appearance?

- Will I lose my teeth? Can they be replaced? How soon?
- If I need to have plastic surgery, when can that be done?
- Will I need to see a specialist for help with my speech?
- When can I get back to my normal activities?

Radiation therapy (also called radiotherapy) is the use of high-energy rays to damage cancer cells and stop them from growing. Like surgery, radiation therapy is local therapy; it affects only the cells in the treated area. The energy may come from a large machine (external radiation). It can also come from radioactive materials placed directly into or near the tumor (internal radiation). Radiation therapy is sometimes used instead of surgery for small tumors in the mouth. Patients with large tumors may need both surgery and radiation therapy.

Radiation therapy may be given before or after surgery. Before surgery, radiation can shrink the tumor so that it can be removed. Radiation after surgery is used to destroy cancer cells that may remain.

For external radiation therapy, the patient goes to the hospital or clinic each day for treatments. Usually, treatment is given 5 days a week for 5 to 6 weeks. This schedule helps protect healthy tissues by dividing the total amount of radiation into small doses.

Implant radiation therapy puts tiny seeds containing radioactive material directly into the tumor or in tissue near it. Generally, an implant is left in place for several days, and the patient will stay in the hospital in a private room.

The length of time nurses and other caregivers, as well as visitors, can spend with the patient will be limited. The implant is removed before the patient goes home.

Before radiation therapy, a patient may want to ask the doctor these questions:

- When will the treatments begin? When will they end?
- How will I feel during therapy?
- What can I do to take care of myself during therapy?
- Can I continue my normal activities?
- How will my mouth and face look afterward?
- Will I need a special diet? For how long?
- If my mouth becomes dry, what can I do about it?

Chemotherapy is the use of drugs to kill cancer cells. Researchers are looking for effective drugs or drug combinations to treat oral cancer. They are also exploring ways to combine chemotherapy with other forms of cancer treatment to help destroy the tumor and prevent the disease from spreading.

Clinical Trials

Researchers are developing treatment methods that are more effective against oral cancer, and they are also finding ways to reduce side effects of treatment. When laboratory research shows that a new method has promise, doctors use it to treat cancer patients in clinical trials. These trials are designed to answer scientific questions about the new approach and to find out whether it is both safe and effective. Patients who take part in clinical trials make an important contribution to medical science and may have the first chance to benefit from improved treatment methods.

Clinical trials to study new treatments for oral cancer are under way in hospitals throughout the country. Some trials involve ways to shrink or destroy the primary tumor. In others, scientists are testing ways to prevent the cancer from coming back in the mouth or spreading to other parts of the body. Still others involve treatments to slow or stop cancer that has already spread.

Researchers are studying the timing of treatments and new ways to combine various types of treatment. For example, they are trying to increase the effectiveness of radiation therapy by giving treatments twice a day instead of once a day. They are also working with hyperthermia (heat) and with drugs called radiosensitizers to try to make cancer cells more sensitive to radiation. Researchers are also using drugs to help protect normal cells from radiation damage. In addition, they are exploring various new anticancer drugs and drug combinations.

People who have had oral cancer have an increased risk of getting a new cancer of the mouth or another part of the head or neck. Doctors are trying to find ways to prevent these new cancers. Some research has shown that a substance related to vitamin A may prevent a new cancer from developing in someone who has already been successfully treated for oral cancer.

Oral cancer patients who are interested in taking part in a trial should talk with their doctor. They may want to read "Taking Part in Clinical Trials: What Cancer Patients Need To Know," a booklet that explains what treatment studies are and outlines some of their possible benefits and risks. One way to learn about clinical trials is through PDQ®, a computerized resource developed by the National Cancer Institute. PDQ® contains information about cancer treatment and an up-to-date list of trials all over the country. The Cancer Information Service, at 1-800-4-CANCER, can provide PDQ® information to patients and the public.

Side Effects of Treatment

It is hard to limit the effects of cancer treatment so that only cancer cells are removed or destroyed. Because healthy cells and tissues may also be damaged, treatment often causes side effects.

The side effects of cancer treatment vary. They depend mainly on the type and extent of the treatment and the specific area being treated. Also, each person reacts differently. Some side effects are temporary; others are permanent. Doctors try to plan the patient's therapy to keep side effects to a minimum. They also watch patients very carefully so they can help with any problems that occur.

Surgery to remove a small tumor in the mouth usually does not cause any lasting problems. For a larger tumor, however, the surgeon may need to remove part of the palate, tongue, or jaw. Such surgery is likely to change the patient's ability to chew, swallow, or talk. The patient may also look different. After surgery, the patient's face may be swollen. This swelling usually goes away within a few weeks. However, removing lymph nodes can slow the flow of lymph, which may collect in the tissues; this swelling may last for a long time.

Before starting radiation therapy, a patient should see a dentist who is familiar with the changes this therapy can cause in the mouth. Radiation therapy can make the mouth sore. It can also cause changes in the saliva and may reduce the amount of saliva, making it hard to chew and swallow. Because saliva normally protects the teeth, mouth dryness can promote tooth decay. Good mouth care can help keep the teeth and gums healthy and can make the patient feel more comfortable. The health care team may suggest the use of a special kind of toothbrush or mouthwash. The dentist usually suggests a special fluoride program to keep the teeth healthy. To help relieve mouth dryness, the health care team may suggest the use of artificial saliva and other methods to keep the mouth moist. Mouth dryness from radiation therapy goes away in some patients, but it can be permanent.

Weight loss can be a serious problem for patients being treated for oral cancer because a sore mouth may make eating difficult. Your doctor may suggest ways to maintain a healthy diet. In many cases, it helps to have food and beverages in very small amounts. Many patients find that eating several small meals and snacks during the day works better than trying to have three large meals. Often, it is easier to eat soft, bland foods that have been moistened with sauces or gravies; thick soups, puddings, and high protein milkshakes are nourishing and easy to swallow. It may be helpful to prepare other foods in a blender. The doctor may also suggest special liquid dietary supplements for patients who have trouble chewing. Drinking lots of fluids helps keep the mouth moist and makes it easier to eat.

Some patients are able to wear their dentures during radiation therapy. Many, however, will not be able to wear dentures for up to a year after treatment. Because the tissues in the mouth that support the denture may change during or after treatment, dentures may no longer fit properly. After treatment is over, a patient may need to have dentures refitted or replaced.

Radiation therapy can also cause sores in the mouth and cracked and peeling lips. These usually heal in the weeks after treatment is completed. Often, good mouth care can help prevent these sores. Dentures should not be worn until the sores have healed.

During radiation therapy, patients may become very tired, especially in the later weeks of treatment. Resting is important, but doctors usually advise their patients to try to stay reasonably active. Patients should match their activities to their energy level. It's common for radiation to cause the skin in the treated area to become red and dry, tender, and itchy. Toward the end of treatment, the skin may become moist and weepy. There may be permanent darkening or bronzing of the skin in the treated area. This area should be exposed to the air as much as possible but should also be protected from the sun. Good skin care is important at this time, but patients should not use any lotions or creams without the doctor's advice. Men may lose all or part of their beard, but facial hair generally grows back after treatment is done.

Usually, men shave with an electric razor during treatment to prevent cuts that may lead to infection. Most effects of radiation therapy on the skin are temporary. The area will heal when the treatment is over.

The side effects of chemotherapy depend on the drugs that are given. In general, anticancer drugs affect rapidly growing cells, such as blood cells that fight infection, cells that line the mouth and the digestive tract, and cells in hair follicles. As a result, patients may have side effects such as lower resistance to infection, loss of appetite, nausea, vomiting, or mouth sores. They also may have less energy and may lose their hair.

The side effects of cancer treatment are different for each person, and they may even be different from one treatment to the next. Doctors, nurses, and dietitians can explain the side effects of cancer treatment and can suggest ways to deal with them.

Rehabilitation

Rehabilitation is a very important part of treatment for patients with oral cancer. The goals of rehabilitation depend on the extent of the disease and the treatment a patient has received. The health care team makes every effort to help the patient return to normal activities as soon as possible.

Rehabilitation may include dietary counseling, surgery, a dental prosthesis, speech therapy, and other services. Sometimes, a patient needs reconstructive and plastic surgery to rebuild the bones or tissues of the mouth. If this is not possible, a prosthodontist may be able to make an artificial dental and/or facial part (prosthesis). Patients may need special training to use the device.

Speech therapy generally begins as soon as possible for a patient who has trouble speaking after treatment. Often, a speech therapist visits the patient in the hospital to plan therapy and teach speech exercises. Speech therapy usually continues after the patient returns home.

Follow-Up Care

Regular follow-up exams are very important for anyone who has been treated for oral cancer. The physician and the dentist watch the patient closely to check the healing process and to look for signs that the cancer may have returned. Patients with mouth dryness from radiation therapy should have dental exams three times a year.

The patient may need to see a dietitian if weight loss or eating problems continue. Most doctors urge their oral cancer patients to stop using tobacco and alcohol to reduce the risk of developing a new cancer.

Support for Cancer Patients

Living with a serious disease isn't easy. Cancer patients and those who care about them face many problems and challenges. Finding the strength to cope with these difficulties is easier when people have helpful information and support services.

Cancer patients may worry about holding a job, caring for their family, or starting new relationships. Worries about tests, treatments, hospital stays, and medical bills are common. Doctors, nurses, and other members of the health care team can help calm fears and ease confusion about treatment, working, or daily activities. Also, meeting with a nurse, social worker, counselor, or member of the clergy can be helpful for patients who want to talk about their feelings or discuss their concerns.

Friends and relatives, especially those who have had personal experience with cancer, can be very supportive. Also, many patients find it helpful to discuss their concerns with others who are facing similar problems. Cancer patients often get together in support groups, where they can share what they have learned about cancer and its treatment and about coping with the disease. It is important to keep in mind, however, that each patient is different. Treatments and ways of dealing with cancer that work for one person may not be right for another—even if they both have the same kind of cancer. It is always a good idea to discuss the advice of friends and family members with the doctor.

Often, a social worker at the hospital or clinic can suggest groups that can help with rehabilitation, emotional support, financial aid, transportation, or home care.

What the Future Holds

Patients and their families are naturally concerned about what the future holds. Sometimes they use statistics to try to figure out whether the patient will be cured or how long he or she will live. It is important to remember, however, that statistics are averages based on large numbers of patients. They cannot be used to predict what will happen to a certain patient because no two cancer patients are alike. The doctor who takes care of the patient knows his or her medical history and is in the best position to discuss the person's outlook (prognosis).

People should feel free to ask the doctor about their chance of recovery, but not even the doctor knows for sure what will happen. When doctors talk about surviving cancer, they may use the term remission rather than cure. Even though many patients with oral cancer recover completely, doctors use this term because oral cancer can recur.

Causes and Prevention

Scientists at hospitals and medical centers all across the country are studying this disease to learn more about what causes it and how

445

to prevent it. Doctors do know that no one can catch cancer from another person: it is not contagious.

Two known causes of oral cancer are tobacco and alcohol use. Tobacco use—smoking cigarettes, cigars, or pipes; chewing tobacco; or dipping snuff—accounts for 80 to 90 percent of oral cancers. A number of studies have shown that cigar and pipe smokers have the same risk as cigarette smokers. Studies indicate that smokeless tobacco users are at particular risk of developing oral cancer. For long-time users, the risk is much greater, making the use of snuff or chewing tobacco among young people a special concern.

People who stop using tobacco—even after many years of use—can greatly reduce their risk of oral cancer. Special counseling or self-help groups may be useful for those who are trying to give up tobacco. Some hospitals have groups for people who want to quit. Also, the Cancer Information Service and the American Cancer Society may have information about groups in local areas to help people quit using tobacco.

Chronic and/or heavy use of alcohol also increases the risk of oral cancer, even for people who do not use tobacco. However, people who use both alcohol and tobacco have an especially high risk of oral cancer. Scientists believe that these substances increase each other's harmful effects.

Cancer of the lip can be caused by exposure to the sun. The risk can be avoided with the use of a lotion or lip balm containing a sunscreen. Wearing a hat with a brim can also block the sun's harmful rays. Pipe smokers are especially prone to cancer of the lip.

Some studies have shown that many people who develop oral cancer have a history of leukoplakia, a whitish patch inside the mouth. The causes of leukoplakia are not well understood, but it is commonly associated with heavy use of tobacco and alcohol. The condition often occurs in irritated areas, such as the gums and mouth lining of smokeless tobacco users and the lower lip of pipe smokers.

Another condition, erythroplakia, appears as a red patch in the mouth. Erythroplakia occurs most often in people 60 to 70 years of age. Early diagnosis and treatment of leukoplakia and erythroplakia are important because cancer may develop in these patches.

People who think they might be at risk for developing oral cancer should discuss this concern with their doctor or dentist, who may be able to suggest ways to reduce the risk and plan an appropriate schedule for checkups.

Section 50.2

Spit Tobacco and Oral Cancer

"Spitting into the Wind: The Facts about Dip and Chew" is published by
the National Institute of Dental and Craniofacial Research (NIDCR)/
National Oral Health Information Clearinghouse, January 2000. Available online at www.nidcr.nih.gov/health/pubs/chew/main.htm; accessed
May 2003.

A lot of athletes get hooked before they know the facts about dip
and chew. They don't know that spit tobacco:

- is highly addictive

- contains nicotine

- doesn't help performance

- is not a safe alternative to cigarettes

Addiction is one tough opponent. It doesn't take long to get hooked.
In fact, you get more nicotine from spit tobacco than from cigarettes.
To get unhooked, you have to know what you're up against and you
need a game plan. Once you're hooked, it's hard to keep lid on this
addiction.

There are no benefits of using spit tobacco. In a Major League Baseball poll, not one player who used dip or chew said that the tobacco
improved his game or sharpened his reflexes.

Scientists agree. Spit tobacco does not improve athletic performance.

What's really in it for you?

- Nicotine (addictive drug)

- Polonium 210 (nuclear waste)

- Formaldehyde (embalming fluid)

- Cancer-causing chemicals

- Radioactive elements

These are just some of the ingredients in dip and chew. Spit tobacco is not a safe alternative to cigarettes. The toxic chemicals can damage your gums. They also can cause cancer.

The Truth about Dip and Chew

Even if you don't know the harm dip and chew can do, your body does.

Cancer is like a bomb! You don't know when it will go off. Up to a certain point, if you quit, your body can heal itself, but the longer you use spit tobacco, the bigger your risk of getting cancer. You don't have to dip for 30 years to get cancer! Quit while you're still ahead of the game.

Don't let it be too late. Chewing tobacco and snuff can cause mouth and throat cancer. There are some athletes who have developed mouth cancer after only 6 or 7 years of using spit tobacco. It's hard to cure because it spreads fast.

If not caught right away, major surgery is often needed to take out parts of your mouth, jaw, and tongue.

Check your mouth often. Look closely at places where you hold the tobacco. See your doctor or dentist right away if you have:

- a sore that bleeds easily and doesn't heal
- a lump or thickening anywhere in your mouth or neck
- soreness or swelling that doesn't go away
- trouble chewing, swallowing, or moving your tongue or jaw

Stay in the Game

Your doctor, dentist, trainer, or coach can help you quit. The best way to quit is to have a plan.

For a free copy of a guide to help you quit and quitting advice, call 1-800-4-CANCER.

Chapter 51

Lip and Oral Cavity Cancer

What Is Cancer of the Lip and Oral Cavity?

Cancer of the lip and oral cavity is a disease in which cancer (malignant) cells are found in the tissues of the lip or mouth. The oral cavity includes the front two thirds of the tongue, the upper and lower gums (the gingiva), the lining of the inside of the cheeks and lips (the buccal mucosa), the bottom (floor) of the mouth under the tongue, the bony top of the mouth (the hard palate), and the small area behind the wisdom teeth (the retromolar trigone).

Cancers of the head and neck are most often found in people who are over the age of 45. Cancer of the lip is more common in men than in women, and is more likely to develop in people with light-colored skin who have been in the sun a lot. Cancer of the oral cavity is more common in people who chew tobacco or smoke pipes.

A doctor should be seen if a person finds a lump in the lip, mouth, or gums, finds a sore in the mouth that doesn't heal, or has bleeding or pain in the mouth. Another sign of a cancer of the mouth or gums is when dentures no longer fit well. Often lip and oral cavity cancers are found by dentists when examining the teeth.

If there are symptoms, a doctor will examine the mouth using a mirror and lights. The doctor may order x-rays of the mouth. If tissue that is not normal is found, the doctor will need to cut out a small

PDQ® Cancer Information Summary. National Cancer Institute; Bethesda, MD. Lip and Oral Cavity Cancer (PDQ®): Treatment—Patient. Updated 08/2002. Available at: http://cancer.gov. Accessed May 2003.

piece and look at it under the microscope to see if there are any cancer cells. This is called a biopsy. The patient will be given a substance to take feeling away from the area for a short time (a local anesthetic) so no pain is felt. The doctor will also feel the throat for lumps.

The chance of recovery (prognosis) depends on where the cancer is in the lip or mouth, whether the cancer is just in the lip or mouth or has spread to other tissues (the stage), and the patient's general state of health.

Stage of Cancer of the Lip and Oral Cavity

Once cancer of the lip and oral cavity is found, more tests will be done to find out if cancer cells have spread to other parts of the body. This is called staging. A doctor needs to know the stage of the disease to plan treatment. The following stages are used for cancer of the lip and oral cavity:

Stage I

The cancer is no more than 2 centimeters (about 1 inch) and has not spread to lymph nodes in the area (lymph nodes are small bean-shaped structures that are found throughout the body; they produce and store infection-fighting cells).

Stage II

The cancer is more than 2 centimeters, but less than 4 centimeters (less than 2 inches), and has not spread to lymph nodes in the area.

Stage III

Either of the following may be true:

- The cancer is more than 4 centimeters.
- The cancer is any size but has spread to only one lymph node on the same side of the neck as the cancer. The lymph node that contains cancer measures no more than 3 centimeters (just over one inch).

Stage IV

Any of the following may be true:

- The cancer has spread to tissues around the lip and oral cavity. The lymph nodes in the area may or may not contain cancer.

- The cancer is any size and has spread to more than one lymph node on the same side of the neck as the cancer, to lymph nodes on one or both sides of the neck, or to any lymph node that measures more than 6 centimeters (over 2 inches).

- The cancer has spread to other parts of the body.

Recurrent

Recurrent disease means that the cancer has come back (recurred) after it has been treated. It may come back in the lip and oral cavity or in another part of the body.

How Cancer of the Lip and Oral Cavity Is Treated

There are treatments for all patients with cancer of the lip and oral cavity. Two kinds of treatment are used:

- Surgery (taking out the cancer)

- Radiation therapy (using high-dose x-rays or other high-energy rays to kill cancer cells)

- Chemotherapy (using drugs to kill cancer cells) is being tested in clinical trials.

Surgery is a common treatment of cancer of the lip and oral cavity. The doctor may remove the cancer and some of the healthy tissue around the cancer. The doctor may also remove the lymph nodes in the neck (lymph node dissection).

Radiation therapy uses high-energy x-rays to kill cancer cells and shrink tumors. Radiation may come from a machine outside the body (external radiation therapy) or from putting materials that produce radiation (radioisotopes) through thin plastic tubes or needles in the area where the cancer cells are found (internal radiation therapy). If smoking is stopped before radiation therapy is started, the patient has a better chance of surviving longer.

Chemotherapy uses drugs to kill cancer cells. Chemotherapy may be taken by pill, or it may be put into the body by a needle in a vein or muscle. Chemotherapy is called a systemic treatment because the drug enters the bloodstream, travels through the body, and can kill cancer cells throughout the body.

If the doctor removes all the cancer that can be seen at the time of the operation, the patient may be given chemotherapy after surgery to kill any cancer cells that are left. Chemotherapy given after an operation to a person who has no cancer cells that can be seen is called adjuvant chemotherapy. Chemotherapy given before surgery to try and shrink the cancer so it can be removed is called neoadjuvant chemotherapy.

Hyperthermia is a new treatment being tested in certain patients. It uses a special machine to heat the body for a certain period of time to kill cancer cells. Because cancer cells are often more sensitive to heat than normal cells, the cancer cells die and the cancer shrinks.

Because the lips and mouth are needed to eat and talk, a patient may need special help adjusting to the side effects of the cancer and its treatment. The doctor will consult with several kinds of doctors who can help determine the best treatment for the patient. Trained medical staff can also help a patient recover from treatment and adjust to new ways of eating and talking. A patient may need plastic surgery or help learning to eat and speak if a large part of the lip or mouth is taken out.

Treatment by Stage

Treatment of cancer of the lip and oral cavity depends on where the cancer is, the stage of the disease, and the patient's age and overall health.

Standard treatment may be considered because of its effectiveness in patients in past studies, or participation in a clinical trial may be considered. Not all patients are cured with standard therapy and some standard treatments may have more side effects than are desired. For these reasons, clinical trials are designed to find better ways to treat cancer patients and are based on the most up-to-date information. Clinical trials are ongoing in many parts of the country for patients with cancer of the lip and oral cavity.

To learn more about clinical trials, call the Cancer Information Service at (800) 4-CANCER (800-422-6237); TTY at (800) 332-8615.

Stage I Lip and Oral Cavity Cancer

Treatment depends on where the cancer is in the lip or mouth.

Lip Cancer

If the cancer is in the lip, treatment may be one of the following:

1. Surgery.
2. Radiation therapy.

Tongue Cancer

If the cancer is in the tongue, treatment may be one of the following:

1. Surgery.
2. Surgery followed by radiation therapy to the neck.
3. Radiation therapy to the mouth and the neck.

Buccal Mucosa Cancer

If the cancer is in the lining of the inside of the cheeks and lips (buccal mucosa), treatment may be one of the following:

1. Surgery.
2. Radiation therapy.

Floor of the Mouth Cancer

If the cancer is in the bottom (floor) of the mouth, treatment may be one of the following:

1. Surgery.
2. Radiation therapy.

Lower Gum Cancer

If the cancer is in the lower gums (gingiva), treatment may be one of the following:

1. Surgery.
2. Radiation therapy.

Retromolar Trigone Cancer

If the cancer is in the small area behind the wisdom teeth (retromolar trigone), treatment may be one of the following:

1. Surgery to remove part of the jawbone.
2. Radiation therapy followed (if needed) by surgery.

Upper Gums and Hard Palate Cancer

If the cancer is in the upper gums (gingiva) or the top bony part of the mouth (hard palate), treatment may be one of the following:

1. Surgery.
2. Surgery followed by radiation therapy.

Stage II Lip and Oral Cavity Cancer

Treatment depends on where the cancer is in the lip or mouth.

Lip Cancer

If the cancer is in the lip, treatment may be one of the following:

1. Surgery.
2. External and/or internal radiation therapy.

Tongue Cancer

If the cancer is in the tongue, treatment may be one of the following:

1. Radiation therapy.
2. Surgery and radiation therapy.

Buccal Mucosa Cancer

If the cancer is in the lining of the inside of the cheeks and lips (buccal mucosa), treatment may be one of the following:

1. Radiation therapy.
2. Surgery.
3. Surgery plus radiation therapy.

Floor of the Mouth Cancer

If the cancer is in the bottom (floor) of the mouth, treatment may be one of the following:

1. Surgery.
2. Radiation therapy.
3. Surgery followed by internal or external radiation therapy.

Lower Gum Cancer

If the cancer is in the lower gums (gingiva), treatment may be one of the following:

1. Surgery.
2. Radiation therapy.

Retromolar Trigone Cancer

If the cancer is in the small space behind the wisdom teeth (retromolar trigone), treatment may be one of the following:

1. Surgery to remove part of the jawbone.
2. Radiation therapy followed (if needed) by surgery.

Upper Gum or Hard Palate Cancer

If the cancer is in the upper gums or the top bony part of the mouth (hard palate), treatment will probably be surgery followed by radiation therapy.

Stage III Lip and Oral Cavity Cancer

Treatment depends on where the cancer is in the lip or mouth. In addition to the treatments listed below, a patient will probably have radiation therapy to the neck with or without surgery to remove lymph nodes in the neck (lymph node dissection).

Lip Cancer

If the cancer is in the lip, treatment may be one of the following:

1. Surgery to remove the cancer plus internal or external radiation therapy.
2. Radiation therapy.
3. A clinical trial of chemotherapy followed by surgery or radiation therapy.
4. A clinical trial of surgery followed by chemotherapy.
5. A clinical trial of surgery, radiation therapy, and chemotherapy.
6. A clinical trial of a new radiation therapy technique (superfractionated).

455

Tongue Cancer

If the cancer is in the tongue, treatment may be one of the following:

1. External beam with or without internal radiation therapy.
2. Surgery followed by radiation therapy.

Buccal Mucosa Cancer

If the cancer is in the lining of the inside of the cheeks and lips (buccal mucosa), treatment may be one of the following:

1. Surgery to remove the cancer and the tissue around it.
2. Radiation therapy.
3. Surgery plus radiation therapy.
4. A clinical trial of chemotherapy followed by surgery or radiation therapy.
5. A clinical trial of surgery followed by chemotherapy.
6. A clinical trial of surgery, radiation therapy, and chemotherapy.

Floor of the Mouth Cancer

If the cancer is in the bottom (floor) of the mouth, treatment may be one of the following:

1. Surgery to remove the cancer and lymph nodes in the neck.
2. Part of the jawbone may also be removed if necessary.
3. External beam therapy with or without internal radiation therapy.
4. A clinical trial of chemotherapy followed by surgery or radiation therapy.
5. A clinical trial of fractionated (smaller doses) radiation therapy.

Lower Gum Cancer

If the cancer is in the lower gums (gingiva), treatment will probably be radiation therapy given before or after surgery to remove the cancer.

Retromolar trigone cancer

If the cancer is in the small space behind the wisdom teeth (retromolar trigone), treatment may be one of the following:

1. Surgery followed by radiation therapy.
2. A clinical trial of chemotherapy followed by surgery or radiation therapy.
3. A clinical trial of surgery followed by chemotherapy.
4. A clinical trial of fractionated (smaller doses) radiation therapy.

Upper Gum or Hard Palate Cancer

If the cancer is in the top part of the gums (gingiva) or the top bony part of the mouth (the hard palate), treatment may be one of the following:

1. Radiation therapy.
2. Surgery plus radiation therapy.

For all stage III lip and oral cavity cancers, clinical trials are testing chemotherapy combined with radiation therapy.

Stage IV Lip and Oral Cavity Cancer

Treatment depends on where the cancer is in the lip or mouth. In addition to the treatments listed below, a patient will probably have radiation therapy to the neck with or without surgery to remove lymph nodes in the neck (lymph node dissection).

Lip Cancer

If the cancer is in the lip, treatment may be one of the following:

1. Surgery to remove the cancer plus internal or external radiation therapy.
2. A clinical trial of radiation therapy.
3. A clinical trial of chemotherapy combined with radiation therapy.
4. A clinical trial of fractionated (smaller doses) radiation therapy.

Tongue Cancer

If the cancer is in the tongue, treatment may be one of the following:

1. Surgery to remove the tongue and the voicebox (larynx) below it followed by radiation therapy.
2. Radiation therapy to relieve symptoms.
3. A clinical trial of chemotherapy combined with radiation therapy.
4. A clinical trial of fractionated (smaller doses) radiation therapy.

Buccal Mucosa Cancer

If the cancer is in the lining of the inside of the cheeks and lips (buccal mucosa), treatment may be one of the following:

1. Surgery to remove the cancer and the tissue around it.
2. Radiation therapy.
3. Surgery plus radiation therapy.
4. A clinical trial of chemotherapy combined with radiation therapy.
5. A clinical trial of fractionated (smaller doses) radiation therapy.

Floor of the Mouth Cancer

If the cancer is in the bottom (floor) of the mouth, treatment may be one of the following:

1. Surgery to remove the cancer followed by radiation therapy.
2. Radiation therapy followed by surgery.
3. A clinical trial of chemotherapy combined with radiation therapy.
4. A clinical trial of fractionated (smaller doses) radiation therapy.

Lower Gum Cancer

If the cancer is in the lower gums (gingiva), treatment may be one of the following:

1. Surgery, radiation therapy, or both.
2. A clinical trial of chemotherapy combined with radiation therapy.

3. A clinical trial of fractionated (smaller doses) radiation therapy.

Retromolar Trigone Cancer

If the cancer is in the small space behind the wisdom teeth (retromolar trigone), treatment may be one of the following:

1. Surgery followed by radiation therapy.
2. A clinical trial of chemotherapy combined with radiation therapy.
3. A clinical trial of fractionated (smaller doses) radiation therapy.

Upper Gum or Hard Palate Cancer

If the cancer is in the top part of the gums (gingiva) or the top bony part of the mouth, treatment may be one of the following:

1. Surgery plus radiation therapy.
2. A clinical trial of chemotherapy combined with radiation therapy.
3. A clinical trial of fractionated (smaller doses) radiation therapy.

Recurrent Lip and Oral Cavity Cancer

Treatment depends on the type of treatment the patient had before. If radiation therapy was given, the patient may have surgery when the cancer comes back. If surgery was used, the patient may have more surgery, radiation therapy, or both.

Patients may want to consider taking part in a clinical trial of new chemotherapy drugs, chemotherapy plus additional radiation therapy, or hyperthermia.

To Learn More

Call

For more information, U.S. residents may call the National Cancer Institute's (NCI's) Cancer Information Service toll-free at (800) 4-CANCER (800-422-6237) Monday through Friday from 9:00 a.m. to 4:30 p.m. Deaf and hard-of-hearing callers with TTY equipment may call (800) 332-8615. The call is free and a trained Cancer Information Specialist is available to answer your questions.

Websites and Organizations

The NCI's Cancer.gov website provides online access to information on cancer, clinical trials, and other websites and organizations that offer support and resources for cancer patients and their families. There are also many other places where people can get materials and information about cancer treatment and services. Local hospitals may have information on local and regional agencies that offer information about finances, getting to and from treatment, receiving care at home, and dealing with problems associated with cancer treatment.

Publications

The NCI has booklets and other materials for patients, health professionals, and the public. These publications discuss types of cancer, methods of cancer treatment, coping with cancer, and clinical trials. Some publications provide information on tests for cancer, cancer causes and prevention, cancer statistics, and NCI research activities. NCI materials on these and other topics may be ordered online or printed directly from the NCI Publications Locator. These materials can also be ordered by telephone from the Cancer Information Service toll-free at (800) 4-CANCER (800-422-6237), TTY at (800) 332-8615.

LiveHelp

The NCI's LiveHelp service, a program available on several of the Institute's websites, provides Internet users with the ability to chat online with an Information Specialist. The service is available from 9:00 a.m. to 10:00 p.m. Eastern time, Monday through Friday. Information Specialists can help Internet users find information on NCI websites and answer questions about cancer.

Write

For more information from the NCI, please write to this address:

NCI Public Inquiries Office
Suite 3036A
6116 Executive Boulevard, MSC8322
Bethesda, MD 20892-8322

Chapter 52

Salivary Gland Cancer

What Is Cancer of the Salivary Gland?

Cancer of the salivary gland is a disease in which cancer (malignant) cells are found in the tissues of the salivary glands. The salivary glands make saliva, the fluid that is released into the mouth to keep it moist and to help dissolve food.

Major clusters of salivary glands are found below the tongue, on the sides of the face just in front of the ears, and under the jawbone. Smaller clusters of salivary glands are found in other parts of the upper digestive tract. The smaller glands are called the minor salivary glands.

Many growths in the salivary glands do not spread to other tissues and are not cancer. These tumors are called benign tumors and are not usually treated the same as cancer.

A doctor should be seen if there is a swelling under the chin or around the jawbone, the face becomes numb, muscles in the face cannot move, or there is pain that does not go away in the face, chin, or neck.

If there are symptoms, a doctor will examine the throat and neck using a mirror and lights. The doctor may order a special x-ray called a computed tomographic or CT scan, which uses a computer to make a picture of the inside of parts of the body.

Another type of scan, called a magnetic resonance imaging or MRI scan, uses magnetic waves to make a picture of the head and may also

PDQ® Cancer Information Summary. National Cancer Institute; Bethesda, MD. Salivary Gland Cancer (PDQ®): Treatment—Patient. Updated 08/2002. Available at: http://cancer.gov. Accessed May 2003.

be ordered. If tissue that is not normal is found, the doctor will need to cut out a small piece and look at it under the microscope to see if there are any cancer cells. This is called a biopsy.

The chance of recovery (prognosis) depends on where the cancer is in the salivary glands, whether the cancer is just in the area where it started or has spread to other tissues (the stage), how the cancer cells look under a microscope (the grade), and the patient's general state of health.

Stages of Cancer of the Salivary Gland

Once cancer of the salivary gland is found, more tests will be done to find out if cancer cells have spread to other parts of the body. This is called staging. A doctor needs to know the stage of the disease to plan treatment. Salivary gland cancers are also classified by grade, which tells how fast the cancer cells grow, based on how the cells look under a microscope. Low-grade cancers grow more slowly than high-grade cancers.

The following stages are used for cancer of the salivary gland:

Stage I

The cancer is no more than 4 centimeters in diameter (about 1 1/2 inches) and has not spread into the tissue around it or to the lymph nodes in the area (lymph nodes are small bean-shaped structures that are found throughout the body; they produce and store infection-fighting cells).

Stage II

Either of the following may be true:

- The cancer is no more than 4 centimeters in diameter and has spread into the skin, soft tissue, bone, or nerve around the gland. The cancer has not spread to lymph nodes in the area.

- The cancer is between 4 and 6 centimeters in diameter (a little over 2 inches) and has not spread into the tissue around it or to lymph nodes in the area.

Stage III

The cancer is no more than 4 centimeters in diameter and has not spread into the skin, soft tissue, bone, or nerve around the gland, but has spread to a single lymph node in the same area.

Stage IV

Any of the following may be true:

- The cancer is more than 6 centimeters in diameter and has spread into the skin, soft tissue, bone, or nerve around the gland. The cancer may or may not have spread to the lymph nodes.

- The cancer is any size and has spread to more than one lymph node on the same side of the neck as the cancer, to lymph nodes on one or both sides of the neck, or to any lymph node and measures more than 6 centimeters in diameter.

- The cancer has spread to other parts of the body.

Recurrent

Recurrent disease means that the cancer has come back (recurred) after it has been treated. It may come back in the salivary gland or in another part of the body.

How Cancer of the Salivary Gland Is Treated

There are treatments for all patients with cancer of the salivary gland. Three kinds of treatment are used:

- Surgery (taking out the cancer).
- Radiation therapy (using high-dose x-rays or other high-energy rays to kill cancer cells).
- Chemotherapy (using drugs to kill cancer cells).

Surgery is often used to remove cancers of the salivary gland. Depending on where the cancer is and how far it has spread, a doctor may need to cut out tissue around the cancer. If cancer has spread to lymph nodes in the neck, the lymph nodes may be removed (lymph node dissection).

Radiation therapy is also a common treatment of cancer of the salivary gland. Radiation therapy uses high-energy x-rays to kill cancer cells and shrink tumors. Radiation may come from a machine outside the body (external radiation therapy) or from putting materials that produce radiation (radioisotopes) through thin plastic tubes in the area where the cancer cells are found (internal radiation therapy).

A special type of radiation therapy using tiny particles called neutrons has been shown to be effective in treating some salivary gland cancers. The use of drugs with the radiation therapy to make cancer cells more sensitive to radiation (radiosensitization) is being tested in clinical trials.

Chemotherapy uses drugs to kill cancer cells. Chemotherapy may be taken by pill, or it may be put into the body by a needle in a vein or muscle. Chemotherapy is called a systemic treatment because the drug enters the bloodstream, travels through the body, and can kill cancer cells throughout the body. Chemotherapy for cancer of the salivary gland is still being tested in clinical trials.

Because the salivary glands help digest food and are close to the jaw, a patient may need special help adjusting to the side effects of the cancer and its treatment. A doctor will consult with several kinds of doctors who can help determine the best treatment. Trained medical staff can also help in recovery from treatment. Plastic surgery may be needed if a large amount of tissue or bone around the salivary glands is taken out.

Treatment by Stage

Treatment of cancer of the salivary gland depends on where the cancer is, the stage of the disease, and the patient's age and overall health.

Standard treatment may be considered because of its effectiveness in patients in past studies, or participation in a clinical trial may be considered. Not all patients are cured with standard therapy and some standard treatments may have more side effects than are desired. For these reasons, clinical trials are designed to find better ways to treat cancer patients and are based on the most up-to-date information. Clinical trials are ongoing in some parts of the country for patients with cancer of the salivary gland. To learn more about clinical trials, call the Cancer Information Service at (800) 4-CANCER (800-422-6237); TTY at (800) 332-8615.

Stage I Salivary Gland Cancer

Treatment depends on whether the cancer is low grade (slow growing) or high grade (fast growing).

If the cancer is low grade, treatment will probably be surgery.

If the cancer is high grade, treatment may be one of the following:

1. Surgery.

2. Surgery followed by radiation therapy.

3. A clinical trial of new chemotherapy drugs.

Stage II Salivary Gland Cancer

Treatment depends on whether the cancer is low grade (slow growing) or high grade (fast growing).

If the cancer is low grade, treatment may be one of the following:

1. Surgery possibly followed by radiation therapy.

2. Chemotherapy (if surgery or radiation is refused or if the cancer does not respond to surgery or radiation therapy).

If the cancer is high grade, treatment may be one of the following:

1. Surgery.

2. Surgery followed by radiation therapy.

3. Radiation therapy.

4. A clinical trial of radiosensitization drugs (drugs given with radiation to make the cancer cells more sensitive to the radiation) or new chemotherapy drugs.

Stage III Salivary Gland Cancer

Treatment depends on whether the cancer is low grade (slow growing) or high grade (fast growing).

If the cancer is low grade, treatment may be one of the following:

1. Surgery possibly followed by radiation therapy.

2. Chemotherapy (if surgery or radiation therapy are refused or if the cancer does not respond to surgery or radiation therapy).

3. A clinical trial of specialized radiation therapy or new chemotherapy drugs.

If the cancer is high grade, treatment may be one of the following:

1. Surgery.

2. Surgery followed by radiation therapy.

3. Radiation therapy.

4. A clinical trial of radiosensitization drugs (drugs given with radiation to make the cancer cells more sensitive to the radiation) given with radiation therapy or chemotherapy.

Stage IV Salivary Gland Cancer

Treatment may be one of the following:

1. Radiation therapy.

2. A clinical trial of chemotherapy with or without radiation therapy.

Recurrent Salivary Gland Cancer

Treatment depends on the type of salivary gland cancer the patient has, where the cancer came back, the treatment the patient had before, and the patient's general health.

Radiation therapy may be given, or a patient may choose to take part in a clinical trial of new treatments.

To Learn More

Call

For more information, U.S. residents may call the National Cancer Institute's (NCI's) Cancer Information Service toll-free at (800) 4-CANCER (800-422-6237) Monday through Friday from 9:00 a.m. to 4:30 p.m. Deaf and hard-of-hearing callers with TTY equipment may call (800) 332-8615. The call is free and a trained Cancer Information Specialist is available to answer your questions.

Websites and Organizations

The NCI's Cancer.gov website provides online access to information on cancer, clinical trials, and other websites and organizations that offer support and resources for cancer patients and their families. There are also many other places where people can get materials and information about cancer treatment and services. Local hospitals may have information on local and regional agencies that offer information about finances, getting to and from treatment, receiving care at home, and dealing with problems associated with cancer treatment.

Publications

The NCI has booklets and other materials for patients, health professionals, and the public. These publications discuss types of cancer, methods of cancer treatment, coping with cancer, and clinical trials. Some publications provide information on tests for cancer, cancer causes and prevention, cancer statistics, and NCI research activities. NCI materials on these and other topics may be ordered online or printed directly from the NCI Publications Locator. These materials can also be ordered by telephone from the Cancer Information Service toll-free at (800) 4-CANCER (800-422-6237), TTY at (800) 332-8615.

Live Help

The NCI's LiveHelp service, a program available on several of the Institute's Web sites, provides Internet users with the ability to chat online with an Information Specialist. The service is available from 9:00 a.m. to 10:00 p.m. Eastern time, Monday through Friday. Information Specialists can help Internet users find information on NCI websites and answer questions about cancer.

Write

For more information from the NCI, please write to this address:

NCI Public Inquiries Office
Suite 3036A
6116 Executive Boulevard, MSC8322
Bethesda, MD 20892-8322

Chapter 53

Sjögren's Syndrome

Sjögren's syndrome is an autoimmune disease—that is, a disease in which the immune system turns against the body's own cells.

In Sjögren's syndrome, the immune system targets moisture-producing glands and causes dryness in the mouth and eyes. Other parts of the body can be affected as well, resulting in a wide range of possible symptoms.

Normally, the immune system works to protect us from disease by destroying harmful invading organisms like viruses and bacteria. In the case of Sjögren's syndrome, disease-fighting cells attack the glands that produce tears and saliva (the lacrimal and salivary glands). Damage to these glands keeps them from working properly and causes dry eyes and dry mouth. In technical terms, dry eyes are called keratoconjunctivitis sicca, or KCS, and dry mouth is called xerostomia. Your doctor may use these terms when talking to you about Sjögren's syndrome.

The disease can affect other glands too, such as those in the stomach, pancreas, and intestines, and can cause dryness in other places that need moisture, such as the nose, throat, airways, and skin.

You might hear Sjögren's syndrome called a rheumatic disease. A rheumatic disease causes inflammation in joints, muscles, skin, or other body tissue, and Sjögren's can do that. The many forms of arthritis,

"Questions and Answers about Sjögren's Syndrome" is published by the National Institute of Arthritis and Musculoskeletal and Skin Diseases, January 2001. Available online at www.niams.nih.gov/hi/topics/sjogrens/index.htm; accessed May 2003.

which often involve inflammation in the joints, among other problems, are examples of rheumatic diseases. Sjögren's is also considered a disorder of connective tissue, which is the framework of the body that supports organs and tissues (joints, muscles, and skin).

Primary versus Secondary Sjögren's Syndrome

Sjögren's syndrome is classified as either primary or secondary disease. Primary Sjögren's occurs by itself, and secondary Sjögren's occurs with another disease. Both are systemic disorders, although the symptoms in primary are more restricted.

In primary Sjögren's syndrome, the doctor can trace the symptoms to problems with the tear and saliva glands. People with primary disease are more likely to have certain antibodies (substances that help fight a particular disease) circulating in their blood than people with secondary disease. These antibodies are called SS-A and SS-B. People with primary Sjögren's are more likely to have antinuclear antibodies (ANAs) in their blood. ANAs are autoantibodies, which are directed against the body.

In secondary Sjögren's syndrome, the person had an autoimmune disease like rheumatoid arthritis or lupus before Sjögren's developed. People with this type tend to have more health problems because they have two diseases, and they are also less likely to have the antibodies associated with primary Sjögren's.

What Are the Symptoms of Sjögren's Syndrome?

The main symptoms are

- Dry eyes—Your eyes may be red and burn and itch. People say it feels like they have sand in their eyes. Also, your vision may be blurry, and bright light, especially fluorescent lighting, might bother you.

- Dry mouth—Dry mouth feels like a mouth full of cotton. It's difficult to swallow, speak, and taste. Your sense of smell can change, and you may develop a dry cough. Also, because you lack the protective effects of saliva, dry mouth increases your chances of developing cavities and mouth infections.

Both primary and secondary Sjögren's syndrome can affect other parts of the body as well, including the skin, joints, lungs, kidneys, blood vessels, and nervous system, and cause symptoms such as:

- Dry skin

- Skin rashes

- Thyroid problems

- Joint and muscle pain

- Pneumonia

- Vaginal dryness

- Numbness and tingling in the extremities

When Sjögren's affects other parts of the body, the condition is called extraglandular involvement because the problems extend beyond the tear and salivary glands. These problems are described in more detail later.

Finally, Sjögren's can cause extreme fatigue that can seriously interfere with daily life.

What Causes Dryness in Sjögren's Syndrome?

In the autoimmune attack that causes Sjögren's, disease-fighting cells called lymphocytes target the glands that produce moisture—primarily the lacrimal (tear) and salivary (saliva) glands. Although no one knows exactly how damage occurs, damaged glands can no longer produce tears and saliva, and eye and mouth dryness result. When the skin, sinuses, airways, and vaginal tissues are affected, dryness occurs in those places, too.

Who Gets Sjögren's Syndrome?

Experts believe 1 to 4 million people have the disease. Most—90 percent—are women. It can occur at any age, but it usually is diagnosed after age 40 and can affect people of all races and ethnic backgrounds. It's rare in children, but it can occur.

What Causes Sjögren's Syndrome?

Researchers think Sjögren's syndrome is caused by a combination of genetic and environmental factors. Several different genes appear to be involved, but scientists are not certain exactly which ones are linked to the disease since different genes seem to play a role in different people. For example, there is one gene that predisposes Caucasians to the disease. Other genes are linked to Sjögren's in people of Japanese, Chinese, and African-American descent. Simply having one of these genes will not cause a person to develop the disease, however. Some sort of trigger must activate the immune system.

Scientists think that the trigger may be a viral or bacterial infection. It might work like this: A person who has a Sjögren's-associated gene gets a viral infection. The virus stimulates the immune system to act, but the gene alters the attack, sending fighter cells (lymphocytes) to the eye and mouth glands. Once there, the lymphocytes attack healthy cells, causing the inflammation that damages the glands and keeps them from working properly. These fighter cells are supposed to die after their attack in a natural process called apoptosis, but in people with Sjögren's syndrome, they continue to attack, causing further damage.

Scientists think that resistance to apoptosis may be genetic. The possibility that the endocrine and nervous systems play a role is also under investigation.

How Is Sjögren's Syndrome Diagnosed?

The doctor will first take a detailed medical history, which includes asking questions about general health, symptoms, family medical history, alcohol consumption, smoking, or use of drugs or medications. The doctor will also do a complete physical exam to check for other signs of Sjögren's.

You may have some tests, too. First, the doctor will want to check your eyes and mouth to see whether Sjögren's is causing your symptoms and how severe the problem is. Then, the doctor may do other tests to see whether the disease is elsewhere in the body as well.

Common eye and mouth tests include the following:

- Schirmer test—This test measures tears to see how the lacrimal gland is working. It can be done in two ways: In Schirmer I, the doctor puts thin paper strips under the lower eyelids and measures the amount of wetness on the paper after 5 minutes. People with Sjögren's usually produce less than 8 millimeters of tears. The Schirmer II test is similar, but the doctor uses a cotton swab to stimulate a tear reflex inside the nose.

- Staining with vital dyes (rose bengal or lissamine green)—The tests show how much damage dryness has done to the surface of the eye. The doctor puts a drop of a liquid containing a dye into the lower eye lid. These drops stain on the surface of the eye, highlighting any areas of injury.

- Slit lamp examination—This test shows how severe the dryness is and whether the outside of the eye is inflamed. An ophthalmologist (eye specialist) uses equipment that magnifies to carefully examine the eye.

- Mouth exam—The doctor will look in the mouth for signs of dryness and to see whether any of the major salivary glands are swollen. Signs of dryness include a dry, sticky mouth; cavities; thick saliva, or none at all; a smooth look to the tongue; redness in the mouth; dry, cracked lips; and sores at the corners of the mouth. The doctor might also try to get a sample of saliva to see how much the glands are producing and to check its quality.

- Salivary gland biopsy of the lip—This test is the best way to find out whether dry mouth is caused by Sjögren's syndrome. The doctor removes tiny minor salivary glands from the inside of the lower lip and examines them under the microscope. If the glands contain lymphocytes in a particular pattern, the test is positive for Sjögren's syndrome.

Because there are many causes of dry eyes and dry mouth, the doctor will take other possible causes into account. Generally, you are considered to have definite Sjögren's if you have dry eyes, dry mouth, and a positive lip biopsy. But the doctor may decide to do additional tests to see whether other parts of the body are affected. These tests may include:

- Routine blood tests—The doctor will take blood samples to check blood count and blood sugar level, and to see how the liver and kidneys are working.

- Immunological tests—These blood tests check for antibodies commonly found in the blood of people with Sjögren's syndrome. For example, *antithyroid antibodies* are created when antibodies migrate out of the salivary glands into the thyroid gland. Antithyroid antibodies cause thyroiditis (inflammation of the thyroid), a common problem in people with Sjögren's. *Immunoglobulins and gamma globulins* are antibodies that everyone has in their blood, but people with Sjögren's usually have too many of them. *Rheumatoid factors* (RFs) are found in the blood of people with rheumatoid arthritis, as well as in people with Sjögren's. Substances known as *cryoglobulins* may be detected; these indicate risk of lymphoma. Similarly, the presence of *antinuclear antibodies* (ANAs) can indicate an autoimmune disorder, including Sjögren's. *Sjögren's antibodies*, called SS-A (or SS-Ro) and SS-B (or SS-La), are specific antinuclear antibodies common in people with Sjögren's. However, you can have Sjögren's without having these ANAs.

- Chest x-ray—Sjögren's can cause inflammation in the lungs, so the doctor may want to take an x-ray to check them.

- Urinalysis—The doctor will probably test a sample of your urine to see how well the kidneys are working.

What Type of Doctor Diagnoses and Treats Sjögren's Syndrome?

Because the symptoms of Sjögren's are similar to those of many other diseases, getting a diagnosis can take time—in fact, the average time from first symptom to diagnosis ranges from 2 to 8 years.

During those years, depending on the symptoms, a person might see a number of doctors, any of whom may diagnose the disease and be involved in treatment. Usually, a rheumatologist (a doctor who specializes in diseases of the joints, muscles, and bones) will coordinate treatment among a number of specialists. Other doctors who may be involved include:

- Allergists
- Dentists
- Dermatologists (skin specialists)
- Gastroenterologists (digestive disease specialists)
- Gynecologists (women's reproductive health specialists)
- Neurologists (nerve and brain specialists)
- Ophthalmologists (eye specialists)
- Otolaryngologists (ear, nose, and throat specialists)
- Pulmonologists (lung specialists)
- Urologist

How Is Sjögren's Syndrome Treated?

Treatment is different for each person, depending on what parts of the body are affected. But in all cases, the doctor will help relieve your symptoms, especially dryness. For example, you can use artificial tears to help with dry eyes and saliva stimulants and mouth lubricants for dry mouth. Treatment for dryness is described in more detail below.

If you have extraglandular involvement, your doctor—or the appropriate specialist—will also treat those problems. Treatment may include nonsteroidal anti-inflammatory drugs for joint or muscle pain, saliva- and mucus-stimulating drugs for nose and throat dryness, and corticosteroids or drugs that suppress the immune system for lung, kidney, blood vessel, or nervous system problems. Hydroxychloroquine, methotrexate, and cyclophosphamide are examples of such immunosuppressants (drugs that suppress the immune system).

What Can I Do about Dry Eyes?

Artificial tears can help. They come in different thicknesses, so you may have to experiment to find the right one. Some drops contain preservatives that might irritate your eyes. Drops without preservatives don't usually bother the eyes. Nonpreserved tears typically come in single-dose packages to prevent contamination with bacteria.

At night, an eye ointment might provide more relief. Ointments are thicker than artificial tears and moisturize and protect the eye for several hours. They may blur your vision, which is why some people prefer to use them while they sleep.

Hydroxypropyl cellulose (Lacrisert®) is a chemical that lubricates the surface of the eye and slows the evaporation of natural tears. It comes in a small pellet that you put in your lower eyelid.

When you add artificial tears, the pellet dissolves and forms a film over your own tears that traps the moisture.

Another alternative is surgery to close the tear ducts that drain tears from the eye. The surgery is called punctal occlusion. For a temporary closure, the doctor inserts collagen or silicone plugs into the ducts. Collagen plugs eventually dissolve, and silicone plugs are permanent until they are removed or fall out. For a longer lasting effect, the doctor can use a laser or cautery to seal the ducts.

General Tips for Eye Care

- Don't use artificial tears that irritate your eyes—try another brand or preparation.

- Nonpreserved drops may be more comfortable.

- Blink several times a minute while reading or working on the computer.

- Protect your eyes from drafts, breezes, and wind.

- Put a humidifier in the rooms where you spend the most time, including the bedroom, or install a humidifier in your heating and air conditioning unit.

- Don't smoke and stay out of smoky rooms.

- Apply mascara only to the tips of your lashes so it doesn't get in your eyes. If you use eyeliner or eye shadow, put it only on the skin above your lashes, not on the sensitive skin under your lashes, close to your eyes.

- Ask your doctor whether any of your medications contribute to dryness and, if so, how to reduce that effect.

What Can I Do about Dry Mouth?

If your salivary glands still produce some saliva, you can stimulate them to make more by chewing gum or sucking on hard candy. However, gum and candy must be sugar free because dry mouth makes you extremely prone to cavities. Take sips of water or another sugar-free drink often throughout the day to wet your mouth, especially when you are eating or talking. Note that you should take sips of water—drinking large amounts of liquid throughout the day will not make your mouth any less dry. It will only make you urinate more often and may strip your mouth of mucus, causing even more dryness. You can soothe dry, cracked lips by using oil- or petroleum-based lip balm or lipstick. If your mouth hurts, the doctor may give you medicine in a mouth rinse, ointment, or gel to apply to the sore areas to control pain and inflammation.

If you produce very little saliva or none at all, your doctor might recommend a saliva substitute. These products mimic some of the properties of saliva, which means they make the mouth feel wet, and if they contain fluoride, they can help prevent cavities. Gel-based saliva substitutes tend to give the longest relief, but all saliva products are limited since you eventually swallow them.

At least two drugs that stimulate the salivary glands to produce saliva are available. These are pilocarpine and cevimeline. The effects last for a few hours, and you can take them three or four times a day. However, they are not suitable for everyone, so talk to your doctor about whether they might help you.

People with dry mouth can easily get mouth infections. Candidiasis, a fungal mouth infection, is one of the most commonly seen in people with Sjögren's. It most often shows up as white patches inside the mouth that you can scrape off, or as red, burning areas in the mouth. Candidiasis is treated with antifungal drugs. Various viruses and bacteria can also cause infections; they're treated with the appropriate antiviral or antibiotic medicines.

The Importance of Oral Hygiene

Natural saliva contains substances that rid the mouth of the bacteria that cause cavities and mouth infections, so good oral hygiene is extremely important when you have dry mouth. Here's what you can do to prevent cavities and infections:

- Visit a dentist at least three times a year to have your teeth examined and cleaned.

- Rinse your mouth with water several times a day. Don't use mouthwash that contains alcohol because alcohol is drying.

- Use fluoride toothpaste to gently brush your teeth, gums, and tongue after each meal and before bedtime. Nonfoaming toothpaste is less drying.

- Floss your teeth every day.

- Avoid sugar. That means choosing sugar-free gum, candy, and soda. If you do eat or drink sugary foods, brush your teeth immediately afterward.

- Look at your mouth every day to check for redness or sores. See a dentist right away if you notice anything unusual or have any mouth pain or bleeding.

- Ask your dentist whether you need to take fluoride supplements, use a fluoride gel at night, or have a protective varnish put on your teeth to protect the enamel.

What Other Parts of the Body Are Involved in Sjögren's Syndrome?

The autoimmune response that causes dry eyes and mouth can cause inflammation throughout the body. People with Sjögren's often have skin, lung, kidney, and nerve problems, as well as disorders of the digestive system and connective tissue. Following are examples of extraglandular problems.

Skin Problems

About half of the people who have Sjögren's have dry skin. Some experience only itching, but it can be severe. Others develop cracked, split skin that can easily become infected. Infection is a risk for people with itchy skin, too, particularly if they scratch vigorously. The skin may darken in infected areas, but it returns to normal when the infection clears up and the scratching stops.

To treat dry skin, apply heavy moisturizing creams and ointments three or four times a day to trap moisture in the skin. Lotions, which are lighter than creams and ointments, aren't recommended because they evaporate quickly and can contribute to dry skin. Also, doctors suggest that you take only a short shower (less than 5 minutes), use a moisturizing soap, pat your skin almost dry, and then cover it with a cream or ointment. If you take baths, it's a good idea to soak for 10 to 15 minutes to give your skin time to absorb moisture. Having a humidifier in the bedroom can help hydrate your skin, too. If these steps don't help the itching, your doctor might recommend that you use a skin cream or ointment containing steroids.

Some patients who have Sjögren's, particularly those who have lupus, are sensitive to sunlight and can get painful burns from even a little sun exposure, such as through a window. So, if you're sensitive to sunlight, you need to wear sunscreen (at least SPF 15) whenever you go outdoors and try to avoid being in the sun for long periods of time.

Vaginal Dryness

Vaginal dryness is common in women with Sjögren's syndrome. Painful intercourse is the most common complaint. A vaginal moisturizer helps retain moisture, and a vaginal lubricant can make intercourse more comfortable. Vaginal moisturizers attract liquid to the dry tissues and are designed for regular use. Vaginal lubricants should be used only for intercourse—they don't moisturize. Oil-based lubricants, such as petroleum jelly, trap moisture and can cause sores and hinder the vagina's natural cleaning process. A water-soluble lubricant is better.

Regular skin creams and ointments relieve dry skin on the outer surface of the vagina (the vulva).

Lung Problems

Dry mouth can cause lung problems. For example, aspiration pneumonia can happen when a person breathes in food instead of swallowing it (dry mouth can keep you from swallowing food properly), and the food gets stuck in the lungs. Pneumonia can also develop when bacteria in the mouth migrate into the lungs and cause infection, or when bacteria get into the lungs and coughing doesn't remove them. (Some people with Sjögren's don't produce enough mucus in the lungs to remove bacteria, and others are too weak to be able to cough.) Pneumonia is treated with various antibiotics, depending on the person and the type of infection. It is important to get treatment for pneumonia to prevent lung abscess (a hole in the lung caused by severe infection).

People with Sjögren's also tend to have lung problems caused by inflammation, such as bronchitis (affecting the bronchial tubes), tracheobronchitis (affecting the windpipe and bronchial tubes), and laryngotracheobronchitis (affecting the voice box, windpipe, and bronchial tubes). Depending on your condition, the doctor may recommend using a humidifier, taking medicines to open the bronchial tubes, or taking corticosteroids to relieve inflammation. Pleurisy is inflammation of the lining of the lungs and is treated with corticosteroids and nonsteroidal anti-inflammatory drugs.

Kidney Problems

The kidneys filter waste products from the blood and remove them from the body through urine. The most common kidney problem in people with Sjögren's is interstitial nephritis, or inflammation of the tissue around the kidney's filters, which can occur even before dry eyes and dry mouth. Inflammation of the filters themselves, called glomerulonephritis, is less common. Some people develop renal tubular acidosis, which means they can't get rid of certain acids through urine. The amount of potassium in their blood drops, causing an imbalance in blood chemicals that can affect the heart, muscles, and nerves.

Often, doctors do not treat these problems unless they start to affect kidney function or cause other health problems. However, they keep a close eye on the problem through regular exams, and will prescribe medicines called alkaline agents to balance blood chemicals when necessary. Corticosteroids or immunosuppressants are used to treat more severe cases.

Nerve Problems

People with Sjögren's syndrome can have nerve problems. When they do, the problem usually involves the peripheral nervous system (PNS), which contains the nerves that control sensation and movement. Involvement of the PNS is increasingly being recognized. Carpal tunnel syndrome, peripheral neuropathy, and cranial neuropathy are examples of peripheral nervous system disorders that occur in people with Sjögren's. In carpal tunnel syndrome, inflamed tissue in the forearm presses against the median nerve, causing pain, numbness, tingling, and sometimes muscle weakness in the thumb and index and middle fingers. In peripheral neuropathy, an immune attack damages nerves in the legs or arms, causing the same symptoms there. (Sometimes nerves are damaged because inflamed blood vessels cut off their blood supply.) In cranial neuropathy, nerve damage causes face pain; loss of feeling in the face, tongue, eyes, ears, or throat; and loss of taste and smell.

Nerve problems are treated with medicines to control pain and, if necessary, with steroids or other drugs to control inflammation.

Digestive Problems

Inflammation in the esophagus, stomach, pancreas, and liver can cause problems like painful swallowing, heartburn, abdominal pain and swelling, loss of appetite, diarrhea, and weight loss. It can also cause hepatitis (inflammation of the liver) and cirrhosis (hardening of the liver). Sjögren's is closely linked to a liver disease called primary biliary cirrhosis (PBC), which causes itching, fatigue, and, eventually, cirrhosis. Many patients with PBC have Sjögren's.

Treatment varies, depending on the problem, but may include pain medicine, anti-inflammatory drugs, steroids, and immunosuppressants.

Connective Tissue Disorders

Connective tissue is the framework of the body that supports organs and tissues. Examples are joints, muscles, bones, skin, blood vessel walls, and the lining of internal organs. Many connective tissue disorders are autoimmune diseases, and several are common among people with Sjögren's.

Polymyositis is an inflammation of the muscles that causes weakness and pain, difficulty moving, and, in some cases, problems breathing and swallowing. If the skin is inflamed too, it's called dermatomyositis. The disease is treated with corticosteroids and immunosuppressants.

In Raynaud's phenomenon, blood vessels in the hands, arms, feet, and legs constrict (narrow) when exposed to cold. The result is pain, tingling, and numbness. When vessels constrict, fingers turn white. Shortly after that, they turn blue because of blood that remained in the tissue pools. When new blood rushes in, the fingers turn red. The problem is treated with medicines that dilate blood vessels. Raynaud's phenomenon usually occurs before dryness of the eyes or mouth.

Rheumatoid arthritis (RA) is severe inflammation of the joints that can eventually deform the surrounding bones (fingers, hands, knees, etc.). RA can also damage muscles, blood vessels, and major organs. Treatment depends on the severity of the pain and swelling and which body parts are involved. It may include physical therapy, aspirin, rest, nonsteroidal anti-inflammatory agents, steroids, or immunosuppressants.

Scleroderma causes the body to accumulate too much collagen, a protein commonly found in the skin. The result is thick, tight skin and damage to muscles, joints, and internal organs such as the esophagus, intestines, lungs, heart, kidneys, and blood vessels. Treatment is aimed at relieving pain and includes drugs, skin softeners, and physical therapy.

Systemic lupus erythematosus (SLE) causes joint and muscle pain, weakness, skin rashes, and, in more severe cases, heart, lung, kidney, and nervous system problems. As with RA, treatment for SLE depends on the symptoms and may include aspirin, rest, steroids, and anti-inflammatory and other drugs, as well as dialysis and high blood pressure medicine.

Vasculitis is an inflammation of the blood vessels, which then become scarred and too narrow for blood to get through to reach the organs. In people with Sjögren's, vasculitis tends to occur in those who also have Raynaud's phenomenon and lung and liver problems.

Autoimmune thyroid disorders are common with Sjögren's. They can appear as either the overactive thyroid of Graves' disease or the underactive thyroid of Hashimoto's. Nearly half of the people with autoimmune thyroid disorder also have Sjögren's, and many people with Sjögren's show evidence of thyroid disease.

Does Sjögren's Syndrome Cause Lymphoma?

About 5 percent of people with Sjögren's develop cancer of the lymph nodes, or lymphoma. The most common symptom of lymphoma is a painless swelling of the lymph nodes in the neck, underarm, or groin. In Sjögren's syndrome, when lymphoma develops it often involves the salivary glands. Persistent enlargement of the salivary glands should be investigated further. Other symptoms may include the following:

- Unexplained fever

481

- Night sweats
- Constant fatigue
- Unexplained weight loss
- Itchy skin
- Reddened patches on the skin

These symptoms are not sure signs of lymphoma. They may be caused by other, less serious conditions, such as the flu or an infection. If you have these symptoms, see a doctor so that any illness can be diagnosed and treated as early as possible.

If you're worried that you might develop lymphoma, talk to your doctor to learn more about the disease, symptoms to watch for, any special medical care you might need, and what you can do to relieve your worry.

Medicines and Dryness

Certain drugs can contribute to eye and mouth dryness. If you take any of the drugs listed below, ask your doctor whether they could be causing symptoms. However, don't stop taking them without asking your doctor—he or she may already have adjusted the dose to help protect you against drying side effects or chosen a drug that's least likely to cause dryness.

Drugs that can cause dryness include:

- Antihistamines
- Decongestants
- Diuretics
- Some antidiarrhea drugs
- Some antipsychotic drugs
- Tranquilizers
- Some blood pressure medicines
- Antidepressants

What Research Is Being Done on Sjögren's Syndrome?

Through basic research on the immune system, autoimmunity, genetics, and connective tissue diseases, researchers continue to learn more about Sjögren's syndrome. As they get a better understanding of the genes involved and which environmental factors trigger disease and how, they'll be able to develop more effective treatments. For example, gene therapy studies suggest that we may someday be able to insert molecules into salivary glands that will control inflammation and prevent their destruction. Other research focuses on how the immune and hormonal systems work in people who have Sjögren's and on the natural history of the disease (learning how it affects people by following those who have it).

Researchers are also looking into the use of the salivary stimulant pilocarpine for dry eyes. Other researchers are testing immune modulating drugs to treat the glandular inflammation. A drug called cevimeline has recently been approved for treating dry mouth. Work on developing an artificial salivary gland is in progress.

The National Institute of Dental and Craniofacial Research is conducting several studies on Sjögren's syndrome designed to help scientists better understand, manage, and treat the disease. Some focus on the disease's natural history, while others test potential new treatments. Talk to your doctor if you'd like more information about these clinical trials.

Note: Brand names included in this booklet are provided as examples only, and their inclusion does not mean that these products are endorsed by the National Institutes of Health or any other government agency. Also, if a particular brand name is not mentioned, this does not mean or imply that the product is unsatisfactory.

Chapter 54

Dry Mouth

What Do I Need to Know about Dry Mouth?

Everyone has a dry mouth once in a while—if they are nervous, upset, or under stress.

But if you have a dry mouth all or most of the time, it can be uncomfortable and can lead to serious health problems.

Dry mouth:

- can cause difficulties in tasting, chewing, swallowing, and speaking

- can increase your chance of developing dental decay and other infections in the mouth

- can be a sign of certain diseases and conditions

- can be caused by certain medications or medical treatments

Dry mouth is not a normal part of aging. So if you think you have dry mouth, see your dentist or physician—there are things you can do to get relief.

National Institute of Dental and Craniofacial Research (NIDCR)/National Oral Health Information Clearinghouse, NIH Publication Number 99-3174, December 1999. Available online at www.nohic.nidcr.nih.gov/pubs/drymouth/dmouth.htm; accessed May 2003.

What Is Dry Mouth?

Dry mouth is the condition of not having enough saliva, or spit, to keep your mouth wet.

Symptoms include:

- a sticky, dry feeling in the mouth
- trouble chewing, swallowing, tasting, or speaking
- a burning feeling in the mouth
- a dry feeling in the throat
- cracked lips
- a dry, tough tongue
- mouth sores
- an infection in the mouth

Why Is Saliva So Important?

Saliva does more than keep the mouth wet.

- It helps digest food
- It protects teeth from decay
- It prevents infection by controlling bacteria and fungi in the mouth
- It makes it possible for you to chew and swallow

Without enough saliva you can develop tooth decay or other infections in the mouth. You also might not get the nutrients you need if you cannot chew and swallow certain foods.

What Causes Dry Mouth?

People get dry mouth when the glands in the mouth that make saliva are not working properly. Because of this, there might not be enough saliva to keep your mouth wet. There are several reasons why these glands (called salivary glands) might not work right.

- Side effects of some medicines. More than 400 medicines can cause the salivary glands to make less saliva. Medicines for high blood pressure and depression often cause dry mouth.

- Disease. Some diseases affect the salivary glands. Sjögren's Syndrome, HIV/AIDS, diabetes, and Parkinson's disease can all cause dry mouth.

- Radiation therapy. The salivary glands can be damaged if they are exposed to radiation during cancer treatment.

- Chemotherapy. Drugs used to treat cancer can make saliva thicker, causing the mouth to feel dry.

- Nerve damage. Injury to the head or neck can damage the nerves that tell salivary glands to make saliva.

What Can Be Done about Dry Mouth?

Dry mouth treatment will depend on what is causing the problem. If you think you have dry mouth, see your dentist or physician. He or she can try to determine what is causing your dry mouth.

- If your dry mouth is caused by medicine, your physician might change your medicine or adjust the dosage.

- If your salivary glands are not working right but can still produce some saliva, your physician or dentist might give you a medicine that helps the glands work better.

- Your physician or dentist might suggest that you use artificial saliva to keep your mouth wet.

What Can I Do?

- Sip water or sugarless drinks often.

- Avoid drinks with caffeine, such as coffee, tea, and some sodas. Caffeine can dry out the mouth.

- Sip water or a sugarless drink during meals. This will make chewing and swallowing easier. It may also improve the taste of food.

- Chew sugarless gum or suck on sugarless hard candy to stimulate saliva flow; citrus, cinnamon, or mint-flavored candies are good choices.

- Don't use tobacco or alcohol. They dry out the mouth.

- Be aware that spicy or salty foods may cause pain in a dry mouth.

- Use a humidifier at night.

Tips for Keeping Your Teeth Healthy

Remember, if you have dry mouth, you need to be extra careful to keep your teeth healthy. Make sure you:

- Gently brush your teeth at least twice a day.

- Floss your teeth every day.

- Use toothpaste with fluoride in it. Most toothpastes sold at grocery and drugstores have fluoride in them.

- Avoid sticky, sugary foods. If you do eat them, brush immediately afterward.

- Visit your dentist for a checkup at least twice a year. Your dentist might give you a special fluoride solution that you can rinse with to help keep your teeth healthy.

Chapter 55

Candidiasis (Thrush)

What Is OPC?

Candidiasis of the mouth and throat, also known as a thrush or oropharyngeal candidiasis (OPC), is a fungal infection that occurs when there is overgrowth of fungus called *Candida. Candida* is normally found on skin or mucous membranes. However, if the environment inside the mouth or throat becomes imbalanced, *Candida* can multiply. When this happens, symptoms of thrush appear.

How Common Is OPC and Who Can Get It?

OPC can affect normal newborns, but it occurs more frequently and more severely in people with weakened immune systems, particularly in persons with AIDS.

What Are the Symptoms of OPC?

People with OPC infection usually have painless, white patches in the mouth. Symptoms of OPC in the esophagus may include pain and difficulty swallowing.

"Oropharyngeal Candidiasis" is published by the Centers for Disease Control and Prevention (CDC), April 2000. Available online at www.cdc.gov/ncidod/dbmd/diseaseinfo/candidiasis_opc_g.htm; accessed May 2003.

How Do I Get OPC?

Most cases of OPC are caused by the person's own *Candida* organisms which normally live in the mouth or digestive tract. A person has symptoms when overgrowth of *Candida* organisms occurs.

How Is OPC Diagnosed?

OPC is diagnosed in two ways. A doctor may take a swab or sample of infected tissue and look at it under a microscope. If there is evidence of *Candida* infection, the sample will be cultured to confirm the diagnosis.

How Is OPC Treated?

Prescription treatments such as oral fluconazole, clotrimazole troches, or nystatin suspension usually provide effective treatment for OPC.

What Will Happen If a Person Does Not Seek Treatment for OPC?

Symptoms, which may be uncomfortable, may persist. In rare cases, invasive candidiasis may occur.

Can Candida-Causing OPC Become Resistant to Treatment?

Overuse of antifungal medications can increase the chance that they will eventually not work (the fungus develops resistance to medications). Therefore, it is important to be sure of the diagnosis from before treating with over-the-counter or other antifungal medications.

Chapter 56

Fever Blisters and Canker Sores

Fever blisters and canker sores are two of the most common disorders of the mouth, causing discomfort and annoyance to millions of Americans. Both cause small sores to develop in or around the mouth, and often are confused with each other. Canker sores, however, occur only inside the mouth—on the tongue and the inside linings of the cheeks, lips, and throat. Fever blisters, also called cold sores, usually occur outside the mouth—on the lips, chin, cheeks, or in the nostrils. When fever blisters do occur inside the mouth, it is usually on the gums or the roof of the mouth. Inside the mouth, fever blisters are smaller than canker sores, heal more quickly, and often begin as a blister.

Both canker sores and fever blisters have plagued mankind for thousands of years. Scientists at the National Institute of Dental and Craniofacial Research, one of the federal government's National Institutes of Health, are seeking ways to better control and ultimately prevent these and other oral disorders.

Fever Blisters

In ancient Rome, an epidemic of fever blisters prompted Emperor Tiberius to ban kissing in public ceremonies. Today fever blisters still occur in epidemic proportions. About 100 million episodes of recurrent

National Institute of Dental and Craniofacial Research (NIDCR), NIH Publication Number 92-247. Available online at www.pueblo.gsa.gov/cic_text/ health/fever-blister/fever-canker.html; accessed May 2003. Revised July 1992; reviewed and revised by David A. Cooke, M.D., on March 4, 2003.

491

fever blisters occur yearly in the United States alone. An estimated 45 to 80 percent of adults and children in this country have had at least one bout with the blisters.

What Causes Fever Blisters?

Fever blisters are caused by a contagious virus called herpes simplex. There are two types of herpes simplex virus. Type 1 usually causes oral herpes, or fever blisters. Type 2 usually causes genital herpes. Although both type 1 and type 2 viruses can infect oral tissues, more than 95 percent of recurrent fever blister outbreaks are caused by the type 1 virus.

Herpes simplex virus is highly contagious when fever blisters are present, and the virus frequently is spread by kissing. Children often become infected by contact with parents, siblings, or other close relatives who have fever blisters.

A child can spread the virus by rubbing his or her cold sore and then touching other children. About 10 percent of oral herpes infections in adults result from oral-genital sex with a person who has active genital herpes (type 2). These infections, however, usually do not result in repeat bouts of fever blisters.

Most people infected with the type 1 herpes simplex virus became infected before they were 10 years old. The virus usually invades the moist membrane cells of the lips, throat, or mouth. In most people, the initial infection causes no symptoms. About 15 percent of patients, however, develop many fluid-filled blisters inside and outside the mouth 3 to 5 days after they are infected with the virus. These may be accompanied by fever, swollen neck glands, and general aches. The blisters tend to merge and then collapse. Often a yellowish crest forms over the sores, which usually heal without scarring within 2 weeks.

The herpes virus, however, stays in the body. Once a person is infected with oral herpes, the virus remains in a nerve located near the cheekbone. It may stay permanently inactive in this site, or it may occasionally travel down the nerve to the skin surface, causing a recurrence of fever blisters. Recurring blisters usually erupt at the outside edge of the lip or the edge of the nostril, but can also occur on the chin, cheeks, or inside the mouth.

The symptoms of recurrent fever blister attacks usually are less severe than those experienced by some people after an initial infection. Recurrences appear to be less frequent after age 35. Many people who have recurring fever blisters feel itching, tingling, or burning in the lip 1 to 3 days before the blister appears.

What Causes a Recurrence of Fever Blisters?

Several factors weaken the body's defenses and trigger an outbreak of herpes. These include emotional stress, fever, illness, injury, and exposure to sunlight. Many women have recurrences only during menstruation. One study indicates that susceptibility to herpes recurrences is inherited. Research is under way to discover exactly how the triggering factors interact with the immune system and the virus to prompt a recurrence of fever blisters.

What Are the Treatments for Fever Blisters?

Currently there is no cure for fever blisters. Some medications can relieve some of the pain and discomfort associated with the sores, however. These include ointments that numb the blisters, antibiotics that control secondary bacterial infections, and ointments that soften the crusts of the sores.

Most cases of fever blisters heal well, without any need for treatment. However, certain people have very severe or frequent recurrences. In these cases, several antiviral medications are available to help. They may be used in one of two ways: as needed when an outbreak occurs, or on a daily basis for prophylaxis. When used as needed, they will shorten an outbreak and reduce the time until healing occurs. When used daily, they will reduce the number of outbreaks that occur per year. Unfortunately, neither form of use eliminates the virus from the body. They are treatments, but not cures.

Three medications have been approved in cream form for topical use on the blisters. These medications are penciclovir (Denavir™), acyclovir (Zovirax™), and docosanol (Abreva™). Abreva is available over the counter; the other medications are prescription drugs.

Three medications have also been approved in oral form for treating fever blister outbreaks. Usually, these are used for more severe and widespread outbreaks. The three medications are acyclovir (Zovirax™ and generic brands), valacyclovir (Valtrex™), and famciclovir (Famvir™). All three are available only by prescription. Dosing regimens and costs vary from drug to drug, but they all appear to be about equally effective.

Is There a Vaccine for Fever Blisters?

Currently there is no vaccine for herpes simplex virus available to the public. Many research laboratories, however, are working on this approach to preventing fever blisters. For example, scientists at the National Institute of Dental and Craniofacial Research and the

National Institute of Allergy and Infectious Diseases have developed a promising experimental herpes vaccine. In tests on laboratory mice, the vaccine has prevented the herpes simplex virus from infecting the animals and establishing itself in the nerves.

Although these findings are encouraging, the scientists must complete more animal studies on the safety and effectiveness of the vaccine before a decision can be made whether to test it in humans. The vaccine would be useful only for those not already infected with herpes simplex virus.

What Can the Patient Do?

If fever blisters erupt, keep them clean and dry to prevent bacterial infections. Eat a soft, bland diet to avoid irritating the sores and surrounding sensitive areas. Be careful not to touch the sores and spread the virus to new sites, such as the eyes or genitals. To make sure you do not infect others, avoid kissing them or touching the sores and then touching another person.

There is good news for people whose fever blister outbreaks are triggered by sunlight. Scientists at the National Institute of Dental and Craniofacial Research have confirmed that sunscreen on the lips can prevent sun-induced recurrences of herpes. They recommend applying the sunscreen before going outside and reapplying it frequently during sun exposure. The researchers used a sunblock with a protection factor of 15 in their studies.

Little is known about how to prevent recurrences of fever blisters triggered by factors other than sunlight. People whose cold sores appear in response to stress should try to avoid stressful situations. Some investigators have suggested adding lysine to the diet or eliminating foods such as nuts, chocolate, seeds, or gelatin. These measures have not, however, been proven effective in controlled studies.

What Research Is Being Done?

Researchers are working on several approaches to preventing or treating fever blisters. As mentioned earlier, they are trying to develop a vaccine against herpes simplex virus.

Basic research on how the immune system interacts with herpes simplex viruses may lead to new therapies for fever blisters. The immune system uses a wide array of cells and chemicals to defend the body against infections. Scientists are trying to identify the immune components that prevent recurrent attacks of oral herpes.

Scientists are also trying to determine the precise form and location of the inactive herpes virus in nerve cells. This information might allow them to design antiviral drugs that can attack the herpes virus while it lies dormant in nerves.

In addition, researchers are trying to understand how sunlight, skin injury, and stress can trigger recurrences of fever blisters. They hope to develop methods for blocking reactivation of the virus.

Canker Sores

Recurrent canker sores afflict about 20 percent of the general population. The medical term for the sores is aphthous stomatitis.

Canker sores are usually found on the movable parts of the mouth such as the tongue or the inside linings of the lips and cheeks. They begin as small oval or round reddish swellings, which usually burst within a day. The ruptured sores are covered by a thin white or yellow membrane and edged by a red halo. Generally, they heal within 2 weeks. Canker sores range in size from an eighth of an inch wide in mild cases to more than an inch wide in severe cases. Severe canker sores may leave scars. Fever is rare, and the sores are rarely associated with other diseases. Usually a person will have only one or a few canker sores at a time.

Most people have their first bout with canker sores between the ages of 10 and 20. Children as young as 2, however, may develop the condition. The frequency of canker sore recurrences varies considerably. Some people have only one or two episodes a year, while others may have a continuous series of canker sores.

What Causes Canker Sores?

The cause of canker sores is not well understood. More than one cause is likely, even for individual patients. Canker sores do not appear to be caused by viruses or bacteria, although an allergy to a type of bacterium commonly found in the mouth may trigger them in some people. The sores may be an allergic reaction to certain foods. In addition, there is research suggesting that canker sores may be caused by a faulty immune system that uses the body's defenses against disease to attack and destroy the normal cells of the mouth or tongue.

British studies show that, in about 20 percent of patients, canker sores are due partly to nutritional deficiencies, especially lack of vitamin B12, folic acid, and iron. Similar studies performed in the United States, however, have not confirmed this finding. In a small percentage of patients, canker sores occur with gastrointestinal problems, such as an inability to digest certain cereals. In these patients, canker sores appear to be part of a generalized disorder of the digestive tract. Patients with Crohn's disease, an uncommon autoimmune disorder of the gastrointestinal tract, often have canker sores as one of the symptoms of this disorder.

Female sex hormones apparently play a role in causing canker sores. Many women have bouts of the sores only during certain phases of their menstrual cycles. Most women experience improvement or remission of their canker sores during pregnancy. Researchers have used hormone therapy successfully in clinical studies to treat some women.

Both emotional stress and injury to the mouth can trigger outbreaks of canker sores, but these factors probably do not cause the disorder.

Who Is Susceptible?

Women are more likely than men to have recurrent canker sores. Genetic studies show that susceptibility to recurrent outbreaks of the sores is inherited in some patients. This partially explains why the disorder is often shared by family members.

What Are the Treatments for Canker Sores?

Most doctors recommend that patients who have frequent bouts of canker sores undergo blood and allergy tests to determine if their sores are caused by a nutritional deficiency, an allergy, or some other preventable cause. Vitamins and other nutritional supplements often prevent recurrences or reduce the severity of canker sores in patients with a nutritional deficiency. Patients with food allergies can reduce the frequency of canker sores by avoiding those foods.

There are several treatments for reducing the pain and duration of canker sores for patients whose outbreaks cannot be prevented. These include numbing ointments such as benzocaine, which are available in drugstores without a prescription. Anti-inflammatory steroid mouth rinses or gels can be prescribed for patients with severe sores.

Mouth rinses containing the antibiotic tetracycline may reduce the unpleasant symptoms of canker sores and speed healing by preventing bacterial infections in the sores. Clinical studies at the National Institute of Dental and Craniofacial Research have shown that rinsing the mouth with tetracycline several times a day usually relieves pain in 24 hours and allows complete healing in 5 to 7 days. The U.S. Food and Drug Administration warns, however, that tetracycline given to pregnant women and young children can permanently stain youngsters' teeth. Both steroid and tetracycline treatments require a prescription and care of a dentist or physician.

Patients with severe recurrent canker sores may need to take steroid or other immunosuppressant drugs orally. These potent drugs can cause many undesirable side effects, and should be used only under the close supervision of a dentist or physician.

What Can the Patient Do?

If you have canker sores, avoid abrasive foods such as potato chips that can stick in the cheek or gum and aggravate the sores. Take care when brushing your teeth not to stab the gums or cheek with a toothbrush bristle. Avoid acidic and spicy foods. Canker sores are not contagious, so patients do not have a worry about spreading them to other people.

What Research Is Being Done?

Researchers are trying to identify the malfunctions in patients' immune systems that make them susceptible to recurrent bouts of canker sores. By analyzing the blood of people with and without canker sores, scientists have found several differences in immune function between the two groups. Whether these differences cause canker sores is not yet known.

Researchers also are developing and testing new drugs designed to treat canker sores. Most of these drugs alter the patients' immune function. Although some of the drugs appear to be effective in treating canker sores in some patients, the data are still inconclusive. Until these drugs are proven to be absolutely safe and effective, they will not be available for general use.

Chapter 57

Halitosis (Bad Breath)

Do you ever worry that you're the only one in the room with bad breath? Well, guess again. Nearly 40,000,000 Americans commonly suffer from bad breath, also known as oral malodor or halitosis. Yet, it is a curable condition that is generally caused by strong foods such as onions or garlic; poor oral health habits; or medical problems such as stomach disorders, an excessive postnasal drip, or bacteria in the mouth. Once you discover the source of the problem, there are a number of ways to keep your mouth free of unpleasant odors.

Oral malodor can be divided into two distinctive categories—transitory and chronic. Transitory refers to food-related malodor that can last as long as 72 hours. Virtually everyone suffers from this condition at one time or another. The second category, chronic, is generally related to oral or general medical problems.

There are three basic sources of bad breath. The first is simple: an unclean mouth. Routine cleaning of teeth and gums will help prevent the build up of plaque—a soft, sticky, almost invisible film made up of harmful bacteria—and in turn help prevent bad breath. Carefully brushing at least two to three times a day, flossing daily, and rinsing your mouth vigorously to remove any loose foods is essential. However, research has found that simply keeping teeth clean is not enough to eliminate oral malodor.

Tongue deplaquing with tongue scrapers—tools exclusively designed for use on the tongue—is as essential for fresh breath as regular brushing. Tongue scrapers provide even pressure that forces bacteria, food debris, and dead cells from the pits and crevices in the tongue that a toothbrush cannot remove.

Second, medical problems can keep breath from smelling fresh. Research studies have found that bad breath has been linked to conditions such as diabetes, stomach disorders, or sinus infections with excessive postnasal drip. Common drugs and medications also can affect breath odor.

Third, lifestyle habits play a major role in the prevention of halitosis. For example, smoking and chewing tobacco can affect breath odor.

Caught without a toothbrush? If you're worried about your breath when your toothbrush isn't available, don't rely on sugar-coated candies or alcohol-laden mouth rinse that can cause more harm than good. Use products that are sugarless and alcohol-free and contain antibacterial agents noted for their effectiveness at controlling oral malodor. Substances such as chlorine dioxide, zinc chloride and essential oils like eucalyptol, menthol, methyl salicylate, and thymol have been shown to fight oral malodor. Other tips for keeping breath fresh include:

- Rinsing your mouth with water after eating if you aren't able to brush

- Chewing a piece of sugarless gum to stimulate saliva flow—nature's own cleanser

- Snacking on celery, carrots, or apples; they tend to clear away loose food and debris during the chewing process

- Eating a balanced diet. A vitamin deficiency may contribute to gum disease and bad breath

Just as important to oral health and fresh breath as consistent home care and healthy lifestyle habits is oral health care delivered by a qualified oral health care professional. Regular oral health care appointments, which include a complete prophylaxis—teeth cleaning above and below the gum line—are essential to maintaining good oral health and fresh breath, so visit your dental hygienist every six months, or as often as she or he recommends.

In addition to helping patients understand the connection between oral health care and overall health, dental hygienists educate patients about proper oral hygiene and treat periodontal disease to prevent the condition from advancing and complicating other diseases.

Chapter 58

Taste and Smell Disorders

Chapter Contents

Section 58.1

Taste Disorders

National Institute on Deafness and Other Communication Disorders, NIH Publication Number 01-3231A, March 2002. Available online at www.nidcd.nih.gov/health/smelltaste/taste.asp; accessed May 2003.

If you experience a taste problem, it is important to remember that you are not alone. More than 200,000 people visit a physician for such a chemosensory problem each year. Many more taste disorders go unreported.

Many people who have taste disorders also notice problems with their sense of smell. If you would like more information about your sense of smell, the chapter Smell and Smell Disorders may answer some of your questions.

How Does Our Sense of Taste Work?

Taste belongs to our chemical sensing system, or the chemosenses. The complex process of tasting begins when tiny molecules released by the substances around us stimulate special cells in the nose, mouth, or throat. These special sensory cells transmit messages through nerves to the brain, where specific tastes are identified.

Gustatory or taste cells react to food and beverages. These surface cells in the mouth send taste information to their nerve fibers. The taste cells are clustered in the taste buds of the mouth, tongue, and throat. Many of the small bumps that can be seen on the tongue contain taste buds.

Another chemosensory mechanism, called the common chemical sense, contributes to appreciation of food flavor. In this system, thousands of nerve endings—especially on the moist surfaces of the eyes, nose, mouth, and throat—give rise to sensations like the sting of ammonia, the coolness of menthol, and the irritation of chili peppers.

We can commonly identify at least five different taste sensations: sweet, sour, bitter, salty, and umami (the taste elicited by glutamate, which is found in chicken broth, meat extracts, and some cheeses). In the mouth, these tastes, along with texture, temperature, and the sensations from the common chemical sense, combine with odors to produce a perception of flavor. It is flavor that lets us know whether we are eating a pear or an apple. Some people are surprised to learn that flavors are recognized mainly through the sense of smell. If you hold your nose while eating chocolate, for example, you will have trouble identifying the chocolate flavor—even though you can distinguish the food's sweetness or bitterness. That is because the distinguishing characteristic of chocolate, for example, what differentiates it from caramel, is sensed largely by its odor.

What Are the Taste Disorders?

The most common true taste complaint is phantom taste perceptions. Additionally, testing may demonstrate a reduced ability to taste sweet, sour, bitter, salty, and umami, which is called hypogeusia. Some people can detect no tastes, called ageusia. True taste loss is rare; perceived loss usually reflects a smell loss, which is often confused with a taste loss.

In other disorders of the chemical senses, the system may misread or distort an odor, a taste, or a flavor. Or a person may detect a foul taste from a substance that is normally pleasant tasting.

What Causes Taste Disorders?

Some people are born with chemosensory disorders, but most develop them after an injury or illness. Upper respiratory infections are blamed for some chemosensory losses, and injury to the head can also cause taste problems.

Loss of taste can also be caused by exposure to certain chemicals such as insecticides and by some medicines. Taste disorders may result from oral health problems and some surgeries (e.g., third molar extraction and middle ear surgery). Many patients who receive radiation therapy for cancers of the head and neck develop chemosensory disorders.

How Are Taste Disorders Diagnosed?

The extent of a chemosensory disorder can be determined by measuring the lowest concentration of a chemical that a person can detect or recognize. A patient may also be asked to compare the tastes of different chemicals or to note how the intensity of a taste grows when a chemical's concentration is increased.

Scientists have developed taste testing in which the patient responds to different chemical concentrations. This may involve a simple sip, spit, and rinse test, or chemicals may be applied directly to specific areas of the tongue.

Are Taste Disorders Serious?

Yes. A person with a taste disorder is challenged not only by quality-of-life issues, but also deprived of an early warning system that most of us take for granted. Taste helps us detect spoiled food or beverages and, for some, the presence of food to which we're allergic. Perhaps more serious, loss of the sense of taste can also lead to depression and a reduced desire to eat.

Abnormalities in chemosensory function may accompany and even signal the existence of several diseases or unhealthy conditions, including obesity, diabetes, hypertension, malnutrition, and some degenerative diseases of the nervous system such as Parkinson's disease, Alzheimer's disease, and Korsakoff's psychosis.

Can Taste Disorders Be Treated?

Yes. If a certain medication is the cause of a taste disorder, stopping or changing the medicine may help eliminate the problem. Some patients, notably those with respiratory infections or allergies, regain their sense of taste when the illness resolves.

Often the correction of a general medical problem can also correct the loss of taste. Occasionally, recovery of the chemosenses occurs spontaneously.

What Research Is Being Done?

The NIDCD supports basic and clinical investigations of chemosensory disorders at institutions across the Nation. Some of these studies are conducted at several chemosensory research centers, where scientists work together to unravel the secrets of taste disorders.

Some of the most recent research on our sense of taste focuses on identifying the key receptors in our taste cells and how they work in order to form a more complete understanding of the gustatory system, particularly how the protein mechanisms in G-protein-coupled receptors work. Advances in this area may have great practical uses, such as the creation of medicines and artificial food products that allow older adults with taste disorders to enjoy food again. Future research may examine how tastes change in both humans and animals. Some of this research will focus on adaptive taste changes over long periods in different animal species, while other research will examine why we accept or have an aversion to different tastes. Beyond this, scientists feel future gustatory research may also investigate how taste affects various processing activities in the brain; specifically, how taste interacts with memory, influences hormonal feedback systems, and its role in the eating decisions and behavior.

Already, remarkable progress has been made in establishing the nature of changes that occur in taste senses with age. It is now known that age takes a much greater toll on smell than on taste. Also, taste cells (along with smell cells) are the only sensory cells that are regularly replaced throughout a person's life span—taste cells usually last about 10 days. Scientists are examining these phenomena that may provide ways to replace damaged sensory and nerve cells.

NIDCD's research program goals for chemosensory sciences include:

- Promoting the regeneration of sensory and nerve cells

- Appreciating the effects of the environment (such as gasoline fumes, chemicals, and extremes of relative humidity and temperature) on taste.

- Preventing the effects of aging.

- Preventing infectious agents and toxins from reaching the brain through the olfactory nerve.

- Developing new diagnostic tests.

- Understanding associations between chemosensory disorders and altered food intake in aging as well as in various chronic illnesses.

- Improving treatment methods and rehabilitation strategies.

What Can I Do to Help Myself?

Proper diagnosis by a trained professional, such as an otolaryngologist, is important. These physicians specialize in disorders of the head and neck, especially those related to the ear, nose, and throat. Diagnosis may lead to treatment of the underlying cause of the disorder. Many types of taste disorders are curable, and for those that are not, counseling is available to help patients cope.

505

Where Can I Find More Information?

If you have any other questions, call the NIDCD Information Clearinghouse. Here are several ways to contact us:

Toll-free: (800) 241-1044
Toll-free TTY: (800) 241-1055
1 Communication Avenue
Bethesda, MD 20892-3456
E-mail: nidcdinfo@nidcd.nih.gov
Internet: http://www.nidcd.nih.gov

Section 58.2

Smell Disorders

National Institute on Deafness and Other Communication Disorders, NIH Publication Number 01-3231, March 2002. Available online at www.nidcd.nih.gov/health/smelltaste/smell.asp; accessed May 2003.

Every year, thousands of people develop problems with their sense of smell. In fact, more than 200,000 people visit a physician each year for help with smell disorders or related problems. If you experience a problem with your sense of smell, call your doctor. This fact sheet explains smell and smell disorders.

Many people who have smell disorders also notice problems with their sense of taste. If you would like more information about your sense of taste, the chapter about taste and taste disorders may answer some of your questions.

How Does Our Sense of Smell Work?

The sense of smell is part of our chemical sensing system, or the chemosenses. Sensory cells in our nose, mouth, and throat have a role in helping us interpret smells, as well as taste flavors. Microscopic molecules released by the substances around us (foods, flowers, etc.)

stimulate these sensory cells. Once the cells detect the molecules they send messages to our brains, where we identify the smell.

Olfactory, or smell nerve cells, are stimulated by the odors around us—the fragrance of a gardenia or the smell of bread baking. These nerve cells are found in a small patch of tissue high inside the nose, and they connect directly to the brain. Our sense of smell is also influenced by something called the common chemical sense. This sense involves nerve endings in our eyes, nose, mouth, and throat, especially those on moist surfaces. Beyond smell and taste, these nerve endings help us sense the feelings stimulated by different substances, such as the eye-watering potency of an onion or the refreshing cool of peppermint.

It's a surprise to many people to learn that flavors are recognized mainly through the sense of smell. Along with texture, temperature, and the sensations from the common chemical sense, the perception of flavor comes from a combination of odors and taste. Without the olfactory cells, familiar flavors like coffee or oranges would be harder to distinguish.

What Are the Smell Disorders?

People who experience smell disorders experience either a loss in their ability to smell or changes in the way they perceive odors. As for loss of the sense of smell, some people have hyposmia, which is when their ability to detect odor is reduced. Other people can't detect odor at all, which is called anosmia. As for changes in the perception of odors, some people notice that familiar odors become distorted. Or, an odor that usually smells pleasant instead smells foul. Still other people may perceive a smell that isn't present at all.

What Causes Smell Disorders?

Smell disorders have many causes, some clearer than others. Most people who develop a smell disorder have recently experienced an illness or an injury. Common triggers are upper respiratory infections and head injuries.

Among other causes of smell disorders are polyps in the nasal cavities, sinus infections, hormonal disturbances, or dental problems. Exposure to certain chemicals, such as insecticides and solvents, and some medicines have also been associated with smell disorders. People with head and neck cancers who receive radiation treatment are also among those who experience problems with their sense of smell.

How Are Smell Disorders Diagnosed?

Doctors and scientists have developed tests to determine the extent and nature of a person's smell disorder. Tests are designed to measure the smallest amount of odor patients can detect as well as their accuracy in identifying different smells. In fact, an easily administered scratch and sniff test allows a person to scratch pieces of paper treated to release different odors, sniff them, and try to identify each odor from a list of possibilities. In this way, doctors can easily determine whether patients have hyposmia, anosmia, or another kind of smell disorder.

Are Smell Disorders Serious?

Yes. Like all of our senses, our sense of smell plays an important part in our lives. The sense of smell often serves as a first warning signal, alerting us to the smoke of a fire or the odor of a natural gas leak and dangerous fumes. Perhaps more important is that our chemosenses are sometimes a signal of serious health problems.

Obesity, diabetes, hypertension, malnutrition, Parkinson's disease, Alzheimer's disease, multiple sclerosis, and Korsakoff's psychosis are all accompanied or signaled by chemosensory problems like smell disorders.

Can Smell Disorders Be Treated?

Yes. Some people experience relief from smell disorders. Since certain medications can cause a problem, adjusting or changing that medicine may ease its effect on the sense of smell. Others recover their ability to smell when the illness causing their olfactory problem resolves. For patients with nasal obstructions such as polyps, surgery can remove the obstructions and restore airflow. Not infrequently, people enjoy a spontaneous recovery because olfactory neurons may regenerate following damage.

What Research Is Being Done?

The NIDCD supports basic and clinical investigations of chemosensory disorders at institutions across the nation. Some of these studies are conducted at several chemosensory research centers, where scientists are making advances that help them understand our olfactory system and may lead to new treatments for smell disorders.

Some of the most recent research into our sense of smell is also the most exciting. Though a complete understanding of the uniquely sophisticated olfactory system is still in progress, recent studies on how receptors recognize odors, together with new technology, have revealed some long-hidden secrets to how the olfactory system manages to detect and discriminate between the many chemical compounds that form odors. Besides uncovering the physical mechanisms our bodies use to accomplish the act of identifying smell, these findings are helping scientists view the system as a model for other molecular sensory systems in the body. Further, scientists are confident that they are now laying the foundation to understanding the finest details about our sense of smell—research that may help them understand how smell affects and interacts with other physiological processes.

Since scientists began studying the olfactory system, much has been discovered about how our chemosenses work, especially in how they're affected by aging. Like other senses in our bodies, our sense of smell can be greatly affected simply by our growing older. In fact, scientists have found that the sense of smell begins to decline after age 60. Women at all ages are generally more accurate than men in identifying odors, although smoking can adversely affect that ability in both men and women.

Another area of discovery has been the olfactory system's reaction to different medications. Like our sense of taste, our sense of smell can be damaged by certain medicine. Surprisingly, other medications, especially those prescribed for allergies, have been associated with an improvement of the sense of smell. Scientists are working to find out why this is so and develop drugs that can be used specifically to help restore the sense of smell to patients who've lost it. Also, smell cells (along with taste cells) are the only sensory cells that are regularly replaced throughout the life span. Scientists are examining these phenomena, which may provide ways to replace these and other damaged sensory and nerve cells.

NIDCD's research program goals for chemosensory sciences include:

- Promoting the regeneration of sensory and nerve cells.

- Appreciating the effects of the environment (such as gasoline fumes, chemicals, and extremes of relative humidity and temperature) on smell and taste.

- Preventing the effects of aging.

509

- Preventing infectious agents and toxins from reaching the brain through the olfactory nerve.

- Developing new diagnostic tests.

- Understanding associations between chemosensory disorders and altered food intake in aging as well as in various chronic illnesses.

- Improving treatment methods and rehabilitation strategies.

What Can I Do to Help Myself?

The best thing you can do is see a doctor. Proper diagnosis by a trained professional, such as an otolaryngologist, is important. These physicians specialize in disorders of the head and neck, especially those related to the ear, nose, and throat. Diagnosis may lead to an effective treatment of the underlying cause of your smell disorder. Many types of smell disorders are curable, and for those that are not, counseling is available to help patients cope.

Where Can I Find More Information?

If you have any other questions, call the NIDCD Information Clearinghouse. Here are several ways to contact us:

Toll-free: (800) 241-1044
Toll-free TTY: (800) 241-1055
1 Communication Avenue
Bethesda, MD 20892-3456
E-mail: nidcdinfo@nidcd.nih.gov
Internet: http://www.nidcd.nih.gov

Part Seven

Current Research in Dental and Oral Health

Chapter 59

Research to Reduce Oral Health Disparities

The National Institute of Dental and Craniofacial Research (NIDCR) announced that it is stepping up the effort to address disparities in our nation's health by funding five new Centers for Research To Reduce Oral Health Disparities. The centers, which are the first step in implementing the Institute's strategic plan for eradicating health disparities (http://www.nidcr.nih.gov/research/health_disp.asp), will identify factors contributing to oral health disparities and develop and test strategies for eliminating them. Each center also will provide training and career development opportunities for scientists in underrepresented groups and others interested in establishing careers in oral health disparities research.

In partnership with the National Center on Minority Health and Health Disparities, NIDCR will provide approximately $7 million per year over a seven-year period to support the centers through cooperative agreements. The new centers—at Boston University, New York University, the University of California at San Francisco, the University of Michigan, and the University of Washington—will focus on a wide variety of populations at risk for oral health disparities. They will partner with other academic health centers, state and local health agencies, community and migrant health centers, and institutions that serve targeted patient populations.

"NIDCR Funds Centers for Research to Reduce Oral Health Disparities" is published by the National Institute of Dental and Craniofacial Research (NIDCR), www.nidcr.nih.gov, October 1, 2001.

"The centers represent a cornerstone of NIDCR's efforts to redress oral health disparities," said NIDCR Director Dr. Lawrence Tabak. "More needs to be done, however, and we are working to identify the remaining gaps and the best ways to fill them. Our overall efforts have been markedly strengthened by our partnership with the National Center on Minority Health and Health Disparities and the wise counsel of its director, Dr. John Ruffin."

The need for the centers is underscored by findings reported in the first-ever Surgeon General's Report on Oral Health, released in May 2000 (http://www.nidcr.nih.gov/sgr/oralhealth.asp). The report identified a "silent epidemic" of dental and oral diseases that disproportionately burden the nation's poor, especially children and the elderly, as well as members of minority racial and ethnic groups. People with disabilities or complex health problems also are at greater risk for oral diseases that can, in turn, further complicate their health. The new centers will address concerns raised in the Surgeon General's report, and also will help meet the goals of the Healthy People 2010 initiative, the national effort coordinated by the U.S. Department of Health and Human Services that aims to improve the health of all Americans and eliminate disparities in health (http://www.health.gov/healthypeople).

"Our partnership with NIDCR has been longstanding and very productive," said Dr. John Ruffin, Director of the National Center on Minority Health and Health Disparities and its predecessor, the Office of Research on Minority Health.

"We are so pleased to join in the promising efforts of the NIDCR by helping to support these centers, which create new opportunities to reduce and ultimately eliminate oral health disparities. They will play a key role across the nation in conducting the research and research training that will establish a solid foundation for future progress."

Northeast Center for Research to Reduce Oral Health Disparities (Boston University)

Despite progress in reducing dental caries, tooth decay remains one of the most common diseases of childhood, particularly among poor children and children from minority racial and ethnic groups. The Northeast Center for Research to Reduce Oral Health Disparities, headed by Dr. Raul Garcia at Boston University School of Dental Medicine, will focus on reducing early childhood caries. Researchers at the center will examine the effects of tooth decay on the quality of life of low-income African American, Asian, Hispanic, and white children, and determine whether severe caries can slow growth.

Additionally, investigators will determine the best ways to involve pediatricians in reducing early childhood caries. They also will conduct studies of children and caregivers from the various racial and ethnic groups to learn more about the oral microbes that trigger tooth decay and how they are transmitted.

The center is a collaborative effort involving Harvard University, The Forsyth Institute in Boston, the Children's National Medical Center in Washington, D.C., and Boston Medical Center.

The New York University Oral Cancer Research for Adolescent and Adult Health Promotion Center (New York University)

Oral cancer, like many diseases, continues to take a disproportionate toll on minorities. African American males suffer the highest incidence of any group in the U.S. mainland. Puerto Rican males residing in Puerto Rico also have a high incidence of the disease. Failure to diagnose oral cancers in their earliest stages is probably the greatest factor contributing to poor treatment outcome. The New York University center, headed by Dr. Ralph Katz, will determine why minorities do not get oral cancer exams that might pick up the earliest signs of the disease. Specifically, they will look at differences in willingness to participate in cancer screening exams among African Americans, Puerto Ricans residing in Puerto Rico, Puerto Ricans residing in the U.S. mainland, and whites. The researchers also will look for ways to alter behavior to reduce risk factors such as tobacco and alcohol use.

Collaborating with the New York University center are Boston University, Howard University, the Johns Hopkins University, the University of Pittsburgh, Tuskegee University, the University of Alabama, the University of Puerto Rico, the Puerto Rico Health Department, and Memorial Sloan Kettering Cancer Center.

Center Addressing Disparities in Children's Oral Health (University of California, San Francisco)

The primary focus of this center, directed by Dr. Jane Weintraub of UCSF (University of California, San Francisco), is the prevention of early childhood caries, particularly among Mexican-, African-, Chinese-, and Filipino-Americans and low-socioeconomic-status whites.

Researchers at the UCSF center will explore factors such as cultural attitudes and other barriers that may prevent parents and caregivers from taking their young children to the dentist. Such knowledge may then be used to influence the development of public policy to reduce these barriers. The researchers also will use individual, community, and statewide data to determine what risk factors most likely lead to early childhood caries to help identify susceptible children. Finally, they will conduct clinical trials to test two interventions to prevent dental disease. The effectiveness of fluoride varnish painted on children's teeth is being evaluated at two diverse sites in San Francisco—the San Francisco General Hospital Family Dental Center and the Chinatown Public Health Center. An additional study evaluates a combination of preventive oral care methods for pregnant women, their infants, and toddlers who live on the U.S.-Mexican border.

Collaborating with UCSF are the San Francisco Department of Public Health, the San Ysidro Community Health Center, a model health care center located near the U.S.-Mexican border, and 12 other agencies and institutions along the West coast.

Detroit Center for Research on Oral Health Disparities (University of Michigan)

The Detroit Center for Research on Oral Health Disparities will work with a Detroit community of low-income African American children and their primary caregivers to promote oral health and reduce disparities. Investigators will seek to answer the question: Why do some low-income African American children and their caregivers have better oral health than others from their same community? The researchers will look at the influence of cultural, biological, and dietary factors on oral health status. Using this information, they will develop an educational campaign targeted at the community to improve oral health. Additionally, the center will evaluate whether children's access to dental services improves when Medicaid is managed like private health insurance.

The Detroit Center for Research on Oral Health Disparities, under the leadership of Dr. Amid Ismail, consists of the University of Michigan's Schools of Dentistry, Public Health, Social Work, and Medicine, the Institute for Social Research, and the University of Detroit-Mercy. Additional collaborators are the Detroit Department of Health, and the Voices of Detroit Initiative, funded by the Kellogg Foundation.

The Northwest/Alaska Center to Reduce Oral Health Disparities (University of Washington)

The Northwest/Alaska center will address the needs of poor, minority, and rural children and their caregivers. These groups include Alaska Natives, Native Americans from the Yakima Indian Nation, Hispanic migrant farm workers, African Americans and Hispanics from the local military bases, Hispanics and Pacific Islanders served by urban hospitals, as well as rural and low-income whites.

Researchers will examine why, within some minority populations, individuals are afraid to go to the dentist, and whether parents and caregivers may be passing on cultural beliefs that lead to dental fear. The researchers will use culturally appropriate approaches to talk about dental fear and will create long-distance learning programs to help people overcome their fear. In other research, scientists will test the theory that there are natural antibodies in epithelial cells lining the mouth that protect against dental caries. They will work with caries-prone children to determine if these children experience a breakdown in such antibody protection.

The Northwest/Alaska Center to Reduce Oral Health Disparities, directed by Dr. Peter Milgrom, represents a collaborative effort of the University of Washington School of Dentistry with the UW School of Medicine and Heritage College, the Alaska Native Tribal Health Consortium, the Yukon-Koskokwim Native Health Corporation, the Yakima Valley Farm Workers Clinic, the Northwest Portland Area Indian Health Board, the Northwest Tribal Epidemiology Center, Washington Dental Services Foundation, and the Medical Assistance Administration.

The National Institute of Dental and Craniofacial Research and the National Center on Minority Health and Health Disparities, which are funding the new centers on oral health disparities, are components of the National Institutes of Health, U.S. Department of Health and Human Services. The NIDCR is the nation's leading supporter of research on oral, dental, and craniofacial health.

Chapter 60

Better Dental Care: Hope from Science and Technology

The challenges for oral health in the twenty-first century are formidable. First and foremost is the need to ensure that all people have access to health care and can acquire the health literacy necessary to make use of health promotion and disease prevention information and activities.

The century offers the promise of a new era for health wrought by the convergence of six cultural movements, any one of which would be sufficient to transform the human condition:

- The biological and biotechnology revolutions.

- A redistribution of the world's people by rapid and sizable migrations within countries and across borders.

- Changing demographics in industrialized as well as developing nations.

- Changing patterns of disease, including the emergence and reemergence of infectious diseases, and changes in the organization of health care.

- Instant worldwide communication through the Internet, cable, satellite, and wireless technology.

U.S. Department of Health and Human Services. Oral Health in America: A Report of the Surgeon General. Rockville, MD: U.S. Department of Health and Human Services, National Institute of Dental and Craniofacial Research, National Institutes of Health, 2000.

519

- A continuing exponential rate of growth in information technology, specifically in computer speed, memory, and complexity.

These global currents are changing the way we live now and will have profound implications for the future of the oral and general health and well-being of all people.

The Past and Present as Prologue

The Pioneers

The history and intellectual activity of the eighteenth and nineteenth centuries set the seeds for the flowering of biology in the twentieth and early twenty-first centuries (Porter 1997). The scientific and technological discoveries of the early anatomists and embryologists—the founders of cell theory and brain research—were followed by the brilliant innovations of Pasteur, Koch, and Ehrlich, who established the new fields of microbiology and immunology. The cumulative achievements of these pioneers set the foundation for the diagnostic and therapeutic science and art of dentistry, medicine, nursing, and pharmacology in the twentieth century.

The seeds were also sown for the convergence of chemistry, physics, and biology in the field of molecular biology, as well as the convergence of Darwinism, fruit fly genetics, and population genetics into the modern evolutionary synthesis. These convergences inspired the current quest to identify all 100,000 genes of the human genome and to assign functional meanings to the motifs that are encoded within them.

Vital Statistics

The growth of the world population and the transcontinental movements of people are proving a dominant force for change. The twentieth century began with increased European and Asian migrations to the United States. By 1900 the U.S. population had reached 90 million residents and the Earth's population was approaching 1 billion people. Life expectancy in the United States was 47 years of age. Acute viral and bacterial infections were the primary causes of infant morbidity and mortality. Being edentulous, or toothless, was a normal expectation for mature adults.

For most of recorded human history and the 100,000 years of human prehistory, life expectancy was very low. Life expectancy at the time of the Roman Empire was approximately 28 years of age. From the beginning of the first millennium A.D. to 1900, each year of history saw an average gain of 3 days in life expectancy. Each year since 1900, however, has seen a gain of 110 days in average life expectancy (Rowe and Kahn 1998). Life expectancy at birth in the United States has increased from 47 years in 1900 to approximately 76 years today. While the entire population of the United States has tripled since 1900, the absolute number of older persons, currently 33 million, has increased elevenfold (Finch and Pike 1996, Rowe and Kahn 1998, p. 4). The U.S. population is 270 million and will reach 300 million in the next few decades. The Earth's population doubled by 1950, doubled again by 1975, and currently is 6 billion.

Health Improvement

Measures such as improved sanitation and housing, prenatal care, immunizations, health education and promotion, community water fluoridation, and dental sealants have greatly improved oral health for the majority of the population. Advances in science and technology, health professional education, the science of public health and clinical practice, and the health literacy of the public will continue to improve the health and well-being of Americans in the coming years (Kevles 1997, Schwartz 1998). Ever larger numbers of senior adults expect to retain a full or nearly complete dentition and to live well into their 70s, 80s, and 90s free of pain and discomfort (Slavkin 1997a).

Diversity of Diseases and Patients

Those seeking care in the decades ahead will present with a wide range of diseases and disorders, unevenly distributed across populations. The very youngest patients include children with complex hereditary or congenital craniofacial defects in need of expert multidisciplinary teams to repair and restore form and function. Early childhood caries, one of the most severe forms of the disease, is especially prevalent among poor children in some racial/ethnic groups in America, such as American Indians and Mexican Americans. Young adults are particularly vulnerable to unintentional and intentional craniofacial injuries. Middle-aged and older generations typically experience chronic diseases affecting the heart or lungs as well as cancers, diabetes, and the various degenerative diseases of joints and bones and the nervous system, all of which may affect or be affected by oral diseases and their treatments.

Transforming Treatments

The cultural movements that are changing the human condition will likely transform treatments for many of the complex disorders just described. The instrumentation used to detect subtle genetic variations in each of the 100,000 genes in the human genome will inexorably reveal which gene or genes are defective in hundreds of inherited and acquired craniofacial diseases or syndromes. On the horizon are promotion measures to enhance health and eliminate exposures to teratogens, as well as surgical techniques to correct the defects in utero, obviating the need for costly multiple surgeries and rehabilitation programs for affected children.

We are entering the golden age of molecular oral health with gene-based diagnostics, therapeutics, and biomaterials. Risk assessment for disease will be based in part on understanding the genetic variations that affect resistance or susceptibility, but also will be determined in part by environmental factors, socioeconomic status, personal behaviors, and lifestyle. The risk for early childhood caries is likely to be determined by a combination of all these factors, as well as cultural beliefs and practices within some populations. Elimination of all infections, whether in the oral cavity or elsewhere, will be seen as a critical part of health promotion.

Prevention of injuries will call for approaches that are both culturally and age sensitive, in addition to the coordinated efforts of policymakers and legislators to mandate protective gear in sports and other safety measures when necessary.

Gene therapy will be applied to treat oral and pharyngeal cancers and also will be used for the oral and systemic delivery of endogenous and synthetic molecules to treat salivary gland disorders, oral infections, and systemic disease. Highly specific drugs will be developed for the management of chronic facial pain such as trigeminal neuralgia and Bell's palsy.

Should additional evidence in the early years of the twenty-first century further indicate that oral infections actually cause some cases of heart disease, pulmonary disease, and stroke, or trigger the birth of premature, low-birth-weight babies, treatment approaches will be radically altered.

Transforming Health Professional Education

The scientific and technological bases of dentistry, medicine, nursing, and pharmacy are expanding rapidly in parallel with the changing demographics of the nation, the public's expectations for an enhanced quality of life, and changes in the management and financing of health care. Health professional schools, often organized around academic health science centers, are responding to these challenges and opportunities.

Students and clinicians alike need to be prepared to adopt evidence-based health care. Today and tomorrow, students must be well versed in epidemiology, biometry, bioinformatics, molecular biology, bioengineering, and much more. In addition, they must be prepared to adopt and implement new preventive strategies and comprehensive and molecular-based diagnostics and therapeutics; to support cost-effective community-based health programs; and to anticipate all the challenges that promotion of health entails. Clinical science or scientific evidence in the new millennium will continue to evolve in molecular dentistry and medicine with attendant opportunities for addressing the social, legal, and ethical implications. We must prepare clinicians for the nuances and complexities of modern clinical research-based results.

The previous chapters of this report provide the documentation that can be used to assess health professional education. Major progress in health promotion, disease prevention, diagnostics, therapy and therapeutics, and the socioeconomic and behavioral factors that influence oral, dental, and craniofacial health will further contribute to the transformation of health professional education.

Transforming Health Care

We are currently witnessing a significant transformation in the financing and management of health care, which is affecting all the health specialties. Care providers are assuming new responsibilities and functions and changing employment patterns. Traditionally, the management of health care has been centered on the providers of services and hospitals. Recently, the center has enlarged to include additional marketplace stakeholders, the purchasers of health care and health care plans, and increasingly all segments of society. The interactions among all these participants will shape health and health care for the foreseeable future.

Risk assessment models are also being developed and used to design treatment options tailored to communities and to individual patients. Increased use of information technology, greater efforts to conduct community needs assessments, and greater emphasis on enhanced quality of life expectations of patients, families, and communities are also in evidence (USDHHS 2000).

The responsibility for oral and craniofacial care involves all health professionals, so coordinated care delivery and reimbursement will be critical. Evidence-based systematic assessments and guidelines will contribute to clinical and public health decision making. In addition, the linkage between health care professions and public health and social service activities will need to be strengthened.

These trends are complemented by greater understanding of the psychosocial-behavioral aspects of oral diseases and disorders. These advances will continue to influence the nation's capacity to address the breadth and depth of diseases and conditions affecting oral health across the life span and their relationship to general health and well-being.

Access to the Internet and increased health and science reporting in print and broadcast media have created a more knowledgeable public motivated to understand the value of healthy choices. However, increasing numbers of patients are also questioning traditional practices and seeking alternative and complementary approaches.

Oral Health—Not Yet for All

Demographers predict that by 2050 there will be no single racial/ethnic majority in the United States. Rather, we will become an increasingly diverse nation with diverse patterns of disease and levels of health. This is especially evident for African American, Latino, Asian and Pacific Islander, and American Indian communities (Pamuk et al. 1998). Disparities in educational advancement, job opportunities, income and wealth, housing and neighborhood characteristics, health access and status, and involvement in the criminal justice system for various subpopulations will remain unless steps are taken to reverse the trends (Council of Economic Advisers 1998).

The proportion of school-aged children who are caries-free in their permanent teeth has more than doubled during the last 20 years. However, in states such as California, Texas, Louisiana, Alabama, Florida, and Georgia the trends are different; fewer than one third of the children are caries-free in their permanent dentition.

One attempt to come to the aid of poor children is the State Children's Health Insurance Program (SCHIP), federal legislation designed to help individual states meet the health needs of children (Council of Economic Advisers 1998, NRC 1998). As of 1998, more than 11 million children in America—1 in 7 children—are estimated to be uninsured. Most of these children live in families with working parents who have jobs that do not provide health insurance and who are unable to purchase health care insurance (NRC 1998). Nationally, 1 in 6 African American children and 1 in 4 Hispanic children are uninsured, compared with 1 in 10 white children (Council of Economic Advisers 1998, NRC 1998). This limited health care access is particularly significant in relation to oral health.

Hope from Science and Technology

The biological and biotechnology revolutions will accelerate, inspiring theory building and new models of miniaturization and speed that can be applied to improve oral health. The Human Genome Project will be completed no later than 2003. The entire human genetic lexicon will be accessible through the Internet. To date, more than several hundred mutated craniofacial regulatory and structural genes have been found to cause abnormal formation of oral, dental, and craniofacial tissues and structures.

In addition, the genomes of many significant viruses, bacteria, yeast, parasites, plants, and animals are currently being deciphered, and these are revolutionizing how we think about biology and human diseases (Bodmer and McKie 1995, Chambers 1995, Collins et al. 1998). At present, research is under way to decipher the genetic lexicon of 60 microbes, 6 of which are important oral pathogenic bacteria or fungi. The evolution of this knowledge will yield innovations in areas from clinical prevention to drug and biomaterials discovery.

Perhaps with the sole exception of trauma, all human diseases have a genetic component. Genetic dentistry and medicine are based on the paradigm that changes or mutations in individual nucleotides within genes or alleles result in variations or polymorphisms. These mutations are either inherited or acquired after birth. For example, inherited mutations in the amelogenin gene located on the human X (and Y) chromosome can produce X-linked dominant or recessive amelogenesis imperfecta, a painful disease characterized by defective tooth enamel (Backman 1997), and mutations in the fibroblast growth factor receptor 2 gene can produce serious craniofacial birth defects such as Crouzon's disease and other syndromes with premature fusion of cranial bones (craniosynostosis) (Cohen 1997). Mutations in a number of transcription factors that regulate development produce other craniofacial syndromes (Slavkin 1999).

The human genome contains approximately 100,000 genes or alleles. The genome consists of 3 billion nucleotides or bases. Mutations changing one or more bases, in one or more genes, can result in diseases or disorders. Many environmental factors termed mutagens, carcinogens, or teratogens can cause mutations in one or more genes resulting in human disease such as neoplastic diseases. The completion of the Human Genome Project in the next 2 years will afford an unprecedented opportunity to advance our understanding of inherited as well as acquired human diseases and disorders.

Scientific discoveries are rapidly defining single-gene mutations, mapping these individual genes in their precise positions on each of the 46 human chromosomes. These findings are being used to diagnose inherited and acquired clinical phenotypes as well as at-risk populations throughout the human life span.

These remarkable advances in human molecular genetics are identifying candidate genes for developing targeted gene-mediated therapeutic approaches to many oral health diseases, ranging from passive immunization for dental caries, induction of new bone and cartilage tissue, and regeneration of periodontal tissues, to the artificial synthesis of saliva for patients suffering from xerostomia [dry mouth].

Gene mutations also define the virulence of microbes (viruses, bacteria, yeasts, and parasites), as well as the fidelity of the human immune system. Microbial as well as human genes are extremely sensitive to environmental stress and can and do mutate, resulting in antibiotic resistance. The genetic variance within microbial genomes such as the genome of the yeast *Candida albicans* may be closely aligned with the host changes associated with immunologically compromised patients. The HIV viral genome is another particularly useful model for considering viral mutation frequency during pathogenesis (Slavkin 1996a). These discoveries provide the foundations for gene-based diagnostics for disease detection; therapeutic drug development; and individual predictors of drug response during the management of chronic facial pain, osteoarthritis as related to temporomandibular joint disease, and osteoporosis associated with periodontal diseases.

We are beginning to understand that polymorphisms (variations) in multiple genes confer susceptibility or resistance to chronic and disabling diseases and disorders such as osteoporosis, periodontal diseases, and temporomandibular disorders (Slavkin 1997b). In these examples, multiple genes and multiple gene-environment and gene-gene interactions are associated with the molecular etiology and pathophysiology of the disease process.

The function of most genes must inevitably be studied and understood at the level of their encoded proteins and protein-protein interactions, for these are the biologically active players of life. An enormous number of genes encode protein information that is highly conserved, that is, found in almost identical form in such diverse organisms as fruit flies and humans. Further scrutiny and analysis have determined that specific motifs encoded in larger domains of each protein serve as the business portion of the protein, binding to a cell surface, aggregating with other proteins, serving to catalyze a chemical reaction, binding to zinc or calcium ions, or serving other crucial functions in cell biology. The functional motifs are also being characterized in terms of structural biology. The scientific and educational communities are building large databases and then mining this information by using sophisticated information technology.

These genomic databases provide remarkable opportunities for the identification, design, and production of a new generation of biomarkers for diagnostics; innovative biomaterials for repair and regeneration; and the development of highly sensitive and specific drugs and vaccines to improve the health of all people (Baum et al. 1998, Slavkin 1996b,c, 1997a). Genomics has emerged as a major driver to realign academic, industry, and government science and technology to foster health, pharmaceutical, biotechnology, agricultural, food, chemical, environmental, energy, and computer science applications (Kaku 1997, Rifkin 1998). Many of these applications profoundly influence oral health (Slavkin 1996d, 1998a,b).

This epic period will also herald the advent of biochemistry on a chip, used in connection with body fluids such as saliva, cells, and tissues to diagnose diseases and disorders. The so-called chip technology will enable identification, quantitation, and complex analyses on surfaces no larger than one-centimeter square coupled to laser optical reader systems and computer-assisted informatics. Prototypes are already available to be tested against samples of saliva, cervical fluids, buccal mucosal cells, and blood (Slavkin 1998b). This technology should revolutionize saliva-based diagnostics and prognostics in oral health. Major progress is also anticipated in bioengineering through nanotechnology, miniaturization, and the innovations of design and fabrication of biomaterials. Anticipated advances include the repair and regeneration of cartilage, bone, muscle, nerve, salivary glands and saliva, and teeth (cementum, dentin, enamel, and periodontal ligament) (Slavkin 1996d, 1998a,b).

Additional scientific progress in the neurosciences will have broad implications for the diagnosis and treatment of diseases and disorders of the craniofacial complex including neuromuscular-related conditions (e.g., facial and dental trauma, bruxism, autism, Mobius syndrome, Bell's palsy, temporomandibular joint disorders, trigeminal neuralgia, Parkinson's disease, and disorders of speech, smell, and taste), the habilitation of craniofacial syndromes, and the management of facial pain.

The field of biomimetics is an example of the translation of human genomics into innovative developments in biotechnology. The idea is to use biological strategies to solve human diseases and disorders, essentially mimicking biological processes in the design and fabrication of new biomaterials to replace body parts or synthesize new drugs or reagents. For example, biological cartilage can now be designed and produced in artificial systems that present three-dimensional forms for nose and ear replacements as required in craniofacial birth defects, head and neck trauma, and oral and pharyngeal cancer patients (Slavkin 1996b, 1998a,b). Another approach is to design and fabricate bioceramics to be used in the replacement of human enamel or dentin on the surfaces of teeth.

A Framework for Oral Health

At the most basic level, local, state, and national health care policies will continue to strive to improve the health status of all Americans. Major reforms will improve public health competency. Enlightened health literacy will continue to influence quality of life expectations. Many social, economic, and political influences will continue to influence local, state, and national priorities for health policies (Isaacs and Knickman 1999). Included in these reforms will be efforts to improve the oral and craniofacial health of the American people.

Oral and craniofacial health issues will continue to be diverse and complex. In this context, two major themes remain: the need and demand for oral and craniofacial health services; and the role, functions, and mix of health professionals (Casamassimo 1996, USDHHS 1998).

First, need and demand will continue to be the two drivers of the health service requirements of our society. Need is an epidemiologically based and clinically derived measure of the amount of disease and adverse conditions that require treatment in order for the population to be healthy. Demand measures a population's health literacy, willingness, and capacity to utilize and finance health services. Public health literacy or competency and proactive oral health education will increase demand as well as delineate functions of oral health professionals for 2000 and beyond. Often, biomedical research advances in terms of new pharmaceuticals, devices, and procedures popularized in the media influence quality of life expectations, demand for health services, and the economy (Pardes et al. 1999). They can also lead to the creation of new types of health providers. Research also has the potential to reduce the need, demand, and costs for health services (McRae 1994). Thus outpatient surgery obviates the need for hospitalization; immunization or antibiotics control infections; and community water fluoridation, other fluorides, dental sealants, and related oral health policies help prevent dental caries.

Second, the major changes in demography, patterns of disease, and management of health care will continue to shape the roles and functions of health professionals. For example, significant increases in the numbers of senior citizens (65 years and older) with chronic facial pain, osteoarthritis, temporomandibular joint disorders, type 2 diabetes, dementia, osteoporosis, and oral and pharyngeal cancers will challenge health care providers for the next 50 years. These conditions will necessitate interdisciplinary and multidisciplinary approaches to care. Coordination of professional care with that of individuals, caregivers, and the community will be needed to control costs and ensure early diagnosis and prompt treatment.

To ensure that all people have access to health care and can acquire the health literacy necessary to make use of oral and craniofacial health promotion and disease prevention information and activities, a complete assessment of the nation's capacity to achieve access for all is warranted. Federal, state, and local government programs, legislation, and regulation; health professional societies and organizations; professional schools, colleges within universities, and K-12 education; patient groups; the private sector; and the larger society have the responsibility to achieve access to oral health care for all.

References

AGD. Saliva: a spitting image of the body. *AGD Impact* 1996;24(8):10–5.

Backman B. Inherited enamel defects. In: Chadwick DJ, Cardew G, editors. *Dental enamel*. London: John Wiley and Sons Ltd; 1997. p. 175–96.

Baum BJ, Atkinson, JC, Baccaglini LJ, et al. The mouth is a gateway to the body; gene therapy in 21st-century dental practice. *Can Dent Assoc J* 1998;26:455–60.

Bodmer W, McKie R. *The book of man: the Human Genome Project and the quest to discover our genetic heritage*. New York: Scribner Publishers; 1995.

Casamassimo P, editor. *Bright futures in practice: oral health.* Arlington (VA): National Center for Education in Maternal and Child Health; 1996.

Chambers DA, editor. DNA: *The double helix: 40 years, prospective and perspective.* New York: New York Academy of Sciences; 1995.

Council of Economic Advisers. *Changing America: indicators of social and economic well-being by race and Hispanic origin.* Washington: Council of Economic Advisers, Office of the President; 1998 1 Sep. Available from: US GPO, Washington, DC.

Cohen MM Jr. Molecular biology of craniosynostosis with special emphasis on fibroblast growth factor receptors. In: Cohen MM Jr, Baum BJ, editors. *Studies in stomatology and craniofacial biology.* Amsterdam: IOS Press; 1997. p. 307–30.

Collins F, Patrinos A, Jordan E, Chakravarti A, Gesteland R, Walters L. New goals for the U.S. Human Genome Project: 1998-2003, *Science* 1998;282:689.

Finch CE, Pike MC. Maximum lifespan predictions from the Gompertz mortality model. *J Gerontol A Biol Med Sci* 1996;51(3): B183–94.

Issacs SL, Knickman JR, editors. *To improve health and health care 2000.* San Francisco: Jossey-Bass Publishers; 1999.

Kaku M. *Visions: how science will revolutionize the 21st century.* New York: Anchor Books, Doubleday; 1997.

Kevles BH. *Naked to the bone.* New Brunswick (NJ): Rutgers University Press; 1997.

Malamud D. Saliva as a diagnostic fluid. *BMJ* 1992;(305):207–8.

Malamud D, Tabak L, editors. Saliva as a diagnostic fluid. *Ann NY Acad Sci* 1993;694.

McRae H. *The world in 2020.* Boston: Harvard Business School Press; 1994.

National Research Council (NRC). *America's children: health insurance and access to care.* Washington: National Academy Press, 1998.

Pamuk E, Makuc D, Heck K, Rueben C, Lochner K. *Socioeconomic status and health chartbook. Health, United States, 1998.* Hyattsville (MD): National Center for Health Statistics; 1998.

Pardes H, Manton KG, Lander ES, Tolley HD, Ullian AD. Palmer H. Effects of medical research on health care and the economy. *Science* 1999;283:36–7.

Porter R. *The greatest benefit to mankind.* New York: W.W. Norton & Company; 1997.

Rifkin J. *The biotech century.* New York: Penguin Putnam; 1998.

Rowe JW, Kahn RL. *Successful aging.* New York: Pantheon Books; 1998. p. 182–3.

Schwartz WB. *Life without disease.* Berkeley: University of California Press; 1998.

Slavkin HC. An update on HIV/AIDS. *J Am Dent Assoc* 1996a;127:1401–4.

Slavkin HC. Biomimetics: replacing body parts is no longer science fiction. *J Am Dent Assoc* 1996b;127:1254–7.

Slavkin HC. Understanding human genetics. *J Am Dent Assoc* 1996c;127:266–7.

Slavkin HC. Basic science is the fuel that drives the engine of biotechnology: a personal science transfer vision for the 21st century. *Tech Health Care* 1996d;4:249–53.

Slavkin HC. Clinical dentistry in the 21st century. *Compendium* 1997a;18(3):212–8.

Slavkin HC. Chronic disabling diseases and disorders. *J Am Dent Assoc* 1997b;128:1583–9.

Slavkin HC. Biomimicry, dental implants and clinical trials. *J Am Dent Assoc* 1998a;129:226–30.

Slavkin HC. Toward molecular based diagnostics for the oral cavity. *J Am Dent Assoc* 1998b;129:1138–43.

Slavkin HC. Possibilities of growth modification: nature versus nurture. In: MacNamara JA Jr, editor. *Growth modification:*

what works, what doesn't and why. Ann Arbor: University of Michigan Press; 1999. p. 1–16.

U.S. Department of Health and Human Services (USDHHS), National Center for Health Statistics (NCHS). 1997 *Healthy People 2000 review.* Hyattsville (MD): U.S. Department of Health and Human Services, National Center for Health Statistics; 1998.

U.S. Department of Health and Human Services (USDHHS). *Healthy People 2010: understanding and improving health.* Washington: U.S. Department of Health and Human Services; 2000. Available from: US GPO, Washington, DC.

Chapter 61

Human Trials Near for Caries Vaccine

Researchers at Boston's Forsyth Institute told the *Boston Globe* in March [2002] that they are close to human trials of a vaccine to combat dental caries.

The *Globe* said the scientists were preparing to meet with companies interested in sponsoring tests of an anticaries vaccine that would be "given to toddlers with a spritz up the nose."

The newspaper quoted Forsyth sources who said the vaccine has been in development for three decades, that it underwent limited tests in humans more than a decade ago, and that it is "designed to kill the bacteria that cause tooth decay," *Streptococcus mutans*.

Such a vaccine "would be terrifically helpful to a huge population in the United States and worldwide," Dr. Dominick P. DePaola, Forsyth president, told the *Globe*.

Earlier trials of the vaccine, the paper noted, involved about 70 young adults who received it either in capsule form or as a topical swabbed on the inner lip. Those given the vaccine accumulated bacteria at a slower rate, the *Globe* reported.

The newspaper also noted that a researcher at the University of Florida, Gainesville, is exploring possible genetic modification of caries-causing bacteria.

Chapter 62

Microscopes Help Endodontists See inside Root Canal

A relatively new addition to the instruments used in dentistry, the operating microscope has been used by medical specialists for decades. Endodontists, the dental specialists who treat problems originating inside the tooth, began experimenting with microscopes almost ten years ago, using them to enhance surgical procedures they perform around the roots of teeth. The microscope helps not only by magnifying the surgical field but also by providing more light. In addition, tiny mirrors no more than one tenth the size of traditional dental mirrors help the endodontist see into places where the human eye alone never could.

When endodontists perform endodontic (or root canal) procedures, the goal is to remove pulp tissue comprised of nerves, blood vessels, and connective tissue from canals inside the teeth. The canals are then cleaned, shaped, and filled with a special material, and the tooth restored, usually with a crown. This procedure saves teeth when their internal tissues have been damaged by serious decay or other trauma. Without a root canal, these teeth would have to be extracted and replaced with expensive bridgework, partials, or implants.

"With the microscope, structures that were once barely detectable are easier to see," says Dr. Richard C. Burns, a San Mateo, California, endodontist and past president of the American Association of Endodontists who also lectures on how the microscope has enhanced his personal practice of endodontics.

In most teeth, a canal containing nerves and blood vessels runs from the center of the crown (the part you can see above the gumline) of the tooth through the root and out into the jaw. Near the end of the root, the canal branches into many smaller canals, almost like a river delta. These smaller branches of the canal can be much easier to see with the microscope.

"After initially using the microscope in surgery, many endodontists discovered that it can also help with diagnosis and nonsurgical endodontic procedures," Dr. Burns reports. "For example, endodontists have used the microscope to find tiny fractures, which are often difficult to detect with traditional diagnostic methods. In addition, very small or unusually positioned canals become easier to see."

Sometimes new infection or injury will cause a tooth that has been treated before to need a second endodontic procedure. Endodontists call this retreating the tooth. To accomplish retreatment, all previous filling material and posts that may have been placed to support a crown must be removed from the tooth. The microscope can help with these procedures as well.

Educators in advanced endodontic training programs are using the microscope, too. Endodontists spend an additional two or more years of training in school after graduating from dental school to become specialists in endodontic procedures. The built-in video capability available on some microscopes allows students in these advanced programs to observe live procedures. Treatments may also be videotaped for later viewing.

Because this technology is just emerging in dentistry, more and more endodontists are seeking training in microscope procedures.

Chapter 63

Scientists Discover First Gene Involved in Gum Overgrowth

Dental researchers have known for decades that some people are born with gums that grow abnormally over their teeth. What they have never known is why?

Now, in this month's [April 2002] issue of the *American Journal of Human Genetics*, dental researchers have their first clue. An international team of scientists reports that it has identified the first gene that, when altered, triggers hereditary gingival fibromatosis, or HGF, the most common of these rare, inherited gum conditions.

Interestingly, the researchers note that the gene, called SOS1, encodes a protein that is known to activate the ras pathway, one of the key growth signals in our cells. The authors say this finding suggests that, when the SOS1 gene is not mutated, its protein and the ras pathway likely are involved in the normal growth of healthy gums, or gingiva, an idea that was previously unknown.

If confirmed, they say, learning how to turn on relevant portions of the pathway, like flipping a biological switch, might help dentists one day regenerate the gingiva naturally in people with receding gums or advanced periodontal disease. Conversely, by switching off the growth signal, dentists could prevent gingival overgrowth, meaning people with HGF might not need to have the excess tissue surgically cut away, now the standard treatment.

National Institute of Dental and Craniofacial Research (NIDCR), www. nidcr.nih.gov, April 1, 2002.

"This is yet another example of the importance of studying rare genetic diseases," said Dr. Thomas Hart, lead author on the study and a scientist at the University of Pittsburgh School of Dental Medicine. "By identifying a gene involved in hereditary gingival fibromatosis, it was possible to uncover a key clue into normal gingival development, a clue that could have important implications for dentistry."

Hart and his colleagues add that the discovery also could have important research implications for the gingival overgrowth that occurs in a number of human syndromes or as a side effect of certain frequently prescribed medications. These medications include: phenytoin for seizures, calcium channel blockers for hypertension, and cyclosporine for autoimmune diseases.

Researchers estimate that gingival overgrowth affects about 15 percent of people who use phenytoin, around 15 percent of those who take calcium channel blockers, and approximately 30 percent of people who use cyclosporine. For organ transplant patients who combine cyclosporine and nifedipine, about 40 percent have gingival overgrowth.

According to Hart, given the dearth of molecular information available on gingival overgrowth, HGF was a good place to start the search for clues. The condition was clearly genetic in origin, and, by the early 1990s, the tools were at hand to more efficiently track down inherited disease genes. What was lacking was a large family somewhere in the world with a long history of HGF, meaning many members of the family shared a gene mutation whose location in the human genome might be trackable.

In 1992, that family entered the picture when a woman walked into the University of Taubate dental clinic in Brazil to have her overgrown gingiva cut away from her teeth. Drs. Deborah Pallos and Jose Roberto Cortelli, after further consultation, correctly determined that the woman had HGF. Then, in close collaboration with Hart and his colleagues in the United States, the Brazilian scientists spent the next few years compiling an initial, 32-member family tree, recording each affected and unaffected member over three generations.

In 1998, after analyzing the DNA from many members of the family, the team reported that those affected shared an irregularity on the short arm of chromosome 2. But the researchers still didn't know exactly where the irregularity was on the short arm. As Hart said, this was no trivial matter.

The segment of the chromosome in question was found to contain 33 genes, any of which could be causing the gingival overgrowth, and they were spread out over nearly 5 million bases, or units, of DNA.

To hasten and narrow their search, the scientists contacted additional family members, collecting DNA samples and performing oral examinations on, in total, 83 family members spanning four generations. Meanwhile, Hart's laboratory sequenced—or arranged in order—the five million bases in the region. By knowing the precise, highly repetitive order of the four possible bases, represented by the letters A, T, C, and G, the scientists hoped that, if needed, they would be able to detect even a single, one-letter typo in the sequence.

As reported in this month's article, the group's careful attention to detail paid off. Hart and colleagues found that the 38 family members with HGF shared a single one-letter change in the sequence of the previously mapped son of sevenless (SOS1) gene. Present in organisms on all rungs of the evolutionary ladder, the SOS1 protein complexes with other molecules in our cells to activate the ras signaling pathway, a much-studied topic in cancer research.

This ancient biochemical signal, once activated and processed, can prompt our cells to grow, differentiate, or even commit suicide, tasks that are essential to life.

Hart said this single nucleotide change scrambled some of the genetic code required to produce a normal SOS1 protein. As a result, family members with HGF have shortened, abnormally shaped SOS1 proteins present in cells throughout their bodies, not just the gingiva. This raises the question of why this mutation would affect the gingiva only. Given the fundamental importance of the ras pathway to life, wouldn't the change in the SOS1 protein lead to birth defects or an inherited susceptibility to tumors throughout the body?

However, according to Hart, family members with HGF do not seem to be susceptible to other developmental abnormalities or cancer. "This might speak to the developmental uniqueness of the gingiva, which clearly has a novel pattern of gene and protein expression. Or, it might speak to the redundancy of signaling systems in our cells as a whole. But we really don't know, though biologically it is an extremely interesting lead that shows the power of genetic approaches in dental research."

Hart's study, which was supported by the NIH's [National Institute of Health's] National Institute of Dental and Craniofacial Research, is being published in the April issue of the *American Journal of Human Genetics*. The paper is titled, "A mutation in the SOS1 gene causes hereditary gingival fibromatosis type I." The authors are: Thomas C. Hart, Yingze Zhang, Michael C. Gorry, P. Suzanne Hart, Margaret Cooper, Mary L. Marazita, Jared M. Marks, Jose R. Cortelli, and Deborah Pallos.

Part Eight

Additional Help
and Information

Chapter 64

Glossary of Dental and Oral Health-Related Terms

Amalgam: An alloy of an element or a metal with mercury. In dentistry, primarily of two types: silver-tin alloy, containing small amounts of copper, zinc and perhaps other metals, and a second type containing more copper (12 to 30% by weight); they are used for restoring teeth and making dies.

Apicoectomy: Surgical removal of a tooth root apex. Also known as a root-end resection.

Bicuspid tooth: A tooth usually having two tubercles or cusps on the grinding surface and a flattened root, single in the lower jaw and upper second premolar, and furrowed in the upper first premolar. There are four premolars in each jaw, two on either side between the canine and the molars; there are no premolars in the deciduous dentition. Also known as a premolar tooth.

Bridge: A restoration of one or more missing teeth which cannot be readily removed by the patient or dentist; it is permanently attached to natural teeth or roots which furnish the primary support to the appliance. Also known as a fixed partial denture or fixed denture.

Candidiasis: Infection of the oral tissues with *Candida albicans*; often an opportunistic infection in humans with AIDS or humans suffering

---

from other conditions that depress the immune system; also common in normal infants who have been treated with antibiotics. Also known as thrush.

Canine tooth: A tooth having a crown of thick conical shape and a long, slightly flattened conical root; there are two canine teeth in each jaw, one on either side adjacent to the distal surface of the lateral incisors, in both the deciduous and the permanent dentition. Also known as an eyetooth.

Cavity: The loss of tooth structure due to dental caries.

Crown: In dentistry, that part of a tooth that is covered with enamel, or an artificial substitute for that part.

Dental abscess: An abscess situated within the alveolar process of the jaws, most often caused by extension of infection from an adjacent nonvital tooth. Also known as alveolar abscess.

Dental caries: A localized, progressively destructive disease of the teeth.

Dental hygienist: A licensed, professional auxiliary in dentistry who is both an oral health educator and clinician, and who uses preventive, therapeutic, and educational methods for the control of oral diseases.

Dental implants: Crowns, bridges, or dentures attached permanently to the jaw by means of metal anchors, most frequently titanium posts.

Dental plaque: The noncalcified accumulation mainly of oral microorganisms and their products that adheres tenaciously to the teeth and is not readily dislodged

Dental prophylaxis: A series of procedures whereby calculus, stain, and other accretions are removed from the clinical crowns of the teeth, and the enamel surfaces are polished. Also known as a dental checkup.

Dental sealant: A dental material usually made from interaction between bisphenol A and glycidyl methacrylate; such sealants are used to seal nonfused, noncarious pits and fissures on surfaces of teeth. Also known as a fissure sealant.

Dentist: A legally qualified practitioner of dentistry.

Dentistry: The healing science and art concerned with the structure and function of the oral-facial complex, and with the prevention, diagnosis, and treatment of deformities, pathoses, and traumatic injuries thereof.

Dentition: The natural teeth, as considered collectively, in the dental arch; may be deciduous, permanent, or mixed.

Denture: An artificial substitute for missing natural teeth and adjacent tissues.

Diphyodont: Possessing two sets of teeth, as occurs in humans and most other mammals.

Edentulous: Toothless, having lost the natural teeth.

Enamel: The hard glistening substance covering the exposed portion of the tooth.

Endodontics: A field of dentistry concerned with the biology and pathology of the dental pulp and periapical tissues, and with the prevention, diagnosis, and treatment of diseases and injuries in these tissues.

Fluoridation: Addition of fluorides to a community water supply, usually about 1 ppm [parts per million], to reduce incidence of dental decay.

Fluorosis: A condition caused by an excessive intake of fluorides (2 or more p.p.m. in drinking water), characterized mainly by mottling, staining, or hypoplasia of the enamel of the teeth, although the skeletal bones are also affected.

Halitosis: A foul odor from the mouth. Also known as bad breath.

Incisor tooth: A tooth with a chisel-shaped crown and a single conical tapering root; there are four of these teeth in the anterior part of each jaw, in both the deciduous and the permanent dentitions.

Malocclusion: Any deviation from a physiologically acceptable contact of opposing dentitions.

Molar tooth: A tooth having a somewhat quadrangular crown with four or five cusps on the grinding surface; the root is bifid in the lower jaw, but there are three conical roots in the upper jaw; there are six molars in each jaw, three on either side behind the premolars in the permanent dentition; in the deciduous dentition there are but four molars in each jaw, two on either side behind the canines.

Nursing bottle caries: Caries and tooth enamel erosion that result from permitting infants and children to go to sleep while sucking intermittently from a bottle of formula, whole milk, or fruit juice. Also known as baby bottle tooth decay.

Oral surgery: the branch of dentistry concerned with the diagnosis and surgical and adjunctive treatment of diseases, injuries, and deformities of the oral and maxillofacial region.

Orthodontics: That branch of dentistry concerned with the correction and prevention of irregularities and malocclusion of the teeth.

Palate: The bony and muscular partition between the oral and nasal cavities.

Pedodontics: The branch of dentistry concerned with the dental care and treatment of children. Also known as pediatric dentistry.

Periodontics: The branch of dentistry concerned with the study of the normal tissues and the treatment of abnormal conditions of the tissues immediately about the teeth.

Pharynx: The upper expanded portion of the digestive tube, between the esophagus below and the mouth and nasal cavities above and in front; it is distinct from the rest of the digestive tube in that it is composed exclusively of skeletal (voluntary) muscle arranged in outer circular and inner longitudinal layers.

Prosthodontics: The science of and art of providing suitable substitutes for the coronal portions of teeth, or for one or more lost or missing teeth and their associated parts, in order that impaired function, appearance, comfort, and health of the patient may be restored.

Pulp: The soft tissue within the pulp cavity, consisting of connective tissue containing blood vessels, nerves and lymphatics, and at the periphery a layer of odontoblasts capable of internal repair of the dentin.

Salivary gland: Any of the saliva-secreting exocrine glands of the oral cavity.

Tartar: A white, brown, or yellow-brown deposit at or below the gingival margin of teeth.

Teething: Eruption or cutting of the teeth, especially of the deciduous teeth.

Temporomandibular: Relating to the temporal bone and the mandible; denoting the joint of the lower jaw.

Tooth: One of the hard conical structures set in the alveoli of the upper and lower jaws, used in mastication and assisting in articulation. A tooth is a dermal structure composed of dentin and encased in cementum on the anatomic root and enamel on its anatomic crown. It consists of a root buried in the alveolus, a neck covered by the gum, and a crown, the exposed portion. In the center is the pulp cavity filled with a connective tissue reticulum containing a jellylike substance (dental pulp) and blood vessels and nerves that enter through an aperture or apertures at the apex of the root. The 20 deciduous teeth or primary teeth appear between the sixth and ninth and the 24th month of life; these exfoliate and are replaced by the 32 permanent teeth appearing between the fifth and seventh year and the 17th to 23rd year. There are four kinds of teeth: incisor, canine, premolar, and molar.

Tooth avulsion: The traumatic separation of a tooth from its alveolus.

Toothache: Pain in a tooth due to the condition of the pulp or periodontal ligament resulting from caries, infection, or trauma.

Uvula of soft palate: A conical projection from the posterior edge of the middle of the soft palate, composed of connective tissue containing a number of racemose glands, and some muscular fibers (uvulae muscle).

Veneer: In dentistry, a layer of tooth-colored material, usually porcelain or composite resin, attached to and covering the surface of a metal crown or natural tooth structure.

Chapter 65

Directory of Dental and Oral Health Organizations

Government Organizations That Provide Information about Oral Health

Centers for Disease Control and Prevention
1600 Clifton Road
Atlanta, GA 30333
Toll-Free: (800) 311-3435
Phone: (404) 639-3534
Website: http://www.cdc.gov

Food and Drug Administration
5600 Fishers Lane
Rockville, MD 20857
Toll-Free: (888) INFO-FDA
 (888-463-6332)
Website: http://www.fda.gov

Health Resources and Services Administration
Parklawn Building
5600 Fishers Lane
Rockville, Maryland 20857
Toll-Free: (888) ASK-HRSA
Website: http://www.hrsa.gov
E-mail: ask@hrsa.gov

National Cancer Institute
Suite 3036A
6116 Executive Boulevard, MSC8322
Bethesda, MD 20892-8322
Toll-Free: (800) 4-CANCER
TTY: (800) 332-8615
Website: http://www.nci.nih.gov

Resources in this chapter were compiled from many sources deemed accurate; all contact information was verified and updated in April 2003.

National Center for Complementary and Alternative Medicine
P.O. Box 7923
Gaithersburg, MD 20898
Toll-Free: (888) 644-6226
Phone: (301) 519-3153
TTY: (866) 464-3615
Fax: (866) 464-3616
Website: http://nccam.nih.gov
E-mail: info@nccam.nih.gov

National Health Information Center
P.O. Box 1133
Washington, DC 20013-1133
Toll-Free: (800) 336-4797
Phone: (301) 565-4167
Fax: (301) 984-4256
Website: http://www.health.gov/nhic
E-mail: info@nhic.org

National Institute of Arthritis and Musculoskeletal and Skin Diseases
National Institutes of Health
1 AMS Circle
Bethesda, Maryland 20892-3675
Toll-Free: (877) 22-NIAMS
Phone: (301) 495-4484
TTY: (301) 565-2966
Fax: (301) 718-6366
Website: http://www.niams.nih.gov
E-mail: niamsinfo@mail.nih.gov

National Institute of Child Health and Human Development
Building 31, Room 2A32
MSC 2425
31 Center Drive
Bethesda, MD 20892-2425
Toll-Free: (800) 370-2943
Website: http://www.nichd.nih.gov
E-mail: NICHDClearinghouse@mail.nih.gov

National Institute of Dental and Craniofacial Research
National Institutes of Health
Bethesda, MD 20892-2190
Phone: (301) 496-4261
Website: http://www.nidcr.nih.gov
E-mail: nidcrinfo@mail.nih.gov

National Institute of Diabetes and Digestive and Kidney Diseases
Building 31, Room 9A04
Center Drive, MSC 2560
Bethesda, MD 20892-2560
Toll Free: (800) 860-8747
Phone: (301) 654-3327
Fax: (301) 907-8906
Website: http://www.niddk.nih.gov
E-mail: NIDDK_Inquiries@nih.gov

National Institute on Aging
Building 31, Room 5C27
31 Center Drive, MSC 2292
Bethesda, MD 20892
Toll-Free: (800) 222-2225
Phone: (301) 496-1752
TTY: (800) 222-4225
Website: http://www.nia.nih.gov
E-mail: webmaster@nia.nih.gov

National Institute on Deafness and Other Communication Disorders
National Institutes of Health
31 Center Drive, MSC 2320
Bethesda, MD 20892-2320
Toll-Free: (800) 241-1044
TTY: (800) 241-1055
Website: http://
www.nidcd.nih.gov
E-mail: nidcdinfo@nidcd.nih.gov

National Library of Medicine
8600 Rockville Pike
Bethesda, MD 20894
Toll-Free: (888) FIND-NLM
(888-346-3656)
Phone: (301) 594-5983
Website: http://www.nlm.nih.gov
E-mail: custserv@nlm.nih.gov

National Oral Health Information Clearinghouse
1 NOHIC Way
Bethesda, MD 20892-3500
Phone: (301) 402-7364
TTY: (301) 656-7581
Fax: (301) 907-8830
Website: http://
www.nohic.nidcr.nih.gov
E-mail: nohic@nidcr.nih.gov

Office of the U.S. Surgeon General
5600 Fishers Lane
Room 18-66
Rockville, MD 20857
Phone: (202) 690-7694
Fax: (202) 690-6960
Website: http://www.surgeon
general.gov/sgoffice.htm

U.S. Administration on Aging
1 Massachusetts Avenue
Suites 4100 and 5100
Washington, DC 20201
Phone: (202) 619-0724
Website: http://www.aoa.gov
E-mail: AoAInfo@aoa.gov

U.S. Department of Health and Human Services
200 Independence Avenue, SW
Washington, DC 20201
Toll-Free: (877) 696-6775
Phone: (202) 619-0257
Website: http://www.hhs.gov

Information Available from the Academy of General Dentistry

Academy of General Dentistry
211 East Chicago Ave.
Chicago, IL 60611
Toll Free: (877) 292-9327
Phone: (312) 440-4300
Website: http://www.agd.org

The Academy of General Dentistry website serves as a consumer resource for current dental health information. Consumers can search more than 300 oral health topics.

SmileLine Online
http://forums.agd.org/agdsmileline

Consumers can receive free dental advice by posting questions on the SmileLine Online, a message board on the Academy's website. Questions are answered within hours by an Academy member.

Find a Dentist
http://www.agd.org/consumer/disclaimermem.html

Find a Dentist provides a listing of member dentists nationwide. When consumers provide a zip code, they will receive a randomly selected list of up to six dentists.

(877) 2X-A-YEAR (877-292-9327)

The Academy sponsors a year-round, toll-free service to help consumers find a general dentist in their area and remind them to visit the dentist twice a year.

Free Oral and Overall Health Brochure
Call (877) 292-9327

Dentalnotes

A quarterly public interest newsletter, *Dentalnotes* can be found in Academy members' offices nationwide. *Dentalnotes* provides dental tips for maintaining good oral health.

Other Private and Nonprofit Organizations That Provide Information about Oral Health

American Academy of Cosmetic Dentistry
5401 World Dairy Drive
Madison, WI 53718
Toll-Free: (800) 543-9220
National Smile Hotline: (866) 848-SMILE
Phone: (608) 222-8583
Fax: (608) 222-9540
Website: http://www.aacd.com
E-mail: info@aacd.com

American Academy of Esthetic Dentistry
401 North Michigan Avenue
Chicago, IL 60611
Phone: (312) 321-5121
Fax: (312) 673-6952
E-mail: aaed@sba.com
Website: http://
www.estheticacademy.org

American Academy of Family Physicians
11400 Tomahawk Creek Parkway
Leawood, KS 66211-2672
Toll-Free: (800) 274-2237
Phone: (913) 906-6000
Website: http://familydoctor.org
E-mail: email@familydoctor.org

American Academy of Pediatric Dentistry
211 East Chicago Avenue, #700
Chicago, IL 60611-2663
Phone: (312) 337-2169
Fax: (312) 337-6329
Website: http://www.aapd.org

American Academy of Pediatrics
141 Northwest Point Boulevard
Elk Grove Village, IL 60007-1098
Phone: (847) 434-4000
Fax: (847) 434-8000
Website: http://www.aap.org
E-mail: kidsdocs@aap.org

American Academy of Periodontology
737 North Michigan Avenue, Suite 800
Chicago, Illinois 60611
Phone: (312) 787-5518
Fax: (312) 787-3670
Website: http://www.perio.org
E-mail: aapsite@perio.org

American Association of Endodontists
211 East Chicago Avenue
Suite 1100
Chicago, IL 60611-2691
Toll-Free: (800) 872-3636
Phone: (312) 266-7255
Toll-Free Fax: (866) 451-9020
Fax: (312) 266-9867
Website: http://www.aae.org
E-mail: info@aae.org

American Association of Oral and Maxillofacial Surgeons
9700 West Bryn Mawr Avenue
Rosemont, IL 60018-5701
Phone: (847) 678-6200
Website: http://www.aaoms.org
E-mail: inquiries@aaoms.org

American Association of Orthodontists
401 North Lindbergh Boulevard
St. Louis, MO 63141-7816
Toll-Free: (800) STRAIGHT
Fax: (314) 997-1745
Website: http://www.braces.org
E-mail: info@aaortho.org

American Association of Women Dentists
645 North Michigan Avenue, #800
Chicago, IL 60611
Toll-Free: (800) 920-2293
Fax: (830) 612-3067
E-mail: info@aawd.org
Website: http:// www.womendentists.org

American College of Prosthodontics
211 East Chicago Avenue
Suite 1000
Chicago, IL 60611
Phone: (312) 573-1260
Fax: (312) 573-1257
Website: http:// www.prosthodontics.org

American Dental Association
211 East Chicago Avenue
Chicago, Illinois 60611
Phone: (312) 440-2500
Fax: (312) 440-7494
Website: http://www.ada.org
E-mail: publicinfo@ada.org

American Dental Hygienists' Association
444 North Michigan Avenue, Suite 3400
Chicago, IL 60611
Phone: (312) 440-8900
Website: http://www.adha.org
E-mail: mail@ahda.net

American Medical Association
515 North State Street
Chicago, Illinois 60610
Toll Free: (800) AMA-3211
Phone: (312) 464-5000
Website: http:// www.ama-assn.org

British Dental Health Foundation
Smile House
2 East Union Street
Rugby
Warwickshire CV22 6AJ
England
Phone: 011 44 870 770 4000
Fax: 011 44 870 770 4010
Website: http:// www.dentalhealth.org.uk
E-mail: mail@dentalhealth.org.uk

Children's Dental Health Project
1990 M Street, NW
Suite 200
Washington, DC 20036
Phone: (202) 833-8288
Fax: (202) 318-0667
Website: http://www.cdhp.org

Dental Health Foundation
520 Third Street
Suite 205
Oakland, CA 94607
Phone: (510) 663-3727
Fax: (510) 663-3733
Website: http://
www.dentalhealthfoundation.org
E-mail: tdhf@pacbell.net

Dental Watch
Website: http://
www.dentalwatch.org
E-mail: sbinfo@quackwatch.org

Oral Health America
410 North Michigan Avenue,
Suite 352
Chicago, IL 60611
Phone: (312) 836-9900
Fax: (312) 836-9986
Website: http://
www.oralhealthamerica.org

Chapter 66

Resources for People with Dental and Oral Disorders

AboutFace USA
P.O. Box 969
Batavia, IL 60510-0969
Toll-Free: (888) 486-1209
Website: http://www.aboutfaceusa.org/Resources3.htm
E-mail: AboutFaceUS@aol.com

Academy of General Dentistry
Phone: (877) 292-9327
Website: http://www.agd.org

The Academy of General Dentistry website serves as a consumer resource for current dental health information. Consumers can search more than 300 oral health topics.

SmileLine Online
http://forums.agd.org/agdsmileline

Consumers can receive free dental advice by posting questions on the SmileLine Online, a message board on the Academy's website. Questions are answered within hours by an Academy member.

Find a Dentist
http://www.agd.org/consumer/disclaimermem.html

Resources in this chapter were compiled from many sources deemed accurate; all contact information was verified and updated in April 2003.

Academy of General Dentistry continued

Find a Dentist provides a listing of member dentists nationwide. When consumers provide a zip code, they will receive a randomly selected list of up to six dentists.

(877) 2X-A-YEAR (877-292-9327)

The Academy sponsors a year-round, toll-free service to help consumers find a general dentist in their area and remind them to visit the dentist twice a year.

Free Oral and Overall Health Brochure
Call (877) 292-9327

Dentalnotes

A quarterly public interest newsletter, *Dentalnotes* can be found in Academy members' offices nationwide. *Dentalnotes* provides dental tips for maintaining good oral health.

American Cleft Palate-Craniofacial Association/Cleft Palate Foundation
104 South Estes Drive, Suite 204
Chapel Hill, NC 27514
Toll-Free: (800) 24-CLEFT
Phone: (919) 933-9044
Website: http://www.cleftline.org/links
E-mail: info@cleftline.org

Animated-Teeth.com
2238 Bluff Boulevard
Columbia, MO 65201
Website: http://www.animated-teeth.com/reference/dental_links.htm
E-mail: info@animated-teeth.com

Arthritis Foundation
P.O. Box 7669
Atlanta, GA 30357-0669
Toll-Free: (800) 283-7800
Website: http://www.arthritis.org

Center for Craniofacial Development and Disorders

Children's Medical and Surgical Center, Room 1004
Johns Hopkins Hospital
600 North Wolfe Street
Baltimore, MD 21287-3914
Phone: (410) 955-4160
Fax: (410) 955-0484
Website: http://www.hopkinsmedicine.org/craniofacial

Children's Craniofacial Association

13140 Coit Road, Suite 307
Dallas, TX 75240
Toll-Free: (800) 535-3643
Phone: (214) 570-8811
Website: http://www.ccakids.com
E-mail: contactCCA@ccakids.com

Dental Alliance for AIDS/HIV Care

Website: http://www.critpath.org/daac

Dental Related Internet Resources

Website: http://www.tensegrity.critpath.org/daac
E-mail: DAACWeb@critpath.org

Dystonia Medical Research Foundation

One East Wacker Drive, Suite 2430
Chicago, Illinois 60601-1905
Toll-Free: (800) 361-8061 (from Canada)
Phone: (312) 755-0198
Fax: (312) 803-0138
Website: http://www.dystonia-foundation.org
E-mail: dystonia@dystonia-foundation.org

FACES: National Craniofacial Association

P.O. Box 11082
Chattanooga, TN 37401
Toll-Free: (800) 332-2373
E-mail: faces@faces-cranio.org
Website: http://www.faces-cranio.org

HIVdent
Medical College of Georgia
Augusta, GA 30912-1400
Toll Free: (800) 221-6437
Phone: (706) 721-3967
Fax: (706) 721-4642
Website: http://www.hivdent.org

Let's Face It
P.O. Box 29972
Bellingham, WA 98228-1972
Phone: (360) 676-7325
Website: http://www.faceit.org/classics.html
Website: http://www.faceit.org/gen_org.html
E-mail: letsfaceit@faceit.org

Kimberly A. Loos, DDS
4110 Moorpark Avenue, Suite B
San Jose, CA 95117
Phone: (408) 985-6779
Fax: (408) 985-6884
Website: http://www.smiledoc.com/dentist/links.html
E-mail: kim@drloos.com

National Cancer Institute
Suite 3036A
6116 Executive Boulevard, MSC8322
Bethesda, MD 20892-8322
Toll-Free: (800) 4-CANCER
TTY: (800) 332-8615
Website: http://www.nci.nih.gov

National Institute of Dental and Craniofacial Research
National Institutes of Health
Bethesda, MD 20892-2190
Phone: (301) 496-4261
Website: http://www.nidcr.nih.gov
E-mail: nidcrinfo@mail.nih.gov

National Oral Health Information Clearinghouse
1 NOHIC Way
Bethesda, MD 20892-3500
Phone: (301) 402-7364
TTY: (301) 656-7581
Fax: (301) 907-8830
Website: http://www.nohic.nidcr.nih.gov/links.html
E-mail: nohic@nidcr.nih.gov

Oral Cancer Foundation
3419 Via Lido, # 205
New Port Beach, CA 92663
Phone: (949) 646-8000
Fax: (949) 496-3331
Website: http://www.oralcancer.org
E-mail: info@oralcancerfoundation.org

Sjögren's Syndrome Foundation
8120 Woodmont Avenue, Suite 530
Bethesda, MD 20814
Toll-Free: (800) 475-6473
Fax: (301) 718-0322
Website: http://www.sjogrens.com

Special Care Dentistry
211 E. Chicago Ave., Suite 740
Chicago, IL 60611
Phone: (312) 440-2660
Fax: (312) 440-2824
Website: http://www.scdonline.org/Weblinks.htm
E-mail: SCD@SCDonline.org

Support for People with Oral and Head and Neck Cancer
P.O. Box 53
Locust Valley, NY 11560-0053
Toll-Free: (800) 377-0928
Fax: (516) 671-8794
Website: http://www.spohnc.org/resources.html
E-mail: info@spohnc.org

TMJ Association
P.O. Box 26770
Milwaukee, WI 53226-0770
Website: http://www.tmj.org
E-mail: info@tmj.org

TMJ – Jaw Joints and Allied Musculo-Skeletal Disorders Foundation
The Forsyth Institute
140 Fenway
Boston, MA 02115-3799
Phone: (617) 266 2550
Fax: (617) 267 9020
Website: http://www.tmjoints.org
E-mail: tmjoints@aol.com

Wide Smiles: Cleft Lip and Palate Resource
P.O. Box 5153
Stockton, CA 95205-0153
Phone: (209) 942-2812
Fax: (209) 464-1497
Website: http://www.widesmiles.org
E-mail: josmiles@yahoo.com

Chapter 67

Sources for Charitable and Accessible Dental Care

How Can I Find out about Charitable or Low-Cost Dental Care for People in Need?

Assistance programs vary from state to state, so you may want to contact your state dental society to see if there are programs in your area.

Another possible source of lower-cost dental care is a dental school clinic. Generally, dental costs in school clinics are reduced and may include only partial payment for professional services covering the cost of materials and equipment. Your state dental society can tell you if there is a dental school clinic in your area.

Where Can People with Special Needs Obtain Dental Care?

The ADA Council on Access, Prevention and Interprofessional Relations suggests the following tips:

- Inform the dentist about your special health or financial conditions.

- Ask if the dentist has training and/or experience in treating patients with your specific condition.

The text of this chapter is reprinted with permission of the American Dental Association. © 2003 American Dental Association. For additional information, visit www.ada.org. Resources in this chapter were compiled from many sources deemed accurate; all contact information was verified and updated in April 2003.

- Ask if the dentist has an interest in treating patients with your specific condition.

- Find out if the dentist participates in your dental benefit plan (dental insurance program).

- Ask if the dental facility is accessible to the disabled.

In addition, the Council suggests that patients with special needs

- Call or write the dental director at your state department of public health.

- Contact the nearest dental school clinic or hospital dental department, especially if it is affiliated with a major university.

- Contact the Special Care Dentistry (Formerly Federation of Special Care Organizations in Dentistry), the Academy of General Dentistry, and the American Academy of Pediatric Dentistry for a referral.

- Also, the National Oral Health Information Clearinghouse may have useful information.

- Contact the National Foundation of Dentistry for the Handicapped (NFDH), a charitable affiliate of the American Dental Association since 1988. The NFDH, via several programs, facilitates the provision of comprehensive dental care for needy disabled, elderly, and medically compromised individuals.

- Dentists and dental institutions organizing or participating in voluntary projects that care for uninsured and underserved patients will find information and grant opportunities through Volunteers in Health Care (VIH). VIH Program staff are available to assist you at the toll-free number 877-844-8442.

Tips for Choosing a Dentist

How Do You Find a Dentist?

The American Dental Association offers these suggestions:

- Ask family, friends, neighbors, or coworkers for recommendations.

- Ask your family physician or local pharmacist.

- If you're moving, your current dentist may be able to make a recommendation.

- Call or write your local or state dental society. Your local and state dental societies also may be listed in the telephone directory under Dentists or Associations.

- Use ADA.org's ADA Member Directory to search for dentists in your area.

You may want to call or visit more than one dentist before making your decision. Dental care is a very personalized service that requires a good relationship between the dentist and the patient.

What Should I Look for When Choosing a Dentist?

You may wish to consider several dentists before making your decision. During your first visit, you should be able to determine if this is the right dentist for you. Consider the following:

- Is the appointment schedule convenient for you?

- Is the office easy to get to from your home or job?

- Does the office appear to be clean, neat, and orderly?

- Was your medical and dental history recorded and placed in a permanent file?

- Does the dentist explain techniques that will help you prevent dental health problems? Is dental health instruction provided?

- Are special arrangements made for handling emergencies outside of office hours? (Most dentists make arrangements with a colleague or emergency referral service if they are unable to tend to emergencies.)

- Is information provided about fees and payment plans before treatment is scheduled?

You and your dentist are partners in maintaining your oral health. Take time to ask questions and take notes if that will help you remember your dentist's advice.

What Is the Difference between a DDS and a DMD?

The DDS (Doctor of Dental Surgery) and DMD (Doctor of Dental Medicine) are the same degrees. The difference is a matter of semantics. The majority of dental schools award the DDS degree; however, some award a DMD degree. The education and degrees are the same.

Sources for Charitable and Accessible Dental Care

Centers for Medicare and Medicaid Services: State Children's Health Insurance Program
7500 Security Boulevard
Baltimore, MD 21244-1850
Toll-Free: (877) 267-2323
Phone: (410) 786-3000
TTY: (866) 226-1819
Website: http://cms.hhs.gov/schip

Cleft Advocate
Phone: (702) 228-8662
Website: http://www.cleftadvocate.org
E-mail: webmaster@cleftadvocate

Kids in Need of Dentistry
2465 S. Downing, Suite 207
Denver, Colorado 80210
Toll-Free: (877) 544-KIND
Phone: (303) 733-3710
Fax: (303) 733-3670
Website: http://www.kindsmiles.org
E-mail: info@kindsmiles.org

Operation Smile
6435 Tidewater Drive
Norfolk, VA 23509
Phone: (757) 321-7645
Fax: (757) 321-7600
Website: http://www.operationsmile.org
E-mail: webmaster@operationsmile.org

Smile Train
245 5th Avenue, Suite 2201
New York, NY 10016
Toll-Free: (877) KID-SMILE
Phone: (212) 689-9199
Fax: (212) 689-9299
Website: http://www.smiletrain.org
E-mail: info@smiletrain.org

Index

Index

Page numbers followed by 'n' indicate a footnote. Page numbers in *italics* indicate a table or illustration.

569

bulimia *see* eating disorders
Bullers, Anne Christiansen 112n, 119
Burns, Richard C. 535–36
Burrell, Kenneth 96

C

calcium
  children 28–30
  content in foods *30*
calcium channel blockers 538
calculus, described 235
calculus formation 128
California Dental Association, publications
  cosmetic dentistry 374n
  pregnancy 43n
  receding gums 228n
cancer treatment, oral care 402–12
  see also oral cancer
Candida albicans
  described 543
  genetic research 526
candidiasis
  defined 543–44
   see also thrush
  overview 489–90
canine teeth
  defined 10, 544
  depicted *6*
  described 5, 8
  teething 17
canker sores
  described 9
  overview 495–97
cantilever bridge, described 341–42
carbohydrates, dental health 26
cavitational osteopathosis, described 136
cavities
  defined 544
  described 10
  formation 14
  overview 177–79
  painless drilling 220–22
  see also dental caries
CDC *see* Centers for Disease Control and Prevention

cementum
  defined 11
  depicted *7*
  described 5
Center Addressing Disparities in Children's Oral Health, described 515–16
Center for Craniofacial Development and Disorders, contact information 559
Centers for Disease Control and Prevention (CDC)
  contact information 549
  publications
   community water fluoridation 110n
   dental visits 146n
   fluoride 106n
   oropharyngeal candidiasis 489n
   teeth cleaning 148n
   toothbrush care 97n
Centers for Medicare and Medicaid Services: State Children's Health Insurance Program
  contact information 566
  described 524–25
chemotherapy
  lip cancer 452
  oral cancer 441
  oral cavity cancer 452
  salivary gland cancer 464
chemotherapy, oral care 406–10
chewing process, described 8
chewing tobacco, oral cancer 447–48
Chiappelli, Francesco 62
children
  arthritis 391
  bruxism 369–72, 388
  calcium requirements 28–30
  clefts 393–400
  conscious sedation 214–15
  dental caries 24, 521–22
  dental habits 10, 16–17
  dental sealants 163, 166
  dental visits 147
  enamel fluorisis 119–20
  enamel microabrasion 381–82
  fluoride 19, 23, 27, 106–9
  healthy diets 26–28

G

H

Health Reference Series
COMPLETE CATALOG

Adolescent Health Sourcebook

Basic Consumer Health Information about Common Medical, Mental, and Emotional Concerns in Adolescents, Including Facts about Acne, Body Piercing, Mononucleosis, Nutrition, Eating Disorders, Stress, Depression, Behavior Problems, Peer Pressure, Violence, Gangs, Drug Use, Puberty, Sexuality, Pregnancy, Learning Disabilities, and More

Along with a Glossary of Terms and Other Resources for Further Help and Information

Edited by Chad T. Kimball. 658 pages. 2002. 0-7808-0248-9. $78.

"It is written in clear, nontechnical language aimed at general readers. . . . Recommended for public libraries, community colleges, and other agencies serving health care consumers."
— *American Reference Books Annual, 2003*

"Recommended for school and public libraries. Parents and professionals dealing with teens will appreciate the easy-to-follow format and the clearly written text. This could become a 'must have' for every high school teacher." — *E-Streams, Jan '03*

"A good starting point for information related to common medical, mental, and emotional concerns of adolescents." — *School Library Journal, Nov '02*

"This book provides accurate information in an easy to access format. It addresses topics that parents and caregivers might not be aware of and provides practical, useable information." — *Doody's Health Sciences Book Review Journal, Sep-Oct '02*

"Recommended reference source."
— *Booklist, American Library Association, Sep '02*

AIDS Sourcebook, 3rd Edition

Basic Consumer Health Information about Acquired Immune Deficiency Syndrome (AIDS) and Human Immunodeficiency Virus (HIV) Infection, Including Facts about Transmission, Prevention, Diagnosis, Treatment, Opportunistic Infections, and Other Complications, with a Section for Women and Children, Including Details about Associated Gynecological Concerns, Pregnancy, and Pediatric Care

Along with Updated Statistical Information, Reports on Current Research Initiatives, a Glossary, and Directories of Internet, Hotline, and Other Resources

Edited by Dawn D. Matthews. 664 pages. 2003. 0-7808-0631-X. $78.

ALSO AVAILABLE: AIDS Sourcebook, 1st Edition. Edited by Karen Bellenir and Peter D. Dresser. 831 pages. 1995. 0-7808-0031-1. $78.

AIDS Sourcebook, 2nd Edition. Edited by Karen Bellenir. 751 pages. 1999. 0-7808-0225-X. $78.

"Highly recommended."
— *American Reference Books Annual, 2000*

"Excellent sourcebook. This continues to be a highly recommended book. There is no other book that provides as much information as this book provides."
— *AIDS Book Review Journal, Dec-Jan 2000*

"Recommended reference source."
— *Booklist, American Library Association, Dec '99*

"A solid text for college-level health libraries."
— *The Bookwatch, Aug '99*

Cited in *Reference Sources for Small and Medium-Sized Libraries, American Library Association, 1999*

Alcoholism Sourcebook

Basic Consumer Health Information about the Physical and Mental Consequences of Alcohol Abuse, Including Liver Disease, Pancreatitis, Wernicke-Korsakoff Syndrome (Alcoholic Dementia), Fetal Alcohol Syndrome, Heart Disease, Kidney Disorders, Gastrointestinal Problems, and Immune System Compromise and Featuring Facts about Addiction, Detoxification, Alcohol Withdrawal, Recovery, and the Maintenance of Sobriety

Along with a Glossary and Directories of Resources for Further Help and Information

Edited by Karen Bellenir. 613 pages. 2000. 0-7808-0325-6. $78.

"This title is one of the few reference works on alcoholism for general readers. For some readers this will be a welcome complement to the many self-help books on the market. Recommended for collections serving general readers and consumer health collections."
— *E-Streams, Mar '01*

"This book is an excellent choice for public and academic libraries."
— *American Reference Books Annual, 2001*

"Recommended reference source."
— *Booklist, American Library Association, Dec '00*

"Presents a wealth of information on alcohol use and abuse and its effects on the body and mind, treatment, and prevention." — *SciTech Book News, Dec '00*

"Important new health guide which packs in the latest consumer information about the problems of alcoholism." — *Reviewer's Bookwatch, Nov '00*

SEE ALSO Drug Abuse Sourcebook, Substance Abuse Sourcebook

Allergies Sourcebook, 2nd Edition

Basic Consumer Health Information about Allergic Disorders, Triggers, Reactions, and Related Symptoms, Including Anaphylaxis, Rhinitis, Sinusitis, Asthma, Dermatitis, Conjunctivitis, and Multiple Chemical Sensitivity

Along with Tips on Diagnosis, Prevention, and Treatment, Statistical Data, a Glossary, and a Directory of Sources for Further Help and Information

Edited by Annemarie S. Muth. 598 pages. 2002. 0-7808-0376-0. $78.

ALSO AVAILABLE: Allergies Sourcebook, 1st Edition. Edited by Allan R. Cook. 611 pages. 1997. 0-7808-0036-2. $78.

"This book brings a great deal of useful material together. . . . This is an excellent addition to public and consumer health library collections."
— *American Reference Books Annual, 2003*

"This second edition would be useful to laypersons with little or advanced knowledge of the subject matter. This book would also serve as a resource for nursing and other health care professions students. It would be useful in public, academic, and hospital libraries with consumer health collections." — *E-Streams, Jul '02*

Alternative Medicine Sourcebook, 2nd Edition

Basic Consumer Health Information about Alternative and Complementary Medical Practices, Including Acupuncture, Chiropractic, Herbal Medicine, Homeopathy, Naturopathic Medicine, Mind-Body Interventions, Ayurveda, and Other Non-Western Medical Traditions

Along with Facts about such Specific Therapies as Massage Therapy, Aromatherapy, Qigong, Hypnosis, Prayer, Dance, and Art Therapies, a Glossary, and Resources for Further Information

Edited by Dawn D. Matthews. 618 pages. 2002. 0-7808-0605-0. $78.

ALSO AVAILABLE: Alternative Medicine Sourcebook, 1st Edition. Edited by Allan R. Cook. 737 pages. 1999. 0-7808-0200-4. $78.

"Recommended for public, high school, and academic libraries that have consumer health collections. Hospital libraries that also serve the public will find this to be a useful resource." — *E-Streams, Feb '03*

"Recommended reference source."
— *Booklist, American Library Association, Jan '03*

"An important alternate health reference."
— *MBR Bookwatch, Oct '02*

"A great addition to the reference collection of every type of library." — *American Reference Books Annual, 2000*

Alzheimer's Disease Sourcebook, 3rd Edition

Basic Consumer Health Information about Alzheimer's Disease, Other Dementias, and Related Disorders, Including Multi-Infarct Dementia, AIDS Dementia Complex, Dementia with Lewy Bodies, Huntington's Disease, Wernicke-Korsakoff Syndrome (Alcohol-Related Dementia), Delirium, and Confusional States

Along with Information for People Newly Diagnosed with Alzheimer's Disease and Caregivers, Reports Detailing Current Research Efforts in Prevention, Diagnosis, and Treatment, Facts about Long-Term Care Issues, and Listings of Sources for Additional Information

Edited by Karen Bellenir. 524 pages. 1999. 0-7808-0223-3. $78.

ALSO AVAILABLE: Alzheimer's, Stroke & 29 Other Neurological Disorders Sourcebook, 1st Edition. Edited by Frank E. Bair. 579 pages. 1993. 1-55888-748-2. $78.

ALSO AVAILABLE: Alzheimer's Disease Sourcebook, 2nd Edition. Edited by Karen Bellenir. 524 pages. 1999. 0-7808-0223-3. $78.

"Provides a wealth of useful information not otherwise available in one place. This resource is recommended for all types of libraries."
—*American Reference Books Annual, 2000*

"Recommended reference source."
— *Booklist, American Library Association, Oct '99*

SEE ALSO Brain Disorders Sourcebook

Arthritis Sourcebook

Basic Consumer Health Information about Specific Forms of Arthritis and Related Disorders, Including Rheumatoid Arthritis, Osteoarthritis, Gout, Polymyalgia Rheumatica, Psoriatic Arthritis, Spondyloarthropathies, Juvenile Rheumatoid Arthritis, and Juvenile Ankylosing Spondylitis

Along with Information about Medical, Surgical, and Alternative Treatment Options, and Including Strategies for Coping with Pain, Fatigue, and Stress

Edited by Allan R. Cook. 550 pages. 1998. 0-7808-0201-2. $78.

". . . accessible to the layperson."
—*Reference and Research Book News, Feb '99*

Asthma Sourcebook

Basic Consumer Health Information about Asthma, Including Symptoms, Traditional and Nontraditional Remedies, Treatment Advances, Quality-of-Life Aids, Medical Research Updates, and the Role of Allergies, Exercise, Age, the Environment, and Genetics in the Development of Asthma

Along with Statistical Data, a Glossary, and Directories of Support Groups, and Other Resources for Further Information

Edited by Annemarie S. Muth. 628 pages. 2000. 0-7808-0381-7. $78.

"A worthwhile reference acquisition for public libraries and academic medical libraries whose readers desire a quick introduction to the wide range of asthma information."
— *Choice, Association of College & Research Libraries, Jun '01*

"Recommended reference source."
— *Booklist, American Library Association, Feb '01*

"Highly recommended." — *The Bookwatch, Jan '01*

"There is much good information for patients and their families who deal with asthma daily."
— *American Medical Writers Association Journal, Winter '01*

"This informative text is recommended for consumer health collections in public, secondary school, and community college libraries and the libraries of universities with a large undergraduate population."
— *American Reference Books Annual, 2001*

■

Attention Deficit Disorder Sourcebook

Basic Consumer Health Information about Attention Deficit/Hyperactivity Disorder in Children and Adults, Including Facts about Causes, Symptoms, Diagnostic Criteria, and Treatment Options Such as Medications, Behavior Therapy, Coaching, and Homeopathy

Along with Reports on Current Research Initiatives, Legal Issues, and Government Regulations, and Featuring a Glossary of Related Terms, Internet Resources, and a List of Additional Reading Material

Edited by Dawn D. Matthews. 470 pages. 2002. 0-7808-0624-7. $78.

"Recommended reference source."
— *Booklist, American Library Association, Jan '03*

"This book is recommended for all school libraries and the reference or consumer health sections of public libraries." — *American Reference Books Annual, 2003*

■

Back & Neck Disorders Sourcebook

Basic Information about Disorders and Injuries of the Spinal Cord and Vertebrae, Including Facts on Chiropractic Treatment, Surgical Interventions, Paralysis, and Rehabilitation

Along with Advice for Preventing Back Trouble

Edited by Karen Bellenir. 548 pages. 1997. 0-7808-0202-0. $78.

"The strength of this work is its basic, easy-to-read format. Recommended."
— *Reference and User Services Quarterly, American Library Association, Winter '97*

Blood & Circulatory Disorders Sourcebook

Basic Information about Blood and Its Components, Anemias, Leukemias, Bleeding Disorders, and Circulatory Disorders, Including Aplastic Anemia, Thalassemia, Sickle-Cell Disease, Hemochromatosis, Hemophilia, Von Willebrand Disease, and Vascular Diseases

Along with a Special Section on Blood Transfusions and Blood Supply Safety, a Glossary, and Source Listings for Further Help and Information

Edited by Karen Bellenir and Linda M. Shin. 554 pages. 1998. 0-7808-0203-9. $78.

"Recommended reference source."
— *Booklist, American Library Association, Feb '99*

"An important reference sourcebook written in simple language for everyday, non-technical users. "
— *Reviewer's Bookwatch, Jan '99*

■

Brain Disorders Sourcebook

Basic Consumer Health Information about Strokes, Epilepsy, Amyotrophic Lateral Sclerosis (ALS/Lou Gehrig's Disease), Parkinson's Disease, Brain Tumors, Cerebral Palsy, Headache, Tourette Syndrome, and More

Along with Statistical Data, Treatment and Rehabilitation Options, Coping Strategies, Reports on Current Research Initiatives, a Glossary, and Resource Listings for Additional Help and Information

Edited by Karen Bellenir. 481 pages. 1999. 0-7808-0229-2. $78.

"Belongs on the shelves of any library with a consumer health collection." — *E-Streams, Mar '00*

"Recommended reference source."
— *Booklist, American Library Association, Oct '99*

SEE ALSO *Alzheimer's Disease Sourcebook*

■

Breast Cancer Sourcebook

Basic Consumer Health Information about Breast Cancer, Including Diagnostic Methods, Treatment Options, Alternative Therapies, Self-Help Information, Related Health Concerns, Statistical and Demographic Data, and Facts for Men with Breast Cancer

Along with Reports on Current Research Initiatives, a Glossary of Related Medical Terms, and a Directory of Sources for Further Help and Information

Edited by Edward J. Prucha and Karen Bellenir. 580 pages. 2001. 0-7808-0244-6. $78.

"It would be a useful reference book in a library or on loan to women in a support group."
— *Cancer Forum, Mar '03*

"Recommended reference source."
— *Booklist, American Library Association, Jan '02*

"This reference source is highly recommended. It is quite informative, comprehensive and detailed in nature, and yet it offers practical advice in easy-to-read language. It could be thought of as the 'bible' of breast cancer for the consumer."   —E-Streams, Jan '02

"The broad range of topics covered in lay language make the *Breast Cancer Sourcebook* an excellent addition to public and consumer health library collections."
—American Reference Books Annual 2002

"From the pros and cons of different screening methods and results to treatment options, *Breast Cancer Sourcebook* provides the latest information on the subject."
—Library Bookwatch, Dec '01

"This thoroughgoing, very readable reference covers all aspects of breast health and cancer. . . . Readers will find much to consider here. Recommended for all public and patient health collections."
—Library Journal, Sep '01

SEE ALSO *Cancer Sourcebook for Women, Women's Health Concerns Sourcebook*

Breastfeeding Sourcebook

Basic Consumer Health Information about the Benefits of Breastmilk, Preparing to Breastfeed, Breastfeeding as a Baby Grows, Nutrition, and More, Including Information on Special Situations and Concerns Such as Mastitis, Illness, Medications, Allergies, Multiple Births, Prematurity, Special Needs, and Adoption

Along with a Glossary and Resources for Additional Help and Information

Edited by Jenni Lynn Colson. 388 pages. 2002. 0-7808-0332-9. $78.

SEE ALSO *Pregnancy & Birth Sourcebook*

"Particularly useful is the information about professional lactation services and chapters on breastfeeding when returning to work. . . . *Breastfeeding Sourcebook* will be useful for public libraries, consumer health libraries, and technical schools offering nurse assistant training, especially in areas where Internet access is problematic."
—American Reference Books Annual, 2003

Burns Sourcebook

Basic Consumer Health Information about Various Types of Burns and Scalds, Including Flame, Heat, Cold, Electrical, Chemical, and Sun Burns

Along with Information on Short-Term and Long-Term Treatments, Tissue Reconstruction, Plastic Surgery, Prevention Suggestions, and First Aid

Edited by Allan R. Cook. 604 pages. 1999. 0-7808-0204-7. $78.

"This is an exceptional addition to the series and is highly recommended for all consumer health collections, hospital libraries, and academic medical centers."
—E-Streams, Mar '00

"This key reference guide is an invaluable addition to all health care and public libraries in confronting this ongoing health issue."
—American Reference Books Annual, 2000

"Recommended reference source."
—Booklist, American Library Association, Dec '99

SEE ALSO *Skin Disorders Sourcebook*

Cancer Sourcebook, 4th Edition

Basic Consumer Health Information about Major Forms and Stages of Cancer, Featuring Facts about Head and Neck Cancers, Lung Cancers, Gastrointestinal Cancers, Genitourinary Cancers, Lymphomas, Blood Cell Cancers, Endocrine Cancers, Skin Cancers, Bone Cancers, Sarcomas, and Others, and Including Information about Cancer Treatments and Therapies, Identifying and Reducing Cancer Risks, and Strategies for Coping with Cancer and the Side Effects of Treatment

Along with a Cancer Glossary, Statistical and Demographic Data, and a Directory of Sources for Additional Help and Information

Edited by Karen Bellenir. 1,119 pages. 2003. 0-7808-0633-6. $78.

ALSO AVAILABLE: *Cancer Sourcebook, 1st Edition.* Edited by Frank E. Bair. 932 pages. 1990. 1-55888-888-8. $78.

New Cancer Sourcebook, 2nd Edition. Edited by Allan R. Cook. 1,313 pages. 1996. 0-7808-0041-9. $78.

Cancer Sourcebook, 3rd Edition. Edited by Edward J. Prucha. 1,069 pages. 2000. 0-7808-0227-6. $78.

"This title is recommended for health sciences and public libraries with consumer health collections."
—E-Streams, Feb '01

". . . can be effectively used by cancer patients and their families who are looking for answers in a language they can understand. Public and hospital libraries should have it on their shelves."
—American Reference Books Annual, 2001

"Recommended reference source."
—Booklist, American Library Association, Dec '00

Cited in *Reference Sources for Small and Medium-Sized Libraries, American Library Association, 1999*

"The amount of factual and useful information is extensive. The writing is very clear, geared to general readers. Recommended for all levels."   —Choice, Association of College & Research Libraries, Jan '97

SEE ALSO *Breast Cancer Sourcebook, Cancer Sourcebook for Women, Pediatric Cancer Sourcebook, Prostate Cancer Sourcebook*

Cancer Sourcebook for Women, 2nd Edition

Basic Consumer Health Information about Gynecologic Cancers and Related Concerns, Including Cervical Cancer, Endometrial Cancer, Gestational Trophoblastic Tumor, Ovarian Cancer, Uterine Cancer, Vaginal Cancer, Vulvar Cancer, Breast Cancer, and Common Non-Cancerous Uterine Conditions, with Facts about Cancer Risk Factors, Screening and Prevention, Treatment Options, and Reports on Current Research Initiatives

Along with a Glossary of Cancer Terms and a Directory of Resources for Additional Help and Information

Edited by Karen Bellenir. 604 pages. 2002. 0-7808-0226-8. $78.

ALSO AVAILABLE: Cancer Sourcebook for Women, 1st Edition. Edited by Allan R. Cook and Peter D. Dresser. 524 pages. 1996. 0-7808-0076-1. $78.

"An excellent addition to collections in public, consumer health, and women's health libraries."
— American Reference Books Annual, 2003

"Overall, the information is excellent, and complex topics are clearly explained. As a reference book for the consumer it is a valuable resource to assist them to make informed decisions about cancer and its treatments."
— Cancer Forum, Nov '02

"Highly recommended for academic and medical reference collections."
— Library Bookwatch, Sep '02

"This is a highly recommended book for any public or consumer library, being reader friendly and containing accurate and helpful information."
— E-Streams, Aug '02

"Recommended reference source."
— Booklist, American Library Association, Jul '02

SEE ALSO Breast Cancer Sourcebook, Women's Health Concerns Sourcebook

---

Cardiovascular Diseases & Disorders Sourcebook, 1st Edition

SEE Heart Diseases & Disorders Sourcebook, 2nd Edition

Caregiving Sourcebook

Basic Consumer Health Information for Caregivers, Including a Profile of Caregivers, Caregiving Responsibilities and Concerns, Tips for Specific Conditions, Care Environments, and the Effects of Caregiving

Along with Facts about Legal Issues, Financial Information, and Future Planning, a Glossary, and a Listing of Additional Resources

Edited by Joyce Brennfleck Shannon. 600 pages. 2001. 0-7808-0331-0. $78.

"Essential for most collections."
— Library Journal, Apr 1, 2002

"An ideal addition to the reference collection of any public library. Health sciences information professionals may also want to acquire the Caregiving Sourcebook for their hospital or academic library for use as a ready reference tool by health care workers interested in aging and caregiving."
— E-Streams, Jan '02

"Recommended reference source."
— Booklist, American Library Association, Oct '01

Childhood Diseases & Disorders Sourcebook

Basic Consumer Health Information about Medical Problems Often Encountered in Pre-Adolescent Children, Including Respiratory Tract Ailments, Ear Infections, Sore Throats, Disorders of the Skin and Scalp, Digestive and Genitourinary Diseases, Infectious Diseases, Inflammatory Disorders, Chronic Physical and Developmental Disorders, Allergies, and More

Along with Information about Diagnostic Tests, Common Childhood Surgeries, and Frequently Used Medications, with a Glossary of Important Terms and Resource Directory

Edited by Chad T. Kimball. 662 pages. 2003. 0-7808-0458-9. $78.

Colds, Flu & Other Common Ailments Sourcebook

Basic Consumer Health Information about Common Ailments and Injuries, Including Colds, Coughs, the Flu, Sinus Problems, Headaches, Fever, Nausea and Vomiting, Menstrual Cramps, Diarrhea, Constipation, Hemorrhoids, Back Pain, Dandruff, Dry and Itchy Skin, Cuts, Scrapes, Sprains, Bruises, and More

Along with Information about Prevention, Self-Care, Choosing a Doctor, Over-the-Counter Medications, Folk Remedies, and Alternative Therapies, and Including a Glossary of Important Terms and a Directory of Resources for Further Help and Information

Edited by Chad T. Kimball. 638 pages. 2001. 0-7808-0435-X. $78.

"A good starting point for research on common illnesses. It will be a useful addition to public and consumer health library collections."
— American Reference Books Annual 2002

"Will prove valuable to any library seeking to maintain a current, comprehensive reference collection of health resources.... Excellent reference."
— The Bookwatch, Aug '01

"Recommended reference source."
— Booklist, American Library Association, July '01

Communication Disorders Sourcebook

Basic Information about Deafness and Hearing Loss, Speech and Language Disorders, Voice Disorders, Balance and Vestibular Disorders, and Disorders of Smell, Taste, and Touch

Edited by Linda M. Ross. 533 pages. 1996. 0-7808-0077-X. $78.

"This is skillfully edited and is a welcome resource for the layperson. It should be found in every public and medical library." — *Booklist Health Sciences Supplement, American Library Association, Oct '97*

■

Congenital Disorders Sourcebook

Basic Information about Disorders Acquired during Gestation, Including Spina Bifida, Hydrocephalus, Cerebral Palsy, Heart Defects, Craniofacial Abnormalities, Fetal Alcohol Syndrome, and More

Along with Current Treatment Options and Statistical Data

Edited by Karen Bellenir. 607 pages. 1997. 0-7808-0205-5. $78.

"Recommended reference source." — *Booklist, American Library Association, Oct '97*

SEE ALSO *Pregnancy & Birth Sourcebook*

■

Consumer Issues in Health Care Sourcebook

Basic Information about Health Care Fundamentals and Related Consumer Issues, Including Exams and Screening Tests, Physician Specialties, Choosing a Doctor, Using Prescription and Over-the-Counter Medications Safely, Avoiding Health Scams, Managing Common Health Risks in the Home, Care Options for Chronically or Terminally Ill Patients, and a List of Resources for Obtaining Help and Further Information

Edited by Karen Bellenir. 618 pages. 1998. 0-7808-0221-7. $78.

"Both public and academic libraries will want to have a copy in their collection for readers who are interested in self-education on health issues." — *American Reference Books Annual, 2000*

"The editor has researched the literature from government agencies and others, saving readers the time and effort of having to do the research themselves. Recommended for public libraries." — *Reference and User Services Quarterly, American Library Association, Spring '99*

"Recommended reference source." — *Booklist, American Library Association, Dec '98*

Contagious & Non-Contagious Infectious Diseases Sourcebook

Basic Information about Contagious Diseases like Measles, Polio, Hepatitis B, and Infectious Mononucleosis, and Non-Contagious Infectious Diseases like Tetanus and Toxic Shock Syndrome, and Diseases Occurring as Secondary Infections Such as Shingles and Reye Syndrome

Along with Vaccination, Prevention, and Treatment Information, and a Section Describing Emerging Infectious Disease Threats

Edited by Karen Bellenir and Peter D. Dresser. 566 pages. 1996. 0-7808-0075-3. $78.

■

Death & Dying Sourcebook

Basic Consumer Health Information for the Layperson about End-of-Life Care and Related Ethical and Legal Issues, Including Chief Causes of Death, Autopsies, Pain Management for the Terminally Ill, Life Support Systems, Insurance, Euthanasia, Assisted Suicide, Hospice Programs, Living Wills, Funeral Planning, Counseling, Mourning, Organ Donation, and Physician Training

Along with Statistical Data, a Glossary, and Listings of Sources for Further Help and Information

Edited by Annemarie S. Muth. 641 pages. 1999. 0-7808-0230-6. $78.

"Public libraries, medical libraries, and academic libraries will all find this sourcebook a useful addition to their collections." — *American Reference Books Annual, 2001*

"An extremely useful resource for those concerned with death and dying in the United States." — *Respiratory Care, Nov '00*

"Recommended reference source." — *Booklist, American Library Association, Aug '00*

"This book is a definite must for all those involved in end-of-life care." — *Doody's Review Service, 2000*

■

Dental Care & Oral Health Sourcebook, 2nd Edition

Basic Consumer Health Information about Dental Care, Including Oral Hygiene, Dental Visits, Pain Management, Cavities, Crowns, Bridges, Dental Implants, and Fillings, and Other Oral Health Concerns, Such as Gum Disease, Bad Breath, Dry Mouth, Genetic and Developmental Abnormalities, Oral Cancers, Orthodontics, and Temporomandibular Disorders

Along with Updates on Current Research in Oral Health, a Glossary, a Directory of Dental and Oral Health Organizations, and Resources for People with Dental and Oral Health Disorders

Edited by Amy L. Sutton. 609 pages. 2003. 0-7808-0634-4. $78.

"Unique source which will fill a gap in dental sources for patients and the lay public. A valuable reference tool even in a library with thousands of books on dentistry. Comprehensive, clear, inexpensive, and easy to read and use. It fills an enormous gap in the health care literature." —Reference and User Services Quarterly, American Library Association, Summer '98

"Recommended reference source."
—Booklist, American Library Association, Dec '97

Depression Sourcebook

Basic Consumer Health Information about Unipolar Depression, Bipolar Disorder, Postpartum Depression, Seasonal Affective Disorder, and Other Types of Depression in Children, Adolescents, Women, Men, the Elderly, and Other Selected Populations

Along with Facts about Causes, Risk Factors, Diagnostic Criteria, Treatment Options, Coping Strategies, Suicide Prevention, a Glossary, and a Directory of Sources for Additional Help and Information

Edited by Karen Belleni. 602 pages. 2002. 0-7808-0611-5. $78.

"Invaluable reference for public and school library collections alike." —Library Bookwatch, Apr '03

"Recommended for purchase."
—American Reference Books Annual, 2003

Diabetes Sourcebook, 3rd Edition

Basic Consumer Health Information about Type 1 Diabetes (Insulin-Dependent or Juvenile-Onset Diabetes), Type 2 Diabetes (Noninsulin-Dependent or Adult-Onset Diabetes), Gestational Diabetes, Impaired Glucose Tolerance (IGT), and Related Complications, Such as Amputation, Eye Disease, Gum Disease, Nerve Damage, and End-Stage Renal Disease, Including Facts about Insulin, Oral Diabetes Medications, Blood Sugar Testing, and the Role of Exercise and Nutrition in the Control of Diabetes

Along with a Glossary and Resources for Further Help and Information

Edited by Dawn D. Matthews. 622 pages. 2003. 0-7808-0629-8. $78.

ALSO AVAILABLE: Diabetes Sourcebook, 1st Edition. Edited by Karen Bellenir and Peter D. Dresser. 827 pages. 1994. 1-55888-751-2. $78.

Diabetes Sourcebook, 2nd Edition. Edited by Karen Bellenir. 688 pages. 1998. 0-7808-0224-1. $78.

"An invaluable reference." —Library Journal, May '00

Selected as one of the 250 "Best Health Sciences Books of 1999." —Doody's Rating Service, Mar-Apr 2000

"This comprehensive book is an excellent addition for high school, academic, medical, and public libraries. This volume is highly recommended."
—American Reference Books Annual, 2000

"Provides useful information for the general public."
—Healthlines, University of Michigan Health Management Research Center, Sep/Oct '99

". . . provides reliable mainstream medical information . . . belongs on the shelves of any library with a consumer health collection." —E-Streams, Sep '99

"Recommended reference source."
—Booklist, American Library Association, Feb '99

Diet & Nutrition Sourcebook, 2nd Edition

Basic Consumer Health Information about Dietary Guidelines, Recommended Daily Intake Values, Vitamins, Minerals, Fiber, Fat, Weight Control, Dietary Supplements, and Food Additives

Along with Special Sections on Nutrition Needs throughout Life and Nutrition for People with Such Specific Medical Concerns as Allergies, High Blood Cholesterol, Hypertension, Diabetes, Celiac Disease, Seizure Disorders, Phenylketonuria (PKU), Cancer, and Eating Disorders, and Including Reports on Current Nutrition Research and Source Listings for Additional Help and Information

Edited by Karen Bellenir. 650 pages. 1999. 0-7808-0228-4. $78.

ALSO AVAILABLE: Diet & Nutrition Sourcebook, 1st Edition. Edited by Dan R. Harris. 662 pages. 1996. 0-7808-0084-2. $78.

"This book is an excellent source of basic diet and nutrition information." —Booklist Health Sciences Supplement, American Library Association, Dec '00

"This reference document should be in any public library, but it would be a very good guide for beginning students in the health sciences. If the other books in this publisher's series are as good as this, they should all be in the health sciences collections."
—American Reference Books Annual, 2000

"This book is an excellent general nutrition reference for consumers who desire to take an active role in their health care for prevention. Consumers of all ages who select this book can feel confident they are receiving current and accurate information." —Journal of Nutrition for the Elderly, Vol. 19, No. 4, '00

"Recommended reference source."
—Booklist, American Library Association, Dec '99

SEE ALSO Digestive Diseases & Disorders Sourcebook, Eating Disorders Sourcebook, Gastrointestinal Diseases & Disorders Sourcebook, Vegetarian Sourcebook

Digestive Diseases & Disorders Sourcebook

Basic Consumer Health Information about Diseases and Disorders that Impact the Upper and Lower Digestive System, Including Celiac Disease, Constipation,

Crohn's Disease, Cyclic Vomiting Syndrome, Diarrhea, Diverticulosis and Diverticulitis, Gallstones, Heartburn, Hemorrhoids, Hernias, Indigestion (Dyspepsia), Irritable Bowel Syndrome, Lactose Intolerance, Ulcers, and More

Along with Information about Medications and Other Treatments, Tips for Maintaining a Healthy Digestive Tract, a Glossary, and Directory of Digestive Diseases Organizations

Edited by Karen Bellenir. 335 pages. 2000. 0-7808-0327-2. $78.

"This title would be an excellent addition to all public or patient-research libraries."
—American Reference Books Annual, 2001

"This title is recommended for public, hospital, and health sciences libraries with consumer health collections." —E-Streams, Jul-Aug '00

"Recommended reference source."
—Booklist, American Library Association, May '00

SEE ALSO Diet & Nutrition Sourcebook, Eating Disorders Sourcebook, Gastrointestinal Diseases & Disorders Sourcebook

■

Disabilities Sourcebook

Basic Consumer Health Information about Physical and Psychiatric Disabilities, Including Descriptions of Major Causes of Disability, Assistive and Adaptive Aids, Workplace Issues, and Accessibility Concerns

Along with Information about the Americans with Disabilities Act, a Glossary, and Resources for Additional Help and Information

Edited by Dawn D. Matthews. 616 pages. 2000. 0-7808-0389-2. $78.

"It is a must for libraries with a consumer health section." — American Reference Books Annual 2002

"A much needed addition to the Omnigraphics Health Reference Series. A current reference work to provide people with disabilities, their families, caregivers or those who work with them, a broad range of information in one volume, has not been available until now. . . . It is recommended for all public and academic library reference collections." — E-Streams, May '01

"An excellent source book in easy-to-read format covering many current topics; highly recommended for all libraries." — Choice, Association of College and Research Libraries, Jan '01

"Recommended reference source."
—Booklist, American Library Association, Jul '00

■

Domestic Violence & Child Abuse Sourcebook

Basic Consumer Health Information about Spousal/ Partner, Child, Sibling, Parent, and Elder Abuse, Covering Physical, Emotional, and Sexual Abuse, Teen Dating Violence, and Stalking; Includes Information

about Hotlines, Safe Houses, Safety Plans, and Other Resources for Support and Assistance, Community Initiatives, and Reports on Current Directions in Research and Treatment

Along with a Glossary, Sources for Further Reading, and Governmental and Non-Governmental Organizations Contact Information

Edited by Helene Henderson. 1,064 pages. 2001. 0-7808-0235-7. $78.

"Interested lay persons should find the book extremely beneficial. . . . A copy of Domestic Violence and Child Abuse Sourcebook should be in every public library in the United States."
— Social Science & Medicine, No. 56, 2003

"This is important information. The Web has many resources but this sourcebook fills an important societal need. I am not aware of any other resources of this type." — Doody's Review Service, Sep '01

"Recommended for all libraries, scholars, and practitioners." — Choice, Association of College & Research Libraries, Jul '01

"Recommended reference source."
— Booklist, American Library Association, Apr '01

"Important pick for college-level health reference libraries." — The Bookwatch, Mar '01

"Because this problem is so widespread and because this book includes a lot of issues within one volume, this work is recommended for all public libraries."
— American Reference Books Annual, 2001

■

Drug Abuse Sourcebook

Basic Consumer Health Information about Illicit Substances of Abuse and the Diversion of Prescription Medications, Including Depressants, Hallucinogens, Inhalants, Marijuana, Narcotics, Stimulants, and Anabolic Steroids

Along with Facts about Related Health Risks, Treatment Issues, and Substance Abuse Prevention Programs, a Glossary of Terms, Statistical Data, and Directories of Hotline Services, Self-Help Groups, and Organizations Able to Provide Further Information

Edited by Karen Bellenir. 629 pages. 2000. 0-7808-0242-X. $78.

"Containing a wealth of information . . . . This resource belongs in libraries that serve a lower-division undergraduate or community college clientele as well as the general public." — Choice, Association of College and Research Libraries, Jun '01

"Recommended reference source."
— Booklist, American Library Association, Feb '01

"Highly recommended." — The Bookwatch, Jan '01

"Even though there is a plethora of books on drug abuse, this volume is recommended for school, public, and college libraries."
—American Reference Books Annual, 2001

SEE ALSO Alcoholism Sourcebook, Substance Abuse Sourcebook

Ear, Nose & Throat Disorders Sourcebook

Basic Information about Disorders of the Ears, Nose, Sinus Cavities, Pharynx, and Larynx, Including Ear Infections, Tinnitus, Vestibular Disorders, Allergic and Non-Allergic Rhinitis, Sore Throats, Tonsillitis, and Cancers That Affect the Ears, Nose, Sinuses, and Throat

Along with Reports on Current Research Initiatives, a Glossary of Related Medical Terms, and a Directory of Sources for Further Help and Information

Edited by Karen Bellenir and Linda M. Shin. 576 pages. 1998. 0-7808-0206-3. $78.

"Overall, this sourcebook is helpful for the consumer seeking information on ENT issues. It is recommended for public libraries."
—American Reference Books Annual, 1999

"Recommended reference source."
—Booklist, American Library Association, Dec '98

Eating Disorders Sourcebook

Basic Consumer Health Information about Eating Disorders, Including Information about Anorexia Nervosa, Bulimia Nervosa, Binge Eating, Body Dysmorphic Disorder, Pica, Laxative Abuse, and Night Eating Syndrome

Along with Information about Causes, Adverse Effects, and Treatment and Prevention Issues, and Featuring a Section on Concerns Specific to Children and Adolescents, a Glossary, and Resources for Further Help and Information

Edited by Dawn D. Matthews. 322 pages. 2001. 0-7808-0335-3. $78.

"Recommended for health science libraries that are open to the public, as well as hospital libraries. This book is a good resource for the consumer who is concerned about eating disorders." *— E-Streams, Mar '02*

"This volume is another convenient collection of excerpted articles. Recommended for school and public library patrons; lower-division undergraduates; and two-year technical program students." *— Choice, Association of College & Research Libraries, Jan '02*

"Recommended reference source." *— Booklist, American Library Association, Oct '01*

SEE ALSO *Diet & Nutrition Sourcebook, Digestive Diseases & Disorders Sourcebook, Gastrointestinal Diseases & Disorders Sourcebook*

Emergency Medical Services Sourcebook

Basic Consumer Health Information about Preventing, Preparing for, and Managing Emergency Situations, When and Who to Call for Help, What to Expect in the Emergency Room, the Emergency Medical Team, Patient Issues, and Current Topics in Emergency Medicine

Along with Statistical Data, a Glossary, and Sources of Additional Help and Information

Edited by Jenni Lynn Colson. 494 pages. 2002. 0-7808-0420-1. $78.

"Handy and convenient for home, public, school, and college libraries. Recommended." *— Choice, Association of College and Research Libraries, Apr '03*

"This reference can provide the consumer with answers to most questions about emergency care in the United States, or it will direct them to a resource where the answer can be found."
—American Reference Books Annual, 2003

"Recommended reference source."
— Booklist, American Library Association, Feb '03

Endocrine & Metabolic Disorders Sourcebook

Basic Information for the Layperson about Pancreatic and Insulin-Related Disorders Such as Pancreatitis, Diabetes, and Hypoglycemia; Adrenal Gland Disorders Such as Cushing's Syndrome, Addison's Disease, and Congenital Adrenal Hyperplasia; Pituitary Gland Disorders Such as Growth Hormone Deficiency, Acromegaly, and Pituitary Tumors; Thyroid Disorders Such as Hypothyroidism, Graves' Disease, Hashimoto's Disease, and Goiter; Hyperparathyroidism; and Other Diseases and Syndromes of Hormone Imbalance or Metabolic Dysfunction

Along with Reports on Current Research Initiatives

Edited by Linda M. Shin. 574 pages. 1998. 0-7808-0207-1. $78.

"Omnigraphics has produced another needed resource for health information consumers."
—American Reference Books Annual, 2000

"Recommended reference source."
— Booklist, American Library Association, Dec '98

Environmental Health Sourcebook, 2nd Edition

Basic Consumer Health Information about the Environment and Its Effect on Human Health, Including the Effects of Air Pollution, Water Pollution, Hazardous Chemicals, Food Hazards, Radiation Hazards, Biological Agents, Household Hazards, Such as Radon, Asbestos, Carbon Monoxide, and Mold, and Information about Associated Diseases and Disorders, Including Cancer, Allergies, Respiratory Problems, and Skin Disorders

Along with Information about Environmental Concerns for Specific Populations, a Glossary of Related Terms, and Resources for Further Help and Information

Edited by Dawn D. Matthews. 673 pages. 2003. 0-7808-0632-8. $78.

ALSO AVAILABLE: *Environmentally Induced Disorders Sourcebook, 1st Edition.* Edited by Allan R. Cook. 620 pages. 1997. 0-7808-0083-4. $78.

"Recommended reference source."
— Booklist, American Library Association, Sep '98

"This book will be a useful addition to anyone's library." —Choice Health Sciences Supplement, Association of College and Research Libraries, May '98

". . . a good survey of numerous environmentally induced physical disorders . . . a useful addition to anyone's library." —Doody's Health Sciences Book Reviews, Jan '98

". . . provide[s] introductory information from the best authorities around. Since this volume covers topics that potentially affect everyone, it will surely be one of the most frequently consulted volumes in the *Health Reference Series*." —Rettig on Reference, Nov '97

Environmentally Induced Disorders Sourcebook, 1st Edition

SEE *Environmental Health Sourcebook, 2nd Edition*

Ethnic Diseases Sourcebook

Basic Consumer Health Information for Ethnic and Racial Minority Groups in the United States, Including General Health Indicators and Behaviors, Ethnic Diseases, Genetic Testing, the Impact of Chronic Diseases, Women's Health, Mental Health Issues, and Preventive Health Care Services

Along with a Glossary and a Listing of Additional Resources

Edited by Joyce Brennfleck Shannon. 664 pages. 2001. 0-7808-0336-1. $78.

"Recommended for health sciences libraries where public health programs are a priority." —E-Streams, Jan '02

"Not many books have been written on this topic to date, and the *Ethnic Diseases Sourcebook* is a strong addition to the list. It will be an important introductory resource for health consumers, students, health care personnel, and social scientists. It is recommended for public, academic, and large hospital libraries." —American Reference Books Annual 2002

"Recommended reference source." —Booklist, American Library Association, Oct '01

"Will prove valuable to any library seeking to maintain a current, comprehensive reference collection of health resources. . . . An excellent source of health information about genetic disorders which affect particular ethnic and racial minorities in the U.S." —The Bookwatch, Aug '01

Eye Care Sourcebook, 2nd Edition

Basic Consumer Health Information about Eye Care and Eye Disorders, Including Facts about the Diagnosis, Prevention, and Treatment of Common Refractive Problems Such as Myopia, Hyperopia, Astigmatism, and Presbyopia, and Eye Diseases, Including

Glaucoma, Cataract, Age-Related Macular Degeneration, and Diabetic Retinopathy

Along with a Section on Vision Correction and Refractive Surgeries, Including LASIK and LASEK, a Glossary, and Directories of Resources for Additional Help and Information

Edited by Amy L. Sutton. 543 pages. 2003. 0-7808-0635-2. $78.

ALSO AVAILABLE: Ophthalmic Disorders Sourcebook, 1st Edition. Edited by Linda M. Ross. 631 pages. 1996. 0-7808-0081-8. $78.

Family Planning Sourcebook

Basic Consumer Health Information about Planning for Pregnancy and Contraception, Including Traditional Methods, Barrier Methods, Hormonal Methods, Permanent Methods, Future Methods, Emergency Contraception, and Birth Control Choices for Women at Each Stage of Life

Along with Statistics, a Glossary, and Sources of Additional Information

Edited by Amy Marcaccio Keyzer. 520 pages. 2001. 0-7808-0379-5. $78.

"Recommended for public, health, and undergraduate libraries as part of the circulating collection." —E-Streams, Mar '02

"Information is presented in an unbiased, readable manner, and the sourcebook will certainly be a necessary addition to those public and high school libraries where Internet access is restricted or otherwise problematic." —American Reference Books Annual 2002

"Recommended reference source." —Booklist, American Library Association, Oct '01

"Will prove valuable to any library seeking to maintain a current, comprehensive reference collection of health resources. . . . Excellent reference." —The Bookwatch, Aug '01

SEE ALSO *Pregnancy & Birth Sourcebook*

Fitness & Exercise Sourcebook, 2nd Edition

Basic Consumer Health Information about the Fundamentals of Fitness and Exercise, Including How to Begin and Maintain a Fitness Program, Fitness as a Lifestyle, the Link between Fitness and Diet, Advice for Specific Groups of People, Exercise as It Relates to Specific Medical Conditions, and Recent Research in Fitness and Exercise

Along with a Glossary of Important Terms and Resources for Additional Help and Information

Edited by Kristen M. Gledhill. 646 pages. 2001. 0-7808-0334-5. $78.

ALSO AVAILABLE: Fitness & Exercise Sourcebook, 1st Edition. Edited by Dan R. Harris. 663 pages. 1996. 0-7808-0186-5. $78.

"This work is recommended for all general reference collections."
— *American Reference Books Annual 2002*

"Highly recommended for public, consumer, and school grades fourth through college."
— *E-Streams, Nov '01*

"Recommended reference source." — *Booklist, American Library Association, Oct '01*

"The information appears quite comprehensive and is considered reliable. . . . This second edition is a welcomed addition to the series."
— *Doody's Review Service, Sep '01*

"This reference is a valuable choice for those who desire a broad source of information on exercise, fitness, and chronic-disease prevention through a healthy lifestyle." — *American Medical Writers Association Journal, Fall '01*

"Will prove valuable to any library seeking to maintain a current, comprehensive reference collection of health resources. . . . Excellent reference."
— *The Bookwatch, Aug '01*

Food & Animal Borne Diseases Sourcebook

Basic Information about Diseases That Can Be Spread to Humans through the Ingestion of Contaminated Food or Water or by Contact with Infected Animals and Insects, Such as Botulism, E. Coli, Hepatitis A, Trichinosis, Lyme Disease, and Rabies

Along with Information Regarding Prevention and Treatment Methods, and Including a Special Section for International Travelers Describing Diseases Such as Cholera, Malaria, Travelers' Diarrhea, and Yellow Fever, and Offering Recommendations for Avoiding Illness

Edited by Karen Bellenir and Peter D. Dresser. 535 pages. 1995. 0-7808-0033-8. $78.

"Targeting general readers and providing them with a single, comprehensive source of information on selected topics, this book continues, with the excellent caliber of its predecessors, to catalog topical information on health matters of general interest. Readable and thorough, this valuable resource is highly recommended for all libraries."
— *Academic Library Book Review, Summer '96*

"A comprehensive collection of authoritative information." — *Emergency Medical Services, Oct '95*

Food Safety Sourcebook

Basic Consumer Health Information about the Safe Handling of Meat, Poultry, Seafood, Eggs, Fruit Juices, and Other Food Items, and Facts about Pesticides, Drinking Water, Food Safety Overseas, and the Onset, Duration, and Symptoms of Foodborne Illnesses, Including Types of Pathogenic Bacteria, Parasitic Protozoa, Worms, Viruses, and Natural Toxins

Along with the Role of the Consumer, the Food Handler, and the Government in Food Safety; a Glossary, and

Resources for Additional Help and Information

Edited by Dawn D. Matthews. 339 pages. 1999. 0-7808-0326-4. $78.

"This book is recommended for public libraries and universities with home economic and food science programs." — *E-Streams, Nov '00*

"Recommended reference source."
— *Booklist, American Library Association, May '00*

"This book takes the complex issues of food safety and foodborne pathogens and presents them in an easily understood manner. [It does] an excellent job of covering a large and often confusing topic."
— *American Reference Books Annual, 2000*

Forensic Medicine Sourcebook

Basic Consumer Information for the Layperson about Forensic Medicine, Including Crime Scene Investigation, Evidence Collection and Analysis, Expert Testimony, Computer-Aided Criminal Identification, Digital Imaging in the Courtroom, DNA Profiling, Accident Reconstruction, Autopsies, Ballistics, Drugs and Explosives Detection, Latent Fingerprints, Product Tampering, and Questioned Document Examination

Along with Statistical Data, a Glossary of Forensics Terminology, and Listings of Sources for Further Help and Information

Edited by Annemarie S. Muth. 574 pages. 1999. 0-7808-0232-2. $78.

"Given the expected widespread interest in its content and its easy to read style, this book is recommended for most public and all college and university libraries."
— *E-Streams, Feb '01*

"Recommended for public libraries."
— *Reference & User Services Quarterly, American Library Association, Spring 2000*

"Recommended reference source."
— *Booklist, American Library Association, Feb '00*

"A wealth of information, useful statistics, references are up-to-date and extremely complete. This wonderful collection of data will help students who are interested in a career in any type of forensic field. It is a great resource for attorneys who need information about types of expert witnesses needed in a particular case. It also offers useful information for fiction and nonfiction writers whose work involves a crime. A fascinating compilation. All levels." — *Choice, Association of College and Research Libraries, Jan 2000*

"There are several items that make this book attractive to consumers who are seeking certain forensic data. . . . This is a useful current source for those seeking general forensic medical answers."
— *American Reference Books Annual, 2000*

Gastrointestinal Diseases & Disorders Sourcebook

Basic Information about Gastroesophageal Reflux Disease (Heartburn), Ulcers, Diverticulosis, Irritable Bowel Syndrome, Crohn's Disease, Ulcerative Colitis, Diarrhea, Constipation, Lactose Intolerance, Hemorrhoids, Hepatitis, Cirrhosis, and Other Digestive Problems, Featuring Statistics, Descriptions of Symptoms, and Current Treatment Methods of Interest for Persons Living with Upper and Lower Gastrointestinal Maladies

Edited by Linda M. Ross. 413 pages. 1996. 0-7808-0078-8. $78.

". . . very readable form. The successful editorial work that brought this material together into a useful and understandable reference makes accessible to all readers information that can help them more effectively understand and obtain help for digestive tract problems."
— *Choice, Association of College & Research Libraries, Feb '97*

SEE ALSO *Diet & Nutrition Sourcebook, Digestive Diseases & Disorders, Eating Disorders Sourcebook*

Genetic Disorders Sourcebook, 2nd Edition

Basic Consumer Health Information about Hereditary Diseases and Disorders, Including Cystic Fibrosis, Down Syndrome, Hemophilia, Huntington's Disease, Sickle Cell Anemia, and More; Facts about Genes, Gene Research and Therapy, Genetic Screening, Ethics of Gene Testing, Genetic Counseling, and Advice on Coping and Caring

Along with a Glossary of Genetic Terminology and a Resource List for Help, Support, and Further Information

Edited by Kathy Massimini. 768 pages. 2001. 0-7808-0241-1. $78.

ALSO AVAILABLE: *Genetic Disorders Sourcebook, 1st Edition.* Edited by Karen Bellenir. 642 pages. 1996. 0-7808-0034-6. $78.

"Recommended for public libraries and medical and hospital libraries with consumer health collections."
— *E-Streams, May '01*

"Recommended reference source."
— *Booklist, American Library Association, Apr '01*

"Important pick for college-level health reference libraries."
— *The Bookwatch, Mar '01*

"Provides essential medical information to both the general public and those diagnosed with a serious or fatal genetic disease or disorder."
— *Choice, Association of College and Research Libraries, Jan '97*

Head Trauma Sourcebook

Basic Information for the Layperson about Open-Head and Closed-Head Injuries, Treatment Advances, Recovery, and Rehabilitation

Along with Reports on Current Research Initiatives

Edited by Karen Bellenir. 414 pages. 1997. 0-7808-0208-X. $78.

Headache Sourcebook

Basic Consumer Health Information about Migraine, Tension, Cluster, Rebound and Other Types of Headaches, with Facts about the Cause and Prevention of Headaches, the Effects of Stress and the Environment, Headaches during Pregnancy and Menopause, and Childhood Headaches

Along with a Glossary and Other Resources for Additional Help and Information

Edited by Dawn D. Matthews. 362 pages. 2002. 0-7808-0337-X. $78.

"Highly recommended for academic and medical reference collections." — *Library Bookwatch, Sep '02*

Health Insurance Sourcebook

Basic Information about Managed Care Organizations, Traditional Fee-for-Service Insurance, Insurance Portability and Pre-Existing Conditions Clauses, Medicare, Medicaid, Social Security, and Military Health Care

Along with Information about Insurance Fraud

Edited by Wendy Wilcox. 530 pages. 1997. 0-7808-0222-5. $78.

"Particularly useful because it brings much of this information together in one volume. This book will be a handy reference source in the health sciences library, hospital library, college and university library, and medium to large public library."
— *Medical Reference Services Quarterly, Fall '98*

Awarded "Books of the Year Award"
— *American Journal of Nursing, 1997*

"The layout of the book is particularly helpful as it provides easy access to reference material. A most useful addition to the vast amount of information about health insurance. The use of data from U.S. government agencies is most commendable. Useful in a library or learning center for healthcare professional students."
— *Doody's Health Sciences Book Reviews, Nov '97*

Health Reference Series Cumulative Index 1999

A Comprehensive Index to the Individual Volumes of the Health Reference Series, Including a Subject Index, Name Index, Organization Index, and Publication Index

Along with a Master List of Acronyms and Abbreviations

Edited by Edward J. Prucha, Anne Holmes, and Robert Rudnick. 990 pages. 2000. 0-7808-0382-5. $78.

"This volume will be most helpful in libraries that have a relatively complete collection of the Health Reference Series." —American Reference Books Annual, 2001

"Essential for collections that hold any of the numerous *Health Reference Series* titles." — Choice, Association of College and Research Libraries, Nov '00

Healthy Aging Sourcebook

Basic Consumer Health Information about Maintaining Health through the Aging Process, Including Advice on Nutrition, Exercise, and Sleep, Help in Making Decisions about Midlife Issues and Retirement, and Guidance Concerning Practical and Informed Choices in Health Consumerism

Along with Data Concerning the Theories of Aging, Different Experiences in Aging by Minority Groups, and Facts about Aging Now and Aging in the Future; and Featuring a Glossary, a Guide to Consumer Help, Additional Suggested Reading, and Practical Resource Directory

Edited by Jenifer Swanson. 536 pages. 1999. 0-7808-0390-6. $78.

"Recommended reference source." —Booklist, American Library Association, Feb '00

SEE ALSO *Physical & Mental Issues in Aging Sourcebook*

Healthy Children Sourcebook

Basic Consumer Health Information about the Physical and Mental Development of Children between the Ages of 3 and 12, Including Routine Health Care, Preventative Health Services, Safety and First Aid, Healthy Sleep, Dental Care, Nutrition, and Fitness, and Featuring Parenting Tips on Such Topics as Bedwetting, Choosing Day Care, Monitoring TV and Other Media, and Establishing a Foundation for Substance Abuse Prevention

Along with a Glossary of Commonly Used Pediatric Terms and Resources for Additional Help and Information.

Edited by Chad T. Kimball. 648 pages. 2003. 0-7808-0247-0. $78.

Healthy Heart Sourcebook for Women

Basic Consumer Health Information about Cardiac Issues Specific to Women, Including Facts about Major Risk Factors and Prevention, Treatment and Control Strategies, and Important Dietary Issues

Along with a Special Section Regarding the Pros and Cons of Hormone Replacement Therapy and Its Impact on Heart Health, and Additional Help, Including Recipes, a Glossary, and a Directory of Resources

Edited by Dawn D. Matthews. 336 pages. 2000. 0-7808-0329-9. $78.

"A good reference source and recommended for all public, academic, medical, and hospital libraries." — Medical Reference Services Quarterly, Summer '01

"Because of the lack of information specific to women on this topic, this book is recommended for public libraries and consumer libraries." —American Reference Books Annual, 2001

"Contains very important information about coronary artery disease that all women should know. The information is current and presented in an easy-to-read format. The book will make a good addition to any library." —American Medical Writers Association Journal, Summer '00

"Important, basic reference." —Reviewer's Bookwatch, Jul '00

SEE ALSO *Heart Diseases & Disorders Sourcebook, Women's Health Concerns Sourcebook*

Heart Diseases & Disorders Sourcebook, 2nd Edition

Basic Consumer Health Information about Heart Attacks, Angina, Rhythm Disorders, Heart Failure, Valve Disease, Congenital Heart Disorders, and More, Including Descriptions of Surgical Procedures and Other Interventions, Medications, Cardiac Rehabilitation, Risk Identification, and Prevention Tips

Along with Statistical Data, Reports on Current Research Initiatives, a Glossary of Cardiovascular Terms, and Resource Directory

Edited by Karen Bellenir. 612 pages. 2000. 0-7808-0238-1. $78.

ALSO AVAILABLE: *Cardiovascular Diseases & Disorders Sourcebook, 1st Edition.* Edited by Karen Bellenir and Peter D. Dresser. 683 pages. 1995. 0-7808-0032-X. $78.

"This work stands out as an imminently accessible resource for the general public. It is recommended for the reference and circulating shelves of school, public, and academic libraries." —American Reference Books Annual, 2001

"Recommended reference source." —Booklist, American Library Association, Dec '00

"Provides comprehensive coverage of matters related to the heart. This title is recommended for health sciences and public libraries with consumer health collections." — E-Streams, Oct '00

SEE ALSO *Healthy Heart Sourcebook for Women*

Household Safety Sourcebook

Basic Consumer Health Information about Household Safety, Including Information about Poisons, Chemicals, Fire, and Water Hazards in the Home

Along with Advice about the Safe Use of Home Maintenance Equipment, Choosing Toys and Nursery Furni-

ture, Holiday and Recreation Safety, a Glossary, and Resources for Further Help and Information

Edited by Dawn D. Matthews. 606 pages. 2002. 0-7808-0338-8. $78.

"This work will be useful in public libraries with large consumer health and wellness departments."
— American Reference Books Annual, 2003

"As a sourcebook on household safety this book meets its mark. It is encyclopedic in scope and covers a wide range of safety issues that are commonly seen in the home." — E-Streams, Jul '02

■

Immune System Disorders Sourcebook

Basic Information about Lupus, Multiple Sclerosis, Guillain-Barré Syndrome, Chronic Granulomatous Disease, and More

Along with Statistical and Demographic Data and Reports on Current Research Initiatives

Edited by Allan R. Cook. 608 pages. 1997. 0-7808-0209-8. $78.

■

Infant & Toddler Health Sourcebook

Basic Consumer Health Information about the Physical and Mental Development of Newborns, Infants, and Toddlers, Including Neonatal Concerns, Nutrition Recommendations, Immunization Schedules, Common Pediatric Disorders, Assessments and Milestones, Safety Tips, and Advice for Parents and Other Caregivers

Along with a Glossary of Terms and Resource Listings for Additional Help

Edited by Jenifer Swanson. 585 pages. 2000. 0-7808-0246-2. $78.

"As a reference for the general public, this would be useful in any library." — E-Streams, May '01

"Recommended reference source."
— Booklist, American Library Association, Feb '01

"This is a good source for general use."
— American Reference Books Annual, 2001

■

Injury & Trauma Sourcebook

Basic Consumer Health Information about the Impact of Injury, the Diagnosis and Treatment of Common and Traumatic Injuries, Emergency Care, and Specific Injuries Related to Home, Community, Workplace, Transportation, and Recreation

Along with Guidelines for Injury Prevention, a Glossary, and a Directory of Additional Resources

Edited by Joyce Brennfleck Shannon. 696 pages. 2002. 0-7808-0421-X. $78.

"This publication is the most comprehensive work of its kind about injury and trauma."
— American Reference Books Annual, 2003

"This sourcebook provides concise, easily readable, basic health information about injuries. . . . This book is well organized and an easy to use reference resource suitable for hospital, health sciences and public libraries with consumer health collections."
— E-Streams, Nov '02

"Practitioners should be aware of guides such as this in order to facilitate their use by patients and their families." — Doody's Health Sciences Book Review Journal, Sep-Oct '02

"Recommended reference source."
— Booklist, American Library Association, Sep '02

"Highly recommended for academic and medical reference collections." — Library Bookwatch, Sep '02

■

Kidney & Urinary Tract Diseases & Disorders Sourcebook

Basic Information about Kidney Stones, Urinary Incontinence, Bladder Disease, End Stage Renal Disease, Dialysis, and More

Along with Statistical and Demographic Data and Reports on Current Research Initiatives

Edited by Linda M. Ross. 602 pages. 1997. 0-7808-0079-6. $78.

■

Learning Disabilities Sourcebook, 2nd Edition

Basic Consumer Health Information about Learning Disabilities, Including Dyslexia, Developmental Speech and Language Disabilities, Non-Verbal Learning Disorders, Developmental Arithmetic Disorder, Developmental Writing Disorder, and Other Conditions That Impede Learning Such as Attention Deficit/ Hyperactivity Disorder, Brain Injury, Hearing Impairment, Klinefelter Syndrome, Dyspraxia, and Tourette Syndrome

Along with Facts about Educational Issues and Assistive Technology, Coping Strategies, a Glossary of Related Terms, and Resources for Further Help and Information

Edited by Dawn D. Matthews. 621 pages. 2003. 0-7808-0626-3. $78.

ALSO AVAILABLE: Learning Disabilities Sourcebook, 1st Edition. Edited by Linda M. Shin. 579 pages. 1998. 0-7808-0210-1. $78.

"Teachers as well as consumers will find this an essential guide to understanding various syndromes and their latest treatments. [An] invaluable reference for public and school library collections alike."
— Library Bookwatch, Apr '03

Named "Outstanding Reference Book of 1999."
— New York Public Library, Feb 2000

"An excellent candidate for inclusion in a public library reference section. It's a great source of information. Teachers will also find the book useful. Definitely worth reading."
— Journal of Adolescent & Adult Literacy, Feb 2000

"Readable . . . provides a solid base of information regarding successful techniques used with individuals who have learning disabilities, as well as practical suggestions for educators and family members. Clear language, concise descriptions, and pertinent information for contacting multiple resources add to the strength of this book as a useful tool." — *Choice, Association of College and Research Libraries, Feb '99*

"Recommended reference source."
— *Booklist, American Library Association, Sep '98*

"A useful resource for libraries and for those who don't have the time to identify and locate the individual publications." — *Disability Resources Monthly, Sep '98*

Leukemia Sourcebook

Basic Consumer Health Information about Adult and Childhood Leukemias, Including Acute Lymphocytic Leukemia (ALL), Chronic Lymphocytic Leukemia (CLL), Acute Myelogenous Leukemia (AML), Chronic Myelogenous Leukemia (CML), and Hairy Cell Leukemia, and Treatments Such as Chemotherapy, Radiation Therapy, Peripheral Blood Stem Cell and Marrow Transplantation, and Immunotherapy

Along with Tips for Life During and After Treatment, a Glossary, and Directories of Additional Resources

Edited by Joyce Brennfleck Shannon. 587 pages. 2003. 0-7808-0627-1. $78.

Liver Disorders Sourcebook

Basic Consumer Health Information about the Liver and How It Works; Liver Diseases, Including Cancer, Cirrhosis, Hepatitis, and Toxic and Drug Related Diseases; Tips for Maintaining a Healthy Liver; Laboratory Tests, Radiology Tests, and Facts about Liver Transplantation

Along with a Section on Support Groups, a Glossary, and Resource Listings

Edited by Joyce Brennfleck Shannon. 591 pages. 2000. 0-7808-0383-3. $78.

"A valuable resource."
— *American Reference Books Annual, 2001*

"This title is recommended for health sciences and public libraries with consumer health collections."
— *E-Streams, Oct '00*

"Recommended reference source."
— *Booklist, American Library Association, Jun '00*

Lung Disorders Sourcebook

Basic Consumer Health Information about Emphysema, Pneumonia, Tuberculosis, Asthma, Cystic Fibrosis, and Other Lung Disorders, Including Facts about Diagnostic Procedures, Treatment Strategies, Disease Prevention Efforts, and Such Risk Factors as Smoking, Air Pollution, and Exposure to Asbestos, Radon, and Other Agents

Along with a Glossary and Resources for Additional Help and Information

Edited by Dawn D. Matthews. 678 pages. 2002. 0-7808-0339-6. $78.

"This title is a great addition for public and school libraries because it provides concise health information on the lungs."
— *American Reference Books Annual, 2003*

"Highly recommended for academic and medical reference collections." — *Library Bookwatch, Sep '02*

Medical Tests Sourcebook

Basic Consumer Health Information about Medical Tests, Including Periodic Health Exams, General Screening Tests, Tests You Can Do at Home, Findings of the U.S. Preventive Services Task Force, X-ray and Radiology Tests, Electrical Tests, Tests of Blood and Other Body Fluids and Tissues, Scope Tests, Lung Tests, Genetic Tests, Pregnancy Tests, Newborn Screening Tests, Sexually Transmitted Disease Tests, and Computer Aided Diagnoses

Along with a Section on Paying for Medical Tests, a Glossary, and Resource Listings

Edited by Joyce Brennfleck Shannon. 691 pages. 1999. 0-7808-0243-8. $78.

"Recommended for hospital and health sciences libraries with consumer health collections."
— *E-Streams, Mar '00*

"This is an overall excellent reference with a wealth of general knowledge that may aid those who are reluctant to get vital tests performed."
— *Today's Librarian, Jan 2000*

"A valuable reference guide."
— *American Reference Books Annual, 2000*

Men's Health Concerns Sourcebook

Basic Information about Health Issues That Affect Men, Featuring Facts about the Top Causes of Death in Men, Including Heart Disease, Stroke, Cancers, Prostate Disorders, Chronic Obstructive Pulmonary Disease, Pneumonia and Influenza, Human Immunodeficiency Virus and Acquired Immune Deficiency Syndrome, Diabetes Mellitus, Stress, Suicide, Accidents and Homicides; and Facts about Common Concerns for Men, Including Impotence, Contraception, Circumcision, Sleep Disorders, Snoring, Hair Loss, Diet, Nutrition, Exercise, Kidney and Urological Disorders, and Backaches

Edited by Allan R. Cook. 738 pages. 1998. 0-7808-0212-8. $78.

"This comprehensive resource and the series are highly recommended."
— *American Reference Books Annual, 2000*

"Recommended reference source."
— *Booklist, American Library Association, Dec '98*

Mental Health Disorders Sourcebook, 2nd Edition

Basic Consumer Health Information about Anxiety Disorders, Depression and Other Mood Disorders, Eating Disorders, Personality Disorders, Schizophrenia, and More, Including Disease Descriptions, Treatment Options, and Reports on Current Research Initiatives

Along with Statistical Data, Tips for Maintaining Mental Health, a Glossary, and Directory of Sources for Additional Help and Information

Edited by Karen Bellenir. 605 pages. 2000. 0-7808-0240-3. $78.

ALSO AVAILABLE: Mental Health Disorders Sourcebook, 1st Edition. Edited by Karen Bellenir. 548 pages. 1995. 0-7808-0040-0. $78.

"Well organized and well written."
—*American Reference Books Annual, 2001*

"Recommended reference source."
—*Booklist, American Library Association, Jun '00*

Mental Retardation Sourcebook

Basic Consumer Health Information about Mental Retardation and Its Causes, Including Down Syndrome, Fetal Alcohol Syndrome, Fragile X Syndrome, Genetic Conditions, Injury, and Environmental Sources

Along with Preventive Strategies, Parenting Issues, Educational Implications, Health Care Needs, Employment and Economic Matters, Legal Issues, a Glossary, and a Resource Listing for Additional Help and Information

Edited by Joyce Brennfleck Shannon. 642 pages. 2000. 0-7808-0377-9. $78.

"Public libraries will find the book useful for reference and as a beginning research point for students, parents, and caregivers."
—*American Reference Books Annual, 2001*

"The strength of this work is that it compiles many basic fact sheets and addresses for further information in one volume. It is intended and suitable for the general public. This sourcebook is relevant to any collection providing health information to the general public."
—*E-Streams, Nov '00*

"From preventing retardation to parenting and family challenges, this covers health, social and legal issues and will prove an invaluable overview."
—*Reviewer's Bookwatch, Jul '00*

Movement Disorders Sourcebook

Basic Consumer Health Information about Neurological Movement Disorders, Including Essential Tremor, Parkinson's Disease, Dystonia, Cerebral Palsy, Huntington's Disease, Myasthenia Gravis, Multiple Sclerosis, and Other Early-Onset and Adult-Onset Movement Disorders, Their Symptoms and Causes, Diagnostic Tests, and Treatments

Along with Mobility and Assistive Technology Information, a Glossary, and a Directory of Additional Resources

Edited by Joyce Brennfleck Shannon. 655 pages. 2003. 0-7808-0628-X. $78.

Obesity Sourcebook

Basic Consumer Health Information about Diseases and Other Problems Associated with Obesity, and Including Facts about Risk Factors, Prevention Issues, and Management Approaches

Along with Statistical and Demographic Data, Information about Special Populations, Research Updates, a Glossary, and Source Listings for Further Help and Information

Edited by Wilma Caldwell and Chad T. Kimball. 376 pages. 2001. 0-7808-0333-7. $78.

"The book synthesizes the reliable medical literature on obesity into one easy-to-read and useful resource for the general public."
—*American Reference Books Annual 2002*

"This is a very useful resource book for the lay public."
—*Doody's Review Service, Nov '01*

"Well suited for the health reference collection of a public library or an academic health science library that serves the general population." —*E-Streams, Sep '01*

"Recommended reference source."
—*Booklist, American Library Association, Apr '01*

" Recommended pick both for specialty health library collections and any general consumer health reference collection." — *The Bookwatch, Apr '01*

Ophthalmic Disorders Sourcebook, 1st Edition

SEE Eye Care Sourcebook, 2nd Edition

Oral Health Sourcebook

SEE Dental Care & Oral Health Sourcebook, 2nd Edition

Osteoporosis Sourcebook

Basic Consumer Health Information about Primary and Secondary Osteoporosis and Juvenile Osteoporosis and Related Conditions, Including Fibrous Dysplasia, Gaucher Disease, Hyperthyroidism, Hypophosphatasia, Myeloma, Osteopetrosis, Osteogenesis Imperfecta, and Paget's Disease

Along with Information about Risk Factors, Treatments, Traditional and Non-Traditional Pain Management, a Glossary of Related Terms, and a Directory of Resources

Edited by Allan R. Cook. 584 pages. 2001. 0-7808-0239-X. $78.

"This would be a book to be kept in a staff or patient library. The targeted audience is the layperson, but the therapist who needs a quick bit of information on a particular topic will also find the book useful."
—*Physical Therapy, Jan '02*

"This resource is recommended as a great reference source for public, health, and academic libraries, and is another triumph for the editors of Omnigraphics."
—*American Reference Books Annual 2002*

"Recommended for all public libraries and general health collections, especially those supporting patient education or consumer health programs."
—*E-Streams, Nov '01*

"Will prove valuable to any library seeking to maintain a current, comprehensive reference collection of health resources. . . . From prevention to treatment and associated conditions, this provides an excellent survey."
—*The Bookwatch, Aug '01*

"Recommended reference source."
—*Booklist, American Library Association, July '01*

SEE ALSO *Women's Health Concerns Sourcebook*

■

Pain Sourcebook, 2nd Edition

Basic Consumer Health Information about Specific Forms of Acute and Chronic Pain, Including Muscle and Skeletal Pain, Nerve Pain, Cancer Pain, and Disorders Characterized by Pain, Such as Fibromyalgia, Shingles, Angina, Arthritis, and Headaches

Along with Information about Pain Medications and Management Techniques, Complementary and Alternative Pain Relief Options, Tips for People Living with Chronic Pain, a Glossary, and a Directory of Sources for Further Information

Edited by Karen Bellenir. 670 pages. 2002. 0-7808-0612-3. $78.

ALSO AVAILABLE: *Pain Sourcebook, 1st Edition.* Edited by Allan R. Cook. 667 pages. 1997. 0-7808-0213-6. $78.

"A source of valuable information. . . . This book offers help to nonmedical people who need information about pain and pain management. It is also an excellent reference for those who participate in patient education."
—*Doody's Review Service, Sep '02*

"The text is readable, easily understood, and well indexed. This excellent volume belongs in all patient education libraries, consumer health sections of public libraries, and many personal collections."
—*American Reference Books Annual, 1999*

"A beneficial reference." —*Booklist Health Sciences Supplement, American Library Association, Oct '98*

"The information is basic in terms of scholarship and is appropriate for general readers. Written in journalistic style . . . intended for non-professionals. Quite thorough in its coverage of different pain conditions and summarizes the latest clinical information regarding pain treatment." —*Choice, Association of College and Research Libraries, Jun '98*

"Recommended reference source."
—*Booklist, American Library Association, Mar '98*

Pediatric Cancer Sourcebook

Basic Consumer Health Information about Leukemias, Brain Tumors, Sarcomas, Lymphomas, and Other Cancers in Infants, Children, and Adolescents, Including Descriptions of Cancers, Treatments, and Coping Strategies

Along with Suggestions for Parents, Caregivers, and Concerned Relatives, a Glossary of Cancer Terms, and Resource Listings

Edited by Edward J. Prucha. 587 pages. 1999. 0-7808-0245-4. $78.

"An excellent source of information. Recommended for public, hospital, and health science libraries with consumer health collections." —*E-Streams, Jun '00*

"Recommended reference source."
—*Booklist, American Library Association, Feb '00*

"A valuable addition to all libraries specializing in health services and many public libraries."
—*American Reference Books Annual, 2000*

■

Physical & Mental Issues in Aging Sourcebook

Basic Consumer Health Information on Physical and Mental Disorders Associated with the Aging Process, Including Concerns about Cardiovascular Disease, Pulmonary Disease, Oral Health, Digestive Disorders, Musculoskeletal and Skin Disorders, Metabolic Changes, Sexual and Reproductive Issues, and Changes in Vision, Hearing, and Other Senses

Along with Data about Longevity and Causes of Death, Information on Acute and Chronic Pain, Descriptions of Mental Concerns, a Glossary of Terms, and Resource Listings for Additional Help

Edited by Jenifer Swanson. 660 pages. 1999. 0-7808-0233-0. $78.

"This is a treasure of health information for the layperson." — *Choice Health Sciences Supplement, Association of College & Research Libraries, May 2000*

"Recommended for public libraries."
—*American Reference Books Annual, 2000*

"Recommended reference source."
—*Booklist, American Library Association, Oct '99*

SEE ALSO *Healthy Aging Sourcebook*

■

Podiatry Sourcebook

Basic Consumer Health Information about Foot Conditions, Diseases, and Injuries, Including Bunions, Corns, Calluses, Athlete's Foot, Plantar Warts, Hammertoes and Clawtoes, Clubfoot, Heel Pain, Gout, and More

Along with Facts about Foot Care, Disease Prevention, Foot Safety, Choosing a Foot Care Specialist, a Glossary of Terms, and Resource Listings for Additional Information

Edited by M. Lisa Weatherford. 380 pages. 2001. 0-7808-0215-2. $78.

"There is a lot of information presented here on a topic that is usually only covered sparingly in most larger comprehensive medical encyclopedias."

—*American Reference Books Annual 2002*

Pregnancy & Birth Sourcebook

Basic Information about Planning for Pregnancy, Maternal Health, Fetal Growth and Development, Labor and Delivery, Postpartum and Perinatal Care, Pregnancy in Mothers with Special Concerns, and Disorders of Pregnancy, Including Genetic Counseling, Nutrition and Exercise, Obstetrical Tests, Pregnancy Discomfort, Multiple Births, Cesarean Sections, Medical Testing of Newborns, Breastfeeding, Gestational Diabetes, and Ectopic Pregnancy

Edited by Heather E. Aldred. 737 pages. 1997. 0-7808-0216-0. $78.

"A well-organized handbook. Recommended."

—*Choice, Association of College and Research Libraries, Apr '98*

"Recommended reference source."

—*Booklist, American Library Association, Mar '98*

"Recommended for public libraries."

—*American Reference Books Annual, 1998*

SEE ALSO *Congenital Disorders Sourcebook, Family Planning Sourcebook*

Prostate Cancer Sourcebook

Basic Consumer Health Information about Prostate Cancer, Including Information about the Associated Risk Factors, Detection, Diagnosis, and Treatment of Prostate Cancer

Along with Information on Non-Malignant Prostate Conditions, and Featuring a Section Listing Support and Treatment Centers and a Glossary of Related Terms

Edited by Dawn D. Matthews. 358 pages. 2001. 0-7808-0324-8. $78.

"Recommended reference source."

—*Booklist, American Library Association, Jan '02*

"A valuable resource for health care consumers seeking information on the subject. . . .All text is written in a clear, easy-to-understand language that avoids technical jargon. Any library that collects consumer health resources would strengthen their collection with the addition of the *Prostate Cancer Sourcebook*."

—*American Reference Books Annual 2002*

Public Health Sourcebook

Basic Information about Government Health Agencies, Including National Health Statistics and Trends, Healthy People 2000 Program Goals and Objectives, the Centers for Disease Control and Prevention, the Food and Drug Administration, and the National Institutes of Health

Along with Full Contact Information for Each Agency

Edited by Wendy Wilcox. 698 pages. 1998. 0-7808-0220-9. $78.

"Recommended reference source."

—*Booklist, American Library Association, Sep '98*

"This consumer guide provides welcome assistance in navigating the maze of federal health agencies and their data on public health concerns."

—*SciTech Book News, Sep '98*

Reconstructive & Cosmetic Surgery Sourcebook

Basic Consumer Health Information on Cosmetic and Reconstructive Plastic Surgery, Including Statistical Information about Different Surgical Procedures, Things to Consider Prior to Surgery, Plastic Surgery Techniques and Tools, Emotional and Psychological Considerations, and Procedure-Specific Information

Along with a Glossary of Terms and a Listing of Resources for Additional Help and Information

Edited by M. Lisa Weatherford. 374 pages. 2001. 0-7808-0214-4. $78.

"An excellent reference that addresses cosmetic and medically necessary reconstructive surgeries. . . . The style of the prose is calm and reassuring, discussing the many positive outcomes now available due to advances in surgical techniques."

—*American Reference Books Annual 2002*

"Recommended for health science libraries that are open to the public, as well as hospital libraries that are open to the patients. This book is a good resource for the consumer interested in plastic surgery."

—*E-Streams, Dec '01*

"Recommended reference source."

—*Booklist, American Library Association, July '01*

Rehabilitation Sourcebook

Basic Consumer Health Information about Rehabilitation for People Recovering from Heart Surgery, Spinal Cord Injury, Stroke, Orthopedic Impairments, Amputation, Pulmonary Impairments, Traumatic Injury, and More, Including Physical Therapy, Occupational Therapy, Speech/ Language Therapy, Massage Therapy, Dance Therapy, Art Therapy, and Recreational Therapy

Along with Information on Assistive and Adaptive Devices, a Glossary, and Resources for Additional Help and Information

Edited by Dawn D. Matthews. 531 pages. 1999. 0-7808-0236-5. $78.

"This is an excellent resource for public library reference and health collections."

—*American Reference Books Annual, 2001*

"Recommended reference source."

—*Booklist, American Library Association, May '00*

Respiratory Diseases & Disorders Sourcebook

Basic Information about Respiratory Diseases and Disorders, Including Asthma, Cystic Fibrosis, Pneumonia, the Common Cold, Influenza, and Others, Featuring Facts about the Respiratory System, Statistical and Demographic Data, Treatments, Self-Help Management Suggestions, and Current Research Initiatives

Edited by Allan R. Cook and Peter D. Dresser. 771 pages. 1995. 0-7808-0037-0. $78.

"Designed for the layperson and for patients and their families coping with respiratory illness. . . . an extensive array of information on diagnosis, treatment, management, and prevention of respiratory illnesses for the general reader."
— *Choice, Association of College and Research Libraries, Jun '96*

"A highly recommended text for all collections. It is a comforting reminder of the power of knowledge that good books carry between their covers."
— *Academic Library Book Review, Spring '96*

"A comprehensive collection of authoritative information presented in a nontechnical, humanitarian style for patients, families, and caregivers."
— *Association of Operating Room Nurses, Sep/Oct '95*

SEE ALSO Lung Disorders Sourcebook

Sexually Transmitted Diseases Sourcebook, 2nd Edition

Basic Consumer Health Information about Sexually Transmitted Diseases, Including Information on the Diagnosis and Treatment of Chlamydia, Gonorrhea, Hepatitis, Herpes, HIV, Mononucleosis, Syphilis, and Others

Along with Information on Prevention, Such as Condom Use, Vaccines, and STD Education; And Featuring a Section on Issues Related to Youth and Adolescents, a Glossary, and Resources for Additional Help and Information

Edited by Dawn D. Matthews. 538 pages. 2001. 0-7808-0249-7. $78.

ALSO AVAILABLE: Sexually Transmitted Diseases Sourcebook, 1st Edition. Edited by Linda M. Ross. 550 pages. 1997. 0-7808-0217-9. $78.

"Recommended for consumer health collections in public libraries, and secondary school and community college libraries."
— *American Reference Books Annual 2002*

"Every school and public library should have a copy of this comprehensive and user-friendly reference book."
— *Choice, Association of College & Research Libraries, Sep '01*

"This is a highly recommended book. This is an especially important book for all school and public libraries."   — *AIDS Book Review Journal, Jul-Aug '01*

"Recommended reference source."
— *Booklist, American Library Association, Apr '01*

"Recommended pick both for specialty health library collections and any general consumer health reference collection."   — *The Bookwatch, Apr '01*

Skin Disorders Sourcebook

Basic Information about Common Skin and Scalp Conditions Caused by Aging, Allergies, Immune Reactions, Sun Exposure, Infectious Organisms, Parasites, Cosmetics, and Skin Traumas, Including Abrasions, Cuts, and Pressure Sores

Along with Information on Prevention and Treatment

Edited by Allan R. Cook. 647 pages. 1997. 0-7808-0080-X. $78.

". . . comprehensive, easily read reference book."
— *Doody's Health Sciences Book Reviews, Oct '97*

SEE ALSO Burns Sourcebook

Sleep Disorders Sourcebook

Basic Consumer Health Information about Sleep and Its Disorders, Including Insomnia, Sleepwalking, Sleep Apnea, Restless Leg Syndrome, and Narcolepsy

Along with Data about Shiftwork and Its Effects, Information on the Societal Costs of Sleep Deprivation, Descriptions of Treatment Options, a Glossary of Terms, and Resource Listings for Additional Help

Edited by Jenifer Swanson. 439 pages. 1998. 0-7808-0234-9. $78.

"This text will complement any home or medical library. It is user-friendly and ideal for the adult reader."
— *American Reference Books Annual, 2000*

"A useful resource that provides accurate, relevant, and accessible information on sleep to the general public. Health care providers who deal with sleep disorders patients may also find it helpful in being prepared to answer some of the questions patients ask."
— *Respiratory Care, Jul '99*

"Recommended reference source."
— *Booklist, American Library Association, Feb '99*

Sports Injuries Sourcebook, 2nd Edition

Basic Consumer Health Information about the Diagnosis, Treatment, and Rehabilitation of Common Sports-Related Injuries in Children and Adults

Along with Suggestions for Conditioning and Training, Information and Prevention Tips for Injuries Frequently Associated with Specific Sports and Special Populations, a Glossary, and a Directory of Additional Resources

Edited by Joyce Brennfleck Shannon. 614 pages. 2002. 0-7808-0604-2. $78.

ALSO AVAILABLE: Sports Injuries Sourcebook, 1st Edition. Edited by Heather E. Aldred. 624 pages. 1999. 0-7808-0218-7. $78.

Stress-Related Disorders Sourcebook

Basic Consumer Health Information about Stress and Stress-Related Disorders, Including Stress Origins and Signals, Environmental Stress at Work and Home, Mental and Emotional Stress Associated with Depression, Post-Traumatic Stress Disorder, Panic Disorder, Suicide, and the Physical Effects of Stress on the Cardiovascular, Immune, and Nervous Systems

Along with Stress Management Techniques, a Glossary, and a Listing of Additional Resources

Edited by Joyce Brennfleck Shannon. 610 pages. 2002. 0-7808-0560-7. $78.

Stroke Sourcebook

Basic Consumer Health Information about Stroke, Including Ischemic, Hemorrhagic, Transient Ischemic Attack (TIA), and Pediatric Stroke, Stroke Triggers and Risks, Diagnostic Tests, Treatments, and Rehabilitation Information

Along with Stroke Prevention Guidelines, Legal and Financial Information, a Glossary, and a Directory of Additional Resources

Edited by Joyce Brennfleck Shannon. 606 pages. 2003. 0-7808-0630-1. $78.

Substance Abuse Sourcebook

Basic Health-Related Information about the Abuse of Legal and Illegal Substances Such as Alcohol, Tobacco, Prescription Drugs, Marijuana, Cocaine, and Heroin; and Including Facts about Substance Abuse Prevention Strategies, Intervention Methods, Treatment and Recovery Programs, and a Section Addressing the Special Problems Related to Substance Abuse during Pregnancy

Edited by Karen Bellenir. 573 pages. 1996. 0-7808-0038-9. $78.

SEE ALSO Alcoholism Sourcebook, Drug Abuse Sourcebook

Surgery Sourcebook

Basic Consumer Health Information about Inpatient and Outpatient Surgeries, Including Cardiac, Vascular, Orthopedic, Ocular, Reconstructive, Cosmetic, Gynecologic, and Ear, Nose, and Throat Procedures and More

Along with Information about Operating Room Policies and Instruments, Laser Surgery Techniques, Hospital Errors, Statistical Data, a Glossary, and Listings of Sources for Further Help and Information

Edited by Annemarie S. Muth and Karen Bellenir. 596 pages. 2002. 0-7808-0380-9. $78.

Transplantation Sourcebook

Basic Consumer Health Information about Organ and Tissue Transplantation, Including Physical and Financial Preparations, Procedures and Issues Relating to Specific Solid Organ and Tissue Transplants, Rehabilitation, Pediatric Transplant Information, the Future of Transplantation, and Organ and Tissue Donation

Along with a Glossary and Listings of Additional Resources

Edited by Joyce Brennfleck Shannon. 628 pages. 2002. 0-7808-0322-1. $78.

Traveler's Health Sourcebook

Basic Consumer Health Information for Travelers, Including Physical and Medical Preparations, Transportation Health and Safety, Essential Information about Food and Water, Sun Exposure, Insect and Snake Bites, Camping and Wilderness Medicine, and Travel with Physical or Medical Disabilities

Along with International Travel Tips, Vaccination Recommendations, Geographical Health Issues, Disease Risks, a Glossary, and a Listing of Additional Resources

Edited by Joyce Brennfleck Shannon. 613 pages. 2000. 0-7808-0384-1. $78.

"Recommended reference source."
— Booklist, American Library Association, Feb '01

"This book is recommended for any public library, any travel collection, and especially any collection for the physically disabled."
—American Reference Books Annual, 2001

Vegetarian Sourcebook

Basic Consumer Health Information about Vegetarian Diets, Lifestyle, and Philosophy, Including Definitions of Vegetarianism and Veganism, Tips about Adopting Vegetarianism, Creating a Vegetarian Pantry, and Meeting Nutritional Needs of Vegetarians, with Facts Regarding Vegetarianism's Effect on Pregnant and Lactating Women, Children, Athletes, and Senior Citizens

Along with a Glossary of Commonly Used Vegetarian Terms and Resources for Additional Help and Information

Edited by Chad T. Kimball. 360 pages. 2002. 0-7808-0439-2. $78.

"Organizes into one concise volume the answers to the most common questions concerning vegetarian diets and lifestyles. This title is recommended for public and secondary school libraries." *— E-Streams, Apr '03*

"Invaluable reference for public and school library collections alike." *— Library Bookwatch, Apr '03*

"The articles in this volume are easy to read and come from authoritative sources. The book does not necessarily support the vegetarian diet but instead provides the pros and cons of this important decision. The *Vegetarian Sourcebook* is recommended for public libraries and consumer health libraries."
— American Reference Books Annual, 2003

Women's Health Concerns Sourcebook

Basic Information about Health Issues That Affect Women, Featuring Facts about Menstruation and Other Gynecological Concerns, Including Endometriosis, Fibroids, Menopause, and Vaginitis; Reproductive Concerns, Including Birth Control, Infertility, and Abortion; and Facts about Additional Physical, Emotional, and Mental Health Concerns Prevalent among Women Such as Osteoporosis, Urinary Tract Disorders, Eating Disorders, and Depression

Along with Tips for Maintaining a Healthy Lifestyle

Edited by Heather E. Aldred. 567 pages. 1997. 0-7808-0219-5. $78.

"Handy compilation. There is an impressive range of diseases, devices, disorders, procedures, and other phys-ical and emotional issues covered . . . well organized, illustrated, and indexed."** *—Choice, Association of College and Research Libraries, Jan '98*

SEE ALSO *Breast Cancer Sourcebook, Cancer Sourcebook for Women, Healthy Heart Sourcebook for Women, Osteoporosis Sourcebook*

Workplace Health & Safety Sourcebook

Basic Consumer Health Information about Workplace Health and Safety, Including the Effect of Workplace Hazards on the Lungs, Skin, Heart, Ears, Eyes, Brain, Reproductive Organs, Musculoskeletal System, and Other Organs and Body Parts

Along with Information about Occupational Cancer, Personal Protective Equipment, Toxic and Hazardous Chemicals, Child Labor, Stress, and Workplace Violence

Edited by Chad T. Kimball. 626 pages. 2000. 0-7808-0231-4. $78.

"As a reference for the general public, this would be useful in any library." *—E-Streams, Jun '01*

"Provides helpful information for primary care physicians and other caregivers interested in occupational medicine. . . . General readers; professionals."
— Choice, Association of College & Research Libraries, May '01

"Recommended reference source."
— Booklist, American Library Association, Feb '01

"Highly recommended." *— The Bookwatch, Jan '01*

Worldwide Health Sourcebook

Basic Information about Global Health Issues, Including Malnutrition, Reproductive Health, Disease Dispersion and Prevention, Emerging Diseases, Risky Health Behaviors, and the Leading Causes of Death

Along with Global Health Concerns for Children, Women, and the Elderly, Mental Health Issues, Research and Technology Advancements, and Economic, Environmental, and Political Health Implications, a Glossary, and a Resource Listing for Additional Help and Information

Edited by Joyce Brennfleck Shannon. 614 pages. 2001. 0-7808-0330-2. $78.

"Named an Outstanding Academic Title."
—Choice, Association of College & Research Libraries, Jan '02

"Yet another handy but also unique compilation in the extensive Health Reference Series, this is a useful work because many of the international publications reprinted or excerpted are not readily available. Highly recommended." *—Choice, Association of College & Research Libraries, Nov '01*

"Recommended reference source."
—Booklist, American Library Association, Oct '01

Teen Health Series

Helping Young Adults Understand, Manage, and Avoid Serious Illness

Diet Information for Teens

Health Tips about Diet and Nutrition

Including Facts about Nutrients, Dietary Guidelines, Breakfasts, School Lunches, Snacks, Party Food, Weight Control, Eating Disorders, and More

Edited by Karen Bellenir. 399 pages. 2001. 0-7808-0441-4. $58.

"Full of helpful insights and facts throughout the book. . . . An excellent resource to be placed in public libraries or even in personal collections."
—*American Reference Books Annual 2002*

"Recommended for middle and high school libraries and media centers as well as academic libraries that educate future teachers of teenagers. It is also a suitable addition to health science libraries that serve patrons who are interested in teen health promotion and education."
—*E-Streams, Oct '01*

"This comprehensive book would be beneficial to collections that need information about nutrition, dietary guidelines, meal planning, and weight control. . . . This reference is so easy to use that its purchase is recommended."
—*The Book Report, Sep-Oct '01*

"This book is written in an easy to understand format describing issues that many teens face every day, and then provides thoughtful explanations so that teens can make informed decisions. This is an interesting book that provides important facts and information for today's teens."
—*Doody's Health Sciences Book Review Journal, Jul-Aug '01*

"A comprehensive compendium of diet and nutrition. The information is presented in a straightforward, plain-spoken manner. This title will be useful to those working on reports on a variety of topics, as well as to general readers concerned about their dietary health."
—*School Library Journal, Jun '01*

Drug Information for Teens

Health Tips about the Physical and Mental Effects of Substance Abuse

Including Facts about Alcohol, Anabolic Steroids, Club Drugs, Cocaine, Depressants, Hallucinogens, Herbal Products, Inhalants, Marijuana, Narcotics, Stimulants, Tobacco, and More

Edited by Karen Bellenir. 452 pages. 2002. 0-7808-0444-9. $58.

"The chapters are quick to make a connection to their teenage reading audience. The prose is straightforward and the book lends itself to spot reading. It should be useful both for practical information and for research, and it is suitable for public and school libraries."
—*American Reference Books Annual, 2003*

"Recommended reference source."
—*Booklist, American Library Association, Feb '03*

"This is an excellent resource for teens and their parents. Education about drugs and substances is key to discouraging teen drug abuse and this book provides this much needed information in a way that is interesting and factual."
—*Doody's Review Service, Dec '02*

Mental Health Information for Teens

Health Tips about Mental Health and Mental Illness

Including Facts about Anxiety, Depression, Suicide, Eating Disorders, Obsessive-Compulsive Disorders, Panic Attacks, Phobias, Schizophrenia, and More

Edited by Karen Bellenir. 406 pages. 2001. 0-7808-0442-2. $58.

"In both language and approach, this user-friendly entry in the *Teen Health Series* is on target for teens needing information on mental health concerns."
—*Booklist, American Library Association, Jan '02*

"Readers will find the material accessible and informative, with the shaded notes, facts, and embedded glossary insets adding appropriately to the already interesting and succinct presentation."
—*School Library Journal, Jan '02*

"This title is highly recommended for any library that serves adolescents and parents/caregivers of adolescents."
—*E-Streams, Jan '02*

"Recommended for high school libraries and young adult collections in public libraries. Both health professionals and teenagers will find this book useful."
—*American Reference Books Annual 2002*

"This is a nice book written to enlighten the society, primarily teenagers, about common teen mental health issues. It is highly recommended to teachers and parents as well as adolescents."
—*Doody's Review Service, Dec '01*

Sexual Health Information for Teens

Health Tips about Sexual Development, Human Reproduction, and Sexually Transmitted Diseases

Including Facts about Puberty, Reproductive Health, Chlamydia, Human Papillomavirus, Pelvic Inflam-

matory Disease, Herpes, AIDS, Contraception, Pregnancy, and More

Edited by Deborah A. Stanley. 391 pages. 2003. 0-7808-0445-7. $58.

Skin Health Information
For Teens
Health Tips about Dermatological Concerns and Skin Cancer Risks

Including Facts about Acne, Warts, Hives, and Other Conditions and Lifestyle Choices, Such as Tanning, Tattooing, and Piercing, That Affect the Skin, Nails, Scalp, and Hair

Edited by Robert Aquinas McNally. 430 pages. 2003. 0-7808-0446-5. $58.

Sports Injuries Information
For Teens
Health Tips about Sports Injuries and Injury Protection

Including Facts about Specific Injuries, Emergency Treatment, Rehabilitation, Sports Safety, Competition Stress, Fitness, Sports Nutrition, Steroid Risks, and More

Edited by Joyce Brennfleck Shannon. 425 pages. 2003. 0-7808-0447-3. $58.

609

Health Reference Series

Adolescent Health Sourcebook

AIDS Sourcebook, 3rd Edition

Alcoholism Sourcebook

Allergies Sourcebook, 2nd Edition

Alternative Medicine Sourcebook,
2nd Edition

Alzheimer's Disease Sourcebook,
3rd Edition

Arthritis Sourcebook

Asthma Sourcebook

Attention Deficit Disorder Sourcebook

Back & Neck Disorders Sourcebook

Blood & Circulatory Disorders
Sourcebook

Brain Disorders Sourcebook

Breast Cancer Sourcebook

Breastfeeding Sourcebook

Burns Sourcebook

Cancer Sourcebook, 4th Edition

Cancer Sourcebook for Women,
2nd Edition

Caregiving Sourcebook

Childhood Diseases & Disorders
Sourcebook

Colds, Flu & Other Common Ailments
Sourcebook

Communication Disorders
Sourcebook

Congenital Disorders Sourcebook

Consumer Issues in Health Care
Sourcebook

Contagious & Non-Contagious
Infectious Diseases Sourcebook

Death & Dying Sourcebook

Dental Care & Oral Health Sourcebook,
2nd Edition

Depression Sourcebook

Diabetes Sourcebook, 3rd Edition

Diet & Nutrition Sourcebook,
2nd Edition

Digestive Diseases & Disorder
Sourcebook

Disabilities Sourcebook

Domestic Violence Sourcebook,
2nd Edition

Drug Abuse Sourcebook

Ear, Nose & Throat Disorders
Sourcebook

Eating Disorders Sourcebook

Emergency Medical Services
Sourcebook

Endocrine & Metabolic Disorders
Sourcebook

Environmentally Health Sourcebook,
2nd Edition

Ethnic Diseases Sourcebook

Eye Care Sourcebook, 2nd Edition

Family Planning Sourcebook

Fitness & Exercise Sourcebook,
2nd Edition

Food & Animal Borne Diseases
Sourcebook

Food Safety Sourcebook

Forensic Medicine Sourcebook

Gastrointestinal Diseases & Disorders
Sourcebook

Genetic Disorders Sourcebook,
2nd Edition

Head Trauma Sourcebook

Headache Sourcebook

Health Insurance Sourcebook

Health Reference Series Cumulative
Index 1999

Healthy Aging Sourcebook

Healthy Children Sourcebook

Healthy Heart Sourcebook for Women